P9-DVV-920

Doping in Elite Sport

The Politics of Drugs in the Olympic Movement

Wayne Wilson and Edward Derse

Editors

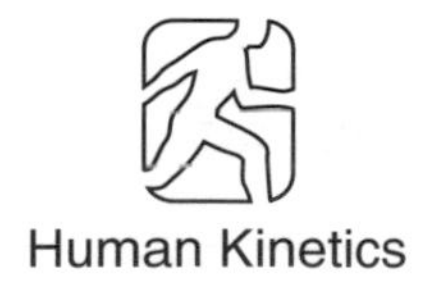

Human Kinetics

Library of Congress Cataloging-in-Publication Data

Doping in elite sport : the politics of drugs in the Olympic movement / Wayne Wilson and Edward Derse, editors.

p. cm.

Includes bibliographical references and index.

ISBN 0-7360-0329-0

1. Doping in sports. 2. Olympics. I. Wilson, Wayne, Ph.D. II. Derse, Ed, 1958-

RC1230 .D76 2001
362.29'088'796--dc21

00-033599

ISBN: 0-7360-0329-0

Acquisitions Editor: Michael S. Bahrke, PhD; **Developmental Editor:** Jennifer Clark; **Assistant Editors:** Derek Campbell and Laurie Stokoe; **Copyeditor:** Kelly Winters; **Proofreader:** Sarah Wiseman; **Indexer:** Marie Rizzo; **Graphic Designer:** Stuart Cartwright; **Graphic Artist:** Kathleen Boudreau-Fuoss; **Photo Manager:** Clark Brooks; **Cover Designer:** Jack W. Davis; **Printer:**Versa Press

Printed in the United States of America 10 9 8 7 6 5 4 3 2 1

Human Kinetics
Web site: www.humankinetics.com

United States: Human Kinetics, P.O. Box 5076, Champaign, IL 61825-5076
800-747-4457
e-mail: humank@hkusa.com

Canada: Human Kinetics, 475 Devonshire Road Unit 100, Windsor, ON N8Y 2L5
800-465-7301 (in Canada only)
e-mail: hkcan@mnsi.net

Europe: Human Kinetics, P.O. Box IW14, Leeds LS16 6TR, United Kingdom
+44 (0)113 278 1708
e-mail: humank@hkeurope.com

Australia: Human Kinetics, 57A Price Avenue, Lower Mitcham, South Australia 5062
08 8277 1555
e-mail: liahka@senet.com.au

New Zealand: Human Kinetics, P.O. Box 105-231, Auckland Central
09-309-1890
e-mail: hkp@ihug.co.nz

Contents

Contributors

R. Craig Kammerer, PhD

David L. Black, PhD, DABFT, DABCC: President and Director, Aegis Sciences, Nashville, TN

Charles E. Yesalis III, ScD: College of Health and Human Development, Pennsylvania State University, University Park, PA

Andrea N. Kopstein, PhD, MPH: Division of Epidemiology and Prevention Research, National Institute on Drug Abuse, Rockville, MD

Michael S. Bahrke, PhD: Human Kinetics, Champaign, IL

Jan Todd, PhD: Department of Kinesiology and Health Education, University of Texas at Austin

Terry Todd, PhD: Department of Kinesiology and Health Education, University of Texas at Austin

Angela J. Schneider, PhD: Faculty of Health Sciences, University of Western Ontario

Robert B. Butcher, PhD: Faculty of Health Sciences, University of Western Ontario

Bruce Kidd: Faculty of Physical Education and Health, University of Toronto

Robert Edelman: Department of History, University of California, San Diego

Susan Brownell: Department of Anthropology, University of Missouri, St. Louis

Tara Magdalinski: Faculty of Arts, University of the Sunshine Coast

John J. MacAloon: Social Sciences Graduate Division, University of Chicago

John Leonard: Executive Director American Swimming Coaches Association; Executive Director World Swimming Coaches Association

John Hoberman: Department of Germanic Studies, University of Texas at Austin

Jim Ferstle: Freelance writer

Foreword

I wear two hats in my life as a sport administrator: one as president of the Amateur Athletic Foundation of Los Angeles, an organization devoted to promoting youth sport, and the other as a vice president of the International Olympic Committee (IOC). The issue of performance-enhancing drugs in sport is a major concern to me in both capacities. In fact, as a leader of both a community-based sport organization and an officer of an elite sport governing body, I am uniquely positioned to understand that the use of drugs in sport truly is pervasive. Furthermore, having a role in both worlds makes me realize what the stakes are in the fight against doping. Creating drug-free competition at the elite level is a worthy goal, in and of itself. The stakes become even higher when one considers that young athletes emulate more mature world-class athletes. Simply put, when famous athletes use steroids and other drugs, kids are more likely to use them too.

The problem of doping in sport remains a persistent one. The IOC began the fight against doping in sport nearly four decades ago, in 1961, with the establishment of its Medical Commission. By 1968, the committee began drug testing at the Olympic Games. Testing has continued ever since and increasingly sophisticated tests have been developed, but the sad truth is that some athletes and officials continue to break the rules.

Neither the IOC nor any other governing body in elite amateur or professional sport has been able to eliminate the problem.

As a number of writers note in *Doping in Elite Sport,* questions and complaints about the current state of doping control reached a head in 1998 following the Tour de France doping scandal. IOC president Juan Antonio Samaranch fueled the controversy with his remarks in a newspaper interview that perhaps the list of banned substances should be reconsidered. The IOC responded by organizing the World Conference on Doping in Sport, in Lausanne, Switzerland, bringing together athletes, sport leaders, and governmental officials.

The Lausanne meetings were revealing in a number of ways. Personally, I was struck by how many people were misinformed about doping control. One of the more common misperceptions, for example, was that the IOC is responsible for all drug testing in international sport. In truth, the IOC can conduct drug testing only during a 16-day period every two years at the Olympic Games and Olympic Winter

Games. The international sport federations and national Olympic committees are responsible for all other athlete testing.

I mention this because two points became abundantly clear in Lausanne. First, any successful effort to control doping will require the cooperation of sport governing bodies, governmental agencies, and athletes. Second, building and maintaining such a coalition will not be easy. At the Lausanne summit, for example, two sport federations resisted adopting the strong sanctions against drug cheats favored by almost everyone else in attendance. The recalcitrant federations feared that European right-to-work laws and the threat of lawsuits would make lengthy sanctions against drug abusers unenforceable. These concerns were not unreasonable, and they illustrated the difficulty of developing truly effective enforcement policies.

Another striking feature of the Lausanne summit was the level of emotion generated by the issue. Before the World Conference on Doping in Sport, many IOC members anticipated that the committee would be the object of intense criticism from many of the invited guests. This proved to be the case. Participants were free to speak their minds and they did so. The confrontational rhetoric seemed to be a source of great titillation for the journalists in attendance. In another sense, though, the strongly expressed desire to change the present order provided the IOC and everyone else present with a clear mandate for meaningful action.

For many IOC members, perhaps the most salient revelation of the Lausanne summit was how adamant many participants were that any agency established to combat drug use have complete autonomy.

We also learned in Lausanne that talk alone will not solve the problem. We listened to speech after speech in Lausanne. But, when all was said and done, it was the IOC, and no one else, that took action, providing $25 million to fund the creation of the World Anti-Doping Agency (WADA). The IOC also spent the next several months enlisting the cooperation of intergovernmental agencies in Europe, Africa, Asia, and Oceania.

WADA began operation in January 2000. How independent WADA should be from the IOC was a contentious issue in Lausanne, and remains so. The present arrangement puts an IOC member in charge of the organization for the first two years. The board eventually will include no more than 35 members, of whom no more than 16 may be appointed by the IOC, national Olympic committees, and international federations. This organizational structure represents a departure from the IOC's original vision as expressed at the Lausanne summit. No doubt it leaves some critics unsatisfied, but I think it is a reasonable compromise that deserves a chance to succeed.

The World Conference on Doping in Sport, in my opinion, was a watershed in the campaign against the use of performance-enhancing drugs in sport. It brought discussion of the topic out into the open. The conference also forced several influential organizations and individuals to invest their reputations in finding a solution to the doping problem.

Success in the fight against doping will not come easily. It will require a broad-based effort by athletes, sport officials, educators, and politicians. There will be setbacks, and total victory may never be achieved. Still, it is a fight worth fighting. The outcome of the battle will have real consequences not only for elite athletes, but also for millions of other athletes who participate in sport, and for spectators who follow sport at every level.

I believe there is a connection between doping in elite sport and drug use among young athletes. As president of the Amateur Athletic Foundation of Los Angeles, an organization that serves youth through sport, I believe it is my responsibility and the responsibility of all of us to succeed in the battle against drugs in sport.

Anita L. DeFrantz

President, Amateur Athletic Foundation of Los Angeles
Vice President, International Olympic Committee

Preface

Doping in Elite Sport is based on papers delivered at a 1998 conference of the same title, which was organized by the Amateur Athletic Foundation of Los Angeles. The 1998 conference critically examined efforts to control doping in international sport. It brought together both critics of the sport establishment and representatives of major sport bodies including the International Olympic Committee (IOC) and the United States Olympic Committee (USOC). Participants included journalists, academicians, former athletes, and sport administrators.

The participants at the conference represented a variety of viewpoints on the doping issue, but most of them could be classified as opponents who did not challenge the basic assumption that doping in sport is pernicious and should be policed. For the most part, the contributors to this book reflect that viewpoint. The weight of opinion in *Doping in Elite Sport* is that efforts to control doping have failed on a number of counts.

Several writers have updated their 1998 papers to reflect important developments in the field. There are also three new papers on the issue. This book, however, remains true to the substance and tenor of the 1998 conference.

Doping in sport engenders strong feelings and strong rhetoric. Much of this derives from a deeply held belief that athletes' use of banned substances threatens the very essence of sport. Sport is a physical competition among athletes, all of whom are subject to the same rules. Every governing body in the Olympic movement bans at least some performance-enhancing drugs. The question of whether doping bans should exist is a valid one, but the fact remains that doping is against the rules and has been for many years. Thus, when athletes use banned substances, they cheat. They gain an unfair advantage over those athletes who choose to follow the rules. In so doing, athletes who use banned substances undermine the foundation that sport, by definition, is based on. When a significant number of athletes (sometimes acting with the tacit or active collusion of coaches and administrators) break or ignore rules, sport is in trouble. For that reason alone, the drug issue is a compelling one.

What makes doping even more interesting is the fact that any discussion of it very quickly leads to and illuminates a number of other important issues in elite sport such as commercialization, governance, nationalism, science, the media, and, of course, athletes' rights and their health. The papers in this book examine doping within a broad framework that encompasses many of these related issues. The book is divided into three parts dealing with the science; the history, ethics, and social context; and the politics of doping and doping control.

Part I, The Science of Doping, begins with Craig Kammerer's article, "What Is Doping and How Is It Detected?" Kammerer provides readers with a basic scientific understanding of how banned substances improve performance and how testers detect drug use. David Black follows with an explanation of the protocols that should be used in drug testing and a critique of the gap between ideals and actual practice. Charles Yesalis, Andrea Kopstein, and Michael Bahrke conclude this section with a discussion of the epidemiology of doping and the difficulty of estimating the extent of the drug use in elite sport with precision.

Jan Todd and Terry Todd begin Part II, The History, Ethics, and Social Context of Doping, by presenting a thorough chronology of doping in sport. The Todds' paper clearly demonstrates that doping is not a new issue and that its impact has been felt throughout sport for several decades.

The doping issue is, at the root, an ethical question. At the same time, ethical interpretations of doping and the policing of doping are determined by the various cultural settings of sport. As of this writing, there are 199 national Olympic committees recognized by the IOC. Any attempt to control doping must take into account the wide range of cultures that sport emerges from. In the next chapter Angela Schneider and Robert Butcher critically evaluate the philosophical basis of doping control. Bruce Kidd, Robert Edelman, and Susan Brownell compare how three very different countries—Canada, Russia, and China—have handled drugs in sport. And Tara Magdalinski analyzes the relationship between the construction of a national identity and Australia's enthusiastic pursuit of doping control as the country prepares to host the Sydney 2000 Olympic Games.

Part III, The Politics of Doping, presents four works. John MacAloon sets the stage by arguing that the IOC's legitimacy and ability to administer the Olympic movement depends on others' perceptions of the committee's sincerity and commitment in its efforts to combat doping. John Leonard, executive director of the World Swimming Coaches Association, offers a scathing indictment of what he characterizes as the failure of international swimming officials to effectively respond to the use of performance-enhancing drugs in the sport. John Hoberman, focusing on the IOC, presents an analysis of the political and financial factors that hinder effective enforcement. The book concludes with journalist Jim Ferstle's account of the February 1999 World Conference on Doping in Sport, including the events leading up to the conference and the policy debates that took place there.

During the preparation of this book, there were several significant events in doping. The 1998 Tour de France was beset by a major drug scandal. Police confiscated drugs, detained riders, and arrested team officials. Shortly thereafter, IOC president Juan Antonio Samaranch touched off a furor when, in a move seen by many as a retreat in the fight against doping, he suggested that the IOC's banned substances list be reevaluated. Irish swimmer Michelle Smith de Bruin, winner of three gold medals at the 1996 Olympic Games, received a lifetime ban from her sport for altering a urine sample during a drug test. In the United States, baseball player Mark McGwire created controversy when he revealed that he regularly used the steroid androstenedione as he chased and ultimately broke Major League Baseball's single-season home run record. McGwire later announced that he had abandoned the use of androstenedione. The IOC, stung by criticisms of President Samaranch's comments, organized a world summit on doping in Lausanne, Switzerland. Meanwhile, several prominent athletes, including the men's 1992 Olympic 100-meter champion Linford Christie, were punished after drug tests revealed traces of nandrolone in their bodies. Many of these episodes played out against a backdrop of a more publicized scandal in 1999 and 2000 that enveloped the IOC and other Olympic groups when it was revealed that some IOC members had accepted bribes from cities wishing to host the Olympic Games. The connection between the bribery scandal and events in the field of doping will be explored in more detail in this book. Suffice it to say here that the scandal severely compromised the credibility of the IOC, and, by implication, the credibility of its anti-doping programs.

The debate over doping has entered a new phase. Any lingering vestiges of naiveté have been eliminated by the events of the past two years. It is clear that doping exists in elite sport. No sport governing body of any significance has eliminated the practice. The continued existence of doping in a social institution that purports to abhor it represents a profound form of corruption.

The response to doping in sport could take a number of forms as sport governing bodies, government agencies, members of the general public, and athletes themselves wrestle with the issue. There may be genuine, well-funded, intense efforts to eradicate the use of banned drugs. Such efforts may or may not succeed. On the other hand, there may be a cynical response that attempts to finesse the issue through public relations strategies designed to allay the concerns of press and public without reducing the use of performance-enhancing drugs. In a more extreme scenario, sport and government officials may simply give up the fight. Or, there may be no uniform course of action among various sport bodies and regulatory agencies. Several models of sport may emerge based on differing responses to the doping issue.

Broader societal pressures undoubtedly will affect the doping debate within sport. If, as one suspects, hormonal therapy, genetic engineering, behavior-altering prescription drugs, and cosmetic surgery become more common, the perception and acceptance of what is "natural" will change accordingly. As we become increasingly tolerant of the use of drugs to improve health and performance in other walks of life, the inevitable question will be, Why not in sport, too? Fifty years from now observers may look back on sport at the turn of the century and wonder what all the fuss was about, much as we now view earlier debates over amateurism.

Whatever scenario transpires, it is clear that the doping issue will be a central component in the evolution of sport. How we define the role of the athlete and the purpose of sport in our lives will be determined to a large extent by how willing or unwilling we are to allow performance-enhancing drugs to intrude in sport.

I
PART

The Science of Doping

1

CHAPTER

What Is Doping and How Is It Detected?

R. Craig Kammerer, PhD

Important Concepts for an Athletic Drug Testing Program

An effective drug testing program involves consideration of these concepts:

- Sample collection
- Regulatory considerations
- Chain of custody
- Laboratory analysis
- Screening
- Confirmation
- Pharmacokinetics
- Drug metabolism
- Drug interactions
- Reports/results

It is important to keep in mind the differences between an effective drug test in an athletic drug program and a therapeutic or other type of clinical test. Clinically, a laboratory test is often effective with a confidence level of more than 80 percent, for several reasons. The clinical test is often taken in context with other tests, a physical exam, presentation of symptoms, discussion of medical history with the attending clinician, and other evaluations to help define the "problem." In athletic drug testing, there is usually only one test (and the corresponding confirmation test), and if the results are not 100 percent accurate (no false-positives and minimal false-negatives), the entire career or reputation and livelihood of the athlete is often lost. In addition to the ethics and moral issues of a false-positive test, the legal ramifications in such a situation are often overwhelming.

History of Drug Use in Sport

Drug testing of humans began in the late 1950s, when, after several European cycling and track races, evidence of drug use was observed. In the 1960 Rome Olympic Games, a cyclist died after apparent amphetamine use. In 1965, Beckett, Tucker, and Moffat (1967), who had developed procedures capable of detecting a number of different stimulants, tested participants of the Tour of Britain Cycle Races. In the 1967 Tour de France, another cyclist died, with amphetamines found both on his person and in his body. Because Professor Beckett was a member of the newly formed International Olympic Committee (IOC) Medical Commission, his procedures were employed on an experimental basis in the 1968 Olympic Games. No testing for anabolic steroids was performed at this time due to the lack of assay procedures. The first "formal" testing for nonsteroidal drugs occurred at the 1972 Munich Olympic Games (Donike and Stratmann, 1974), though there still was no official testing for steroids. The development of complex radioimmunoassay (RIA) screening procedures (Brooks et al., 1979) as well as analytical advances in gas chromatography-mass spectrometry (GC-MS) techniques led to the introduction of tests for anabolic steroids at the 1976 Montreal Olympic Games (Bertrand, Masse, and Dugal, 1978). However, only 275 of the 1,800 total samples could be analyzed for steroids because of the complexity of these procedures.

During both the 1976 Montreal Olympics and the 1980 Moscow Olympics, RIA screening procedures (Brooks, Firth, and Sumner, 1975; Rogozkin, Morozov, and Tchaikovsky, 1979) were used to analyze samples for the presence of anabolic steroids and GCMS analysis was used to confirm positive screening results. Because of the inherent lack of specificity in RIA screening, assays for many of the steroid metabolites (Schänzer, 1996a), whose detection is necessary to infer the presence of anabolic steroids, and because endogenous testosterone was added to the list of banned drugs, GCMS was adopted at the 1984 Olympic Games as both the screening and confirmatory method of analysis of anabolic steroids (Catlin et al., 1987). The method of determining whether or not the testosterone (T) in an athlete's body came from illegal use by the athlete was developed by Donike et al. (1983), based on an earlier study (Baba et al., 1980). The test consisted of measuring both T and its epimeric form (a geometric isomer called epitestosterone; EPIT) in the same sample. Because EPIT is not converted to T in the body to any appreciable extent, and the normal ratio of the quantity of T to the quantity of EPIT [hereinafter called the TEPIT ratio] is approximately in the range of 1:1 for both males and females, administration of T raises this ratio. In 1982, a ratio of over 6:1 was considered evidence of having administered testosterone. Since then, it has been noted that some people have TEPIT ratios that naturally exceed 6:1. As natural exceptions to this threshold of guilt (discussed later) have appeared, the adjusted guidelines now are that a ratio over 6:1 is suspicious, and over 10:1 indicates that the athlete is probably guilty. Further refinement in these guidelines may be forthcoming in the near future.

Drug testing at the 1988 Olympics was summarized by Chung et al. (1990) and Park et al. (1990), but in terms of improved testing procedures, these articles provided little significant new information. In the 1992 Barcelona Olympic Games, the IOC laboratory reported the detection of several banned drugs in the participating athletes; namely, three cases of stimulant medications, two clenbuterol positives, and three TEPIT ratios over 6:1 (between 6:1 and 10:1) (Segura et al., 1995). Samples containing the stimulant drugs and clenbuterol were formally reported for punitive action while the three TEPIT ratios were referred for further study without action against the athletes. A summary of the history of drug abuse in sports is found in the following timeline.

1950s: Drug use seen in competitions: drug controls begin.
1960: Danish cyclist dies at Rome Olympic Games: amphetamine use.
1967: British cyclist dies at Tour de France: amphetamine use.
1967: IOC Medical Commission formed: sub-commission on doping control.
1968: Mexico City Olympic Games; first preliminary drug tests; only nonsteroidal drugs.
1972: Munich Olympic Games: first formal drug control program; preliminary steroid tests.
1976: Montreal Olympic Games: first formal steroid control.
1980: Moscow Olympic Games: no positive drug cases reported.
1984: Los Angeles Olympic Games: control of T; unreported positives.
1988: Seoul Olympic Games: Stanozolol positive; unreported positives.
1992: Barcelona Olympic Games: Clenbuterol positives.
1994: Chinese swimmers found positive for Dihydrotestosterone.
1995: Dope testing pioneer Manfred Donike dies.
1996: Atlanta Olympic Games: Bromantan positives disallowed, and high resolution mass spectrometry (HRMS) results not reported.

Testing Matrix: Blood or Urine

Although a few athletic federations have tried limited blood testing outside Olympic competition, and some experimental blood testing was performed at the Lillehammer Olympic Games, urine is usually the only permitted testing fluid in most testing programs, thus metabolites (final excretion products) are the molecules that must be detected to prove an athlete's drug use. There are several reasons for limiting testing to urine samples. First, athletes (and most athletic federations) feel that taking a blood sample is an unnecessary trauma to the athlete. Second, giving a urine sample does not involve needles or any invasive procedure, the use of which introduces the variables of technique of the staff, possible transmission of disease, and legal and religious considerations. The possibility of using blood for drug testing is not a new idea (Donike, 1976), and in recent years it has again become of interest because of the probable addition of more natural endogenous compounds (such as human growth hormone, or HGH; see discussion later in this chapter) to the banned list. However, the litigious nature of current society (Jacobs and Samuels, 1995) will probably preclude any blood-based drug testing on a wide scale.

An extremely valuable application of the use of blood testing was shown by de la Torre, Segura, and Polettini (1995a,b), with the report that intact T esters have been found in the blood of people who have taken T (usually supplied as an ester of some type in pharmaceutical preparations). Because T esters are *not* found naturally, and are *not* excreted into the urine, the detection of an intact ester proves unequivocally that synthetic T was consumed, which could not have been proven in this manner by a urine test. Thus, the use of blood testing for the verification of T abuse removes any doubt of exogenous supplementation in such a case. Theoretically, however, the use of T skin patches/gels/creams would still circumvent this test, as intact esters would either not be used, or would not survive the passage through the skin to the bloodstream intact. The use of blood for testing for T abuse may be of even greater theoretical interest, given that the first clinical study demonstrating actual benefit of T use for performance in sport has appeared (Bhasin et al., 1996). Also of interest is the work that has been published on the detection of various hormones in blood after T administration (e.g., LH, FSH, 17-hydroxyprogesterone, T, etc.) as well as the use of the ketoconazole suppression test, all of which are being investigated to verify the recent abuse of T (see Carlstroem et al., 1992; Cowan et al., 1991; Kicman et al., 1990; Oftebro et al., 1994; Palonek et al., 1995).

Table 1.1 lists the various classes of banned drugs and methods as currently listed by the IOC. Table 1.2 summarizes examples of each of those classes. Each list details many of the commonly found agents, but these are not intended to be complete lists.

Table 1.3 lists the most common techniques and assay procedures currently in use for the various banned drug classes in a comprehensive athletic drug testing laboratory, which is intended to enforce the IOC-banned drug lists.

Table 1.1 Drug Classes and Methods Banned by the International Olympic Committee

Classes	Methods
1. Stimulants	1. Blood doping
2. Narcotics	2. Manipulation (chemical, physical, or pharmacological)
3. Anabolic steroids and beta$_2$-agonists	
4. Beta blockers	
5. Diuretics	
6. Masking agents	
7. Peptide hormones	

Table 1.2 Examples of Banned Drug Classes

Stimulants

Amphetamine (Dexedrine)
Caffeine
Cocaine
Ephedrine
Fenfluramine
Methamphetamine
Methylephedrine
Phenylpropanolamine
Pseudoephedrine
Strychnine

Anabolic Steroids/β_2-Agonists

Bolasterone
Boldenone (Dehydrotestosterone; Vet.)
Clenbuterol (a β_2-agonist)
Clostebol (Steranabol)
Dehydrochlormethyltestosterone
(Oral-Turinabol; Chlorodianabol)
Dihydrotestosterone (DHT)
Drostanolone
Ethylestrenol
Formebolone
Fluoxymesterone (Halotestin)
Furazabol
Mesterolone (Proviron)
Methandienone (Dianabol)
Methyltestosterone (Metandren)
Mibolerone
Nandrolone (Nortestosterone)
Norethandrolone (Nilevar)
Oxandrolone (Anavar)
Oxymesterone (Oranabol)
Oxymetholone (Anadrol)
Stanozolol (Winstrol)
Stenbolone
Testosterone
Trenbolone

The presence of a urinary testosterone to epitestosterone ratio greater than 6:1 unless there is evidence that this ratio is due to a physiological or pathological condition.

Narcotics*

Ethylmorphine
Hydrocodone (Hycodan)
Methadone
Morphine
Pethidine (Meperidine-Demerol)
Propoxyphene (Darvon)
Methylphenidate (Ritalin)

*Codeine, Dextromethorphan, Dihydrocodeine, Diphenoxylate, and Pholcodine are now allowed.

Beta-Blockers

Acebutolol
Alprenolol (Sinalol)
Atenolol (Tenormin)
Betaxolol
Labetalol
Metoprolol (Lopressor)
Nadolol (Corgard)
Oxprenolol
Propranolol (Inderal)
Sotalol

Diuretics

Acetazolamide
Bendroflurmethiazide
(Naturetin)Bumetanide
Chlorthalidone
Canrenone
Ethacrynic Acid (Edecrin)
Furosemide (Lasix)
Hydrochlorothiazide (Esidrix)
Spironolactone
Triamterene

(continued)

Table 1.2 *(continued)*

Masking Agents	*Peptide Hormones*
Epitestosterone	ACTH (Corticotrophin)
Probenecid	EPO (Erythropoietin)
	HCG (Human Chorionic Gonadotropin)
	HGH (Human Growth Hormone; Somatotrophin)

Table 1.3 Summary of Current Athletic Drug Testing Analytical Methods

Screening Tests	Detection Method
Drugs Method	
1. Volatile Stimulants, Narcotics Extract/No Derivatization	GC-NPD
2. Nonvolatile Stimulants/ß-blockers Deconjugate/Derivatize	GC-NPD or GC-MSD
3. Pemoline and Caffeine Quantitation Extract/ No Derivatization	LC-DAD
4. Diuretics, Probenecid, Mesocarb Extract/No Derivatization	LC-DAD
5. Anabolic Steroids, Free/Unconjugated Extract/Derivatize	GC-MSD
6. Anabolic Steroids, Free and Conjugated Extract/Derivatize	GC-MSD
7. Immunoassays	
A. Amphetamines, Cocaine, Opiates, THC	FPIA, and ELIZA
B. $ß_2$-agonists (Clenbuterol), Corticosteroids	ELIZA
C. HCG, LH	MEIA and ELIZA
D. EPO, HGH	RIA and ELIZA
Confirmation Tests	
Procedures 1, 2, 5, and 6	GC-MSD
Procedures 3, 4	LC-MS or GC-MSD
Procedures 7A, B	GC-MSD
Procedures 7C, D	Under development

Confirmation Methods

Several reviews have appeared regarding anabolic steroid testing (Catlin et al., 1987; Kammerer et al. 1990; Kammerer, 1993; Kammerer, 2000; Schänzer et al., 1996b), so this chapter will now focus on new developments in testing and on methods that may be applied not only to steroids, but also to many other problem drugs.

Gas Chromatography-Mass Spectrometry

During gas chromatographic analysis, a solvent extract of a urine sample is injected into a long column that interacts with the various components of the sample, slowing some components more than others. Under a specified set of conditions, each substance takes a different amount of time to pass through a particular column, and this time, called a retention time (RT), helps to identify it. A mass spectrometer attached to the end of the gas chromatography (GC) column detects substances passed into it by bombarding the molecules with a beam of electrons that fragments the molecules into ionic pieces; these pieces form a kind of "fingerprint" of that particular substance. This spectrum fingerprint of fragment ions, along with the retention time (time spent in the GC column before detection), is unique for each substance. These results are compared with the results from a known reference sample of a substance, and when they match, it is confirmed without a doubt that the substances are the same. In other words, if a certain banned substance is found in an athlete's urine, this test can confirm that the athlete used the drug. Identification without any doubt is confirmed when these data are the same as that collected when the authentic reference substance or sample from a human excretion study is analyzed under the same conditions.

Liquid Chromatography-Mass Spectrometry

Liquid chromatography-mass spectrometry (LCMS) is similar to GCMS, except that the sample is passed through the separation column in the liquid state rather than in the gas phase, and the inert carrier medium, which moves the sample through the separation column, is a liquid instead of a gas.

LCMS is already being used in drug testing laboratories because it has several advantages over traditional GCMS techniques. An LC analysis is usually done at room temperature, whereas GC analysis requires the drug or hormone to be heated or vaporized into a gas. Research by Barron et al. (1996) has reduced or eliminated some of the earlier disadvantages of LCMS analysis, which were poor sensitivity and low sample volume capacity before service, and required maintenance of the instrument. Thus, in the future, LCMS will become increasingly more important in the drug testing lab because of its ability to confirm the presence of most drugs, including the unstable, polar, and large molecular weight natural hormones (HGH, EPO, etc.).

High Resolution Mass Spectrometry

Until recently, high resolution mass spectrometry (HRMS) would not have been an advantage in drug testing, because sensitivity would have been sacrificed for specificity. In addition, the instruments have been extremely expensive ($500,000 and up per instrument). However, costs of these instruments, like those for LCMS instrumentation, have been declining recently, so these instruments may soon be within major lab budget requirements. Because of the improvement in several different electronic and instrumental aspects of HRMS analysis, the technique is now better able to detect some drugs. However, since background signal (also called experimental noise) is also increased with increased sensitivity, the technique may not be of greater value for all substances, because background signal varies with the substance being analyzed (Schänzer et al., 1996a,b; Thieme et al., 1996). HRMS analysis was introduced in the 1996 Atlanta Summer Olympic Games testing program, but the "positives" found with the technique were not formally reported, presumably because of the potential legal problems that would ensue when an athlete tested negative for drugs with the "old" testing methods but then tested positive with the HRMS method. In other words, a database of results must be collected, particularly comparing the two methods on the same samples, in order to validate a result with the "new" HRMS machine. Only after the publication of sufficient results addressing detection limits, any false-negative and false-positive issues, and statistics showing the validity of results will the technique be acceptable both scientifically and legally.

Isotope Ratio Mass Spectrometry

This relatively new technique is being proposed for verification of testosterone positives that could be explained by factors other than drug taking. It is based on the simple fact that the percentage of ^{13}C (a naturally occurring stable-nonradioactive isotope of carbon) found in endogenous testosterone, which is made in the body from dietary components whose carbon sources are plants and animals, is different than the percentage of ^{13}C present in the synthetic testosterone found in a drug preparation. Isotope ratio mass spectrometry (IRMS) analysis can determine the percentage of ^{13}C in the sample, and thus whether it came from a synthetic drug or from the athlete's diet (Aguilera et al., 1996a,b). This differentiation would be valuable, because even though anabolic steroids (AS) are an old class of drugs (Hoberman and Yesalis, 1995), and the ban on athletic abuse of testosterone only occurred in 1983, several different situations (see table 1.4) will raise the TEPIT ratio into the "illegal" range (greater than 6:1), without the athlete ever having taken testosterone. If enough data are published that verify the veracity of the IRMS technique and that it can corroborate whether or not an athlete has taken T, then the technique will be utilized, despite its expense, time, and special equipment needs. It should be emphasized, however, that an IRMS can only be used for isotope ratio analyses, that it cannot be used for other routine assays (such as steroid screening or confirmation tests), and that it costs over

Table 1.4 Possible Reasons for High TEPIT Ratios Without Drug Abuse

1. Alcohol use before test
2. Bacteria growth in sample; high urinary pH
3. Deconjugation conditions used during sample preparation
4. Naturally low EPIT concentration; need to measure absolute levels of T and EPIT
5. Female: monthly cycle fluctuations in TEPIT ratio?
6. Female: birth control pill use effects on TEPIT ratio?
7. Endocrine disease
8. Genetic enzymatic variations

$100,000 per instrument. IRMS may be of value in resolving the "problems" associated with the documented increase in TEPIT ratios after alcohol use (Falk, Palonek, and Björkhem, 1988; Karila et al., 1996): with a fluctuation in the ratio in women apparently caused by many factors (Engelke, Flenker, and Donike, 1996; Engelke, Geyer, and Donike, 1995), an increased TEPIT ratio resulting from experimental conditions during sample preparation (Geyer et al., 1996b), with the possible use of dehydroepiandrosterone (DHEA) (Haning et al., 1991, 1993), or even with simultaneous use of both T and EPIT (Dehennin, 1994); see also table 1.4. However, because of both the complexity and possible sex differences in the metabolism of DHEA (Haning et al., 1991, 1993), it is not clear whether IRMS may be able to distinguish between the use of pharmaceutical and "dietary" DHEA. Thus, despite this last drawback, use of the instrument will increase dramatically in the future, especially if the verification test for T abuse is validated. However, it will add considerable costs to the operation of a laboratory, since this instrument will still be useful only for the relatively small numbers of samples in which a "testosterone problem" is present.

Problem Areas

Several factors make it difficult to determine without a shadow of a doubt that an athlete has abused testosterone.

Testosterone Use

Testosterone is not converted to its 17-epimer, EPIT, in men or women. Testosterone and EPIT exist in approximately equal amounts within males and females, but the absolute quantities in females are at least five-fold lower than those found in males. Thus, theoretically, the TEPIT ratio should not vary much around 1:1 in "normal" humans. After analysis of thousands of TEPIT ratios in both athletes and "other" populations, a ratio of 6:1 was chosen as the threshold indicator of illegal supplementation, which was presumed to account for natural ratio variations.

Since 1983, when T abuse was banned in sport by the IOC Medical Commission, a number of other explanations have been found for "high" TEPIT ratios. Many of these cases are still under investigation, prompting test challenges and lawsuits with incidents of drug positives involving T abuse. These other explanations include those summarized in table 1.4.

An athlete is considered guilty of using testosterone if the TEPIT ratio exceeds 6:1, although in actual practice many organizations will not pursue a "positive" unless it is over 9 or 10:1, because a finite though still low number of cases of TEPIT ratios over 6:1 have been found that did not result from testosterone abuse (Oftebro, 1992; Raynaud et al., 1992, 1993; Garle et al., 1996; Karila et al., 1996). Simultaneous consumption of EPITand T to keep the ratio of the two substances close to the "normal" ratio of 1:1 should not prevent the identification of exogenous T use (Dehennin, 1994), because the laboratories can calculate the ratios of T, as well as the ratios of EPIT, to other endogenous steroids measured during the drug-screening process. These resulting ratios will then change and will be interpreted as atypical by scientists evaluating the data (Dehennin, 1994; Dehennin and Matsumoto, 1993; Norli et al., 1995; Palonek et al., 1995; Geyer et al., 1996a). Laboratories have indeed set reference range values for many endogenous steroid levels and ratios (Donike et al., 1995), but the published data to date is rare. This fact suggests considerable legal problems whenever a positive drug test for the use of an endogenous compound is made public.

Even the published scientific data on the validity of the 6:1 TEPIT ratio as a means to substantiate testosterone abuse are still relatively sparse. This situation confers advantages to the abusers and their lawyers because the independent, peer-reviewed data for the test are not available in quantity sufficient to withstand legal challenge. In other words, there is no specific source in which one may find substantial data on the relationship of TEPIT ratios to sex, age, diet, common drugs taken (cold medications, alcohol, nicotine/tobacco use, caffeine, H_2-receptor antagonists [used for ulcer treatment], birth control pills, etc.). Data on the variation of testosterone levels should also be available for the time of the menstrual cycle, varying bacteria count in the sample, variation in the pH of the sample, and even for the use of other common "permitted" drugs. The data should be on a sufficiently large sample for each category of variable (>10,000) so that there is little chance that a false-positive would occur in the population of athletes that normally attend a summer Olympic Games (usually about 10,000). In other words, control of any natural substance requires the establishment of the "normal" endogenous level in the population and subsequent statistical determination of what constitutes an "abnormal" or abuse level of drug. Although some of these data exist, the quantity is relatively small, and therein lies the legal problem. Catlin, Hatton, and Starcevic (1997) summarized the testosterone testing "problems" and suggested some possible solutions.

To my knowledge, there have been no reported positive cases of T abuse resulting from the use of both EPIT and T. This may be due to the astute use of both

T and EPIT so that urinary levels are not high enough to be conclusive, or because of the anticipated legal issues involved in proving such dual usage. The use of moderate amounts of both T and EPIT will not only prevent the TEPIT ratio from exceeding 6:1 but also will not raise the ratios to other endogenous steroids sufficiently to be conclusive. This situation is analogous to the use of moderate amounts of T, which raises the TEPIT ratio but not over 6:1. Thus, some positive results may not be reported because of the obvious need to protect individuals whose TEPIT ratios or ratios of T and EPIT to other endogenous steroids vary for "natural" reasons and not as a result of drug use. In either case, use of both T and EPIT constitutes a problem in anabolic steroid testing, because they are both endogenous substances and thus illegal levels must be shown to result from the illegal use of those substances and not from normal variations in natural hormones (Dehennin, 1994).

Another strongly rumored method for abusing testosterone is use of the available skin patches (gels) for the application of controlled-release testosterone. A controlled-release preparation delivers the drug into the body on a more consistent, even basis over time, rather than as the larger, more sudden dose that occurs soon after parenteral administration. Consequently, controlled release means a relatively even dosing over a longer time period, usually 8 to 12 hours. Thus, relative to parenteral administration, the use of a sustained-release T preparation will yield a more stable blood level of drug with fewer high fluctuations in drug level, thereby making drug use "safer" than parenteral administration. There is also less chance of exceeding the 6:1 TEPIT ratio with sustained-release preparations (Meikle et al., 1992, 1996). Furthermore, skin (particularly scrotal skin) contains high levels of reductase activity, so T applied to skin is relatively quickly converted to dihydrotestosterone (DHT). Thus, DHT levels could be raised by use of a T skin patch and/or actual consumption of DHT.

A number of female Chinese swimmers were found positive for DHT (Donike et al., 1995; Geyer et al., 1996a) at the world swimming championships in 1994. Their positives were determined by careful comparison of the amount of DHT found in the samples with the amounts of several other endogenous steroids (steroid profile analysis), and reported in the world press (Southan et al., 1992; Kicman et al., 1995; Donike et al., 1995; Coutts et al., 1997). It was clear that those athletes thought that DHT would not be found during testing, and thus usage would probably go undetected.

Illegal use of T by female athletes is more difficult to prove than in male athletes, because absolute levels are much lower in females, and because both the levels of T and EPIT and the TEPIT ratios fluctuate greatly (Karila et al., 1996; Engelke, Flenker, and Donike, 1996; Engelke, Geyer, and Donike, 1995). In addition, there may be a hormonal cycle–dependent TEPIT ratio fluctuation (Engelke, Geyer, and Donike, 1995) and a relatively large increase in TEPIT ratio after alcohol consumption (Falk, Palonek, and Björkhem, 1988; Karila et al., 1996).

Therefore, if the dose of testosterone is carefully chosen and/or combined with sustained-release dosing, significant drug may be used both during training and continuing relatively close to competition time with a very low risk of reaching an illegal TEPIT ratio or positive test. The illegal ratio of TEPIT was chosen such that some drug abuse would be tolerated in order to protect all innocent athletes.

If future experiments prove that the use of IRMS analysis does indeed distinguish between endogenous and exogenous testosterone, or if collection of competition blood specimens is allowed such that the non-endogenous intact testosterone esters may be found when testosterone has been taken, then many of the lab problems in proving testosterone abuse will disappear.

Circumventing Positive Test Results

The following section discusses several methods athletes use to prevent positive test results, despite their abuse of drugs.

Designer Drugs

It is possible but unlikely that an athlete can prevent a positive drug test result by using a substance containing appropriate interfering or masking ion fragments. This prevention is unlikely because laboratories use both the gas chromatographic R.T. and the mass spectrometric fragment ion pattern (spectrum) for declaring a positive, and the chances of an interfering substance possessing both the same R.T. and ion spectrum as the drug are extremely low.

However, designer steroids can be and are being made (Bamberger and Yaeger, 1997; Franke and Berendonk, 1997), which may lead to long-term drug abuse without detection. In addition, when such a drug is initially found in use, before athletes can be penalized for its use, several steps must be taken. The agent must be banned by the various sport federations, the athletes and members must be apprised of such bans, and relevant sanctions must be listed so that all athletes, coaches, trainers, physicians, and other appropriate people are notified. The IOC and the athletic federations usually require evidence that the prohibition of use of an agent is indicated before issuing the ban.

The previously unknown drug bromantan was found in five athletes in the 1996 Atlanta Olympic Games, and the positive cases reported were disallowed by the Court of Arbitration for Sport, because the drug was too new: there was insufficient data, scientific knowledge, and scientific literature available to enforce the ban. A computer search of the world's literature in July 1996 revealed that bromantan was developed in Russia for thermoprotective and stimulant effects and was reportedly to be used in army troops. The only published articles described the compound as a psychostimulant. Its chemical structure was unlike any other known drug (even though one might construe it to be a distant cousin of amantadine, an antiviral drug currently on the market). There was no known metabolic information available in the public scientific literature from 1967 through July 1996.

Rumors were circulating that there was a new drug, which had been abused in the 1992 Barcelona Olympic Games. During screening, the IOC labs began to look in competition samples for a new unknown peak, which was identified by mass spectrometry (MS) as bromantan, before the 1996 Olympic Games.

Old Drugs

Not only the use of new drugs but also new applications for old drugs may occur, and evidently both occurred in recent international sporting events. Cafedrine, a chemical linkage of ephedrine and theophylline, is an old drug and is used after anesthesia to help wake patients. It is a potent stimulant, and *is not* a simple mixture of ephedrine and theophylline (a stimulant related to caffeine), and thus would not yield a positive test for either drug (although theophylline, often used in the treatment of asthma, is not banned at this time). However, cafedrine is a drug for which no metabolic data exists in the published literature, so that its use would be difficult to detect unless a lab knows what to look for by doing an excretion study and the corresponding metabolic identification work. Although not named specifically on any banned list to date, this drug is chemically related to a banned drug (ephedrine), and thus would automatically be banned by the phrase "and related compounds." However, such an "automatic ban by analogy" may not be acceptable to the Court of Arbitration for Sport, given their recent rulings in favor of athletes for use of "new" (bromantan) or recently banned "old" drugs (such as THC, which was found in a 1998 Nagano Olympic Winter Games drug test).

Natural Hormones Other Than Testosterone

Several polypeptide hormones including human growth hormone (HGH), human chorionic gonadotropin (HCG), gonadotropin-releasing hormone (GnRH), insulin, and erythropoietin (EPO) are very likely being abused in competition. HGH, GnRH, and HCG all have anabolic effects in their own rights or stimulate the release of T or other natural anabolic agents (Bradley and Sodeman, 1990; Papadakis et al., 1996; Conn and Crowley, 1994; Laidler et al., 1995). Erythropoietin increases the production of red blood cells, increasing the body's oxygen-carrying capacity (Casoni et al., 1993). It was widely rumored that EPO was abused at the 1996 Atlanta Olympic Games, because no confirmatory lab test was available to enforce the ban, or confirm any potential reported positives (Bamberger and Yaeger, 1997).

Testing for the many polypeptide hormones is difficult because the confirmatory assays for these compounds by MS are not currently developed and validated and thus not available to laboratories yet (HGH, see Kabouris et al., 1996; HCG, see Laidler et al., 1995; Liu and Bowers, 1995, 1996; Stenman et al., 1997; EPO, see Wide et al., 1995; Ekblom, 1996). Besides the fact that the presence of polypeptide hormones is difficult to confirm by a specific assay, all of these compounds are naturally present in all healthy people. Thus, doping control programs must establish what levels of polypeptide hormones are abnormal or indicative of abuse and what levels are normal. A considerable database is needed to confirm the normal concentration range for each of these natural components and to determine what variations occur for a variety of "natural" causes. Endogenous HCG levels are minute or often undetectable in men (except in certain cases of malignancy). Levels of HCG are higher in women; shortly after conception, the levels become huge because this compound is a placental hormone and is the basis of a commonly used pregnancy test. Consequently, an athlete accused of HCG abuse can counter with contentions of illness or pregnancy. No one knows whether these "reasonable" excuses will work for an athlete who has abused these drugs.

Athletes take many other endogenous natural agents to achieve a variety of effects, such as release of endogenous growth hormone, enhanced fat burning, and enhanced normal testosterone levels and synthesis (Conn and Crowley, 1994; Laidler et al., 1995). It is important that the athlete take due care in using new or experimental drugs or dosages that significantly exceed therapeutic levels. Although no scientific proof has appeared, recent deaths that were presumably due to the abuse of erythropoietin emphasize this point (Leith, 1991).

Use of Other Substances

Many other substances have become popular for either their purported anabolic effects, their effects on endogenous anabolic substances, or stimulant effects. Examples include

- Zeranol,
- Clenbuterol,
- Deprenyl,
- Creatine,
- Bicarbonate, and
- Mesocarb/Sydnocarb.

Zeranol is a nonsteroidal but potent anabolic agent commonly used to fatten cattle (Roche and Davis, 1972). The USOC has banned Zeranol because of its anabolic activity. When an athlete consumes beef that contains Zeranol, low levels of the drug could be detected. Also, because Zeranol has no structural similarity to any other anabolic steroid and is not chemically a steroid, the legal issues surrounding a positive case are unclear.

Clenbuterol, a B_2-receptor agonist commonly used to treat asthma in Europe, but not approved for medical use in the United States to date, has been shown in animal studies to increase skeletal muscle mass and reduce body fat (Maltin et al., 1987; Satchell, 1996). Widespread abuse of this drug by athletes, including reported positives in the 1992 Barcelona Olympic Games (Segura et al., 1995) has kept it on most banned lists. A mass spectroscopic method for the detection of clenbuterol and analogues, which also can be used as a confirmation assay, has appeared (Doerge et al., 1995). The labs can detect use of the drug, but because the drug is used at very low dosage, and used only during training prior to competition, it is not known whether use of the drug has been totally deterred.

Deprenyl, a monoamine oxidase inhibitor that was approved in the United States for treatment of Parkinson's disease in 1990, is probably used by athletes for its stimulatory effects. However, this drug is converted to methamphetamine and

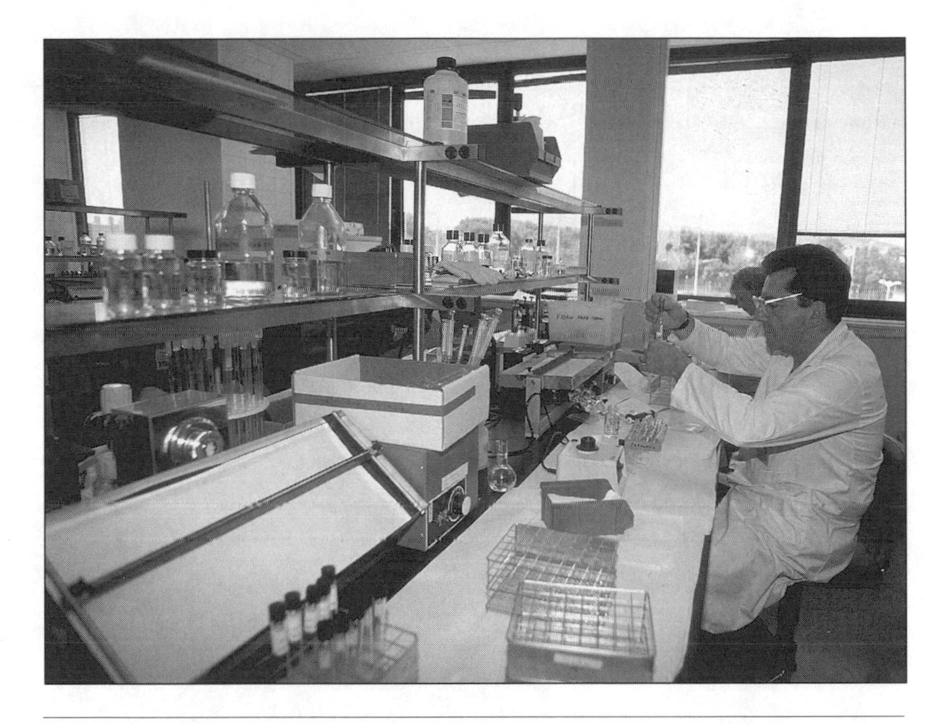

The drug testing center at the 1992 Barcelona Olympic Games. The testing lab reported five positive tests during the Games.
© Simon Bruty/Allsport

amphetamine in man, so any athlete taking this drug will undoubtedly be convicted of methamphetamine/amphetamine use (Heinonen, 1994). Legal problems could ensue if a lab reports amphetamine use when deprenyl was used.

Creatine supplementation is claimed to be widespread (Volek and Kraemer, 1996). Creatine is a simple nitrogenous compound that is found in most meat at about 0.5 percent by weight and is also made in the body. Creatine appears to help maintain the supply of energy, rapidly depleted during strenuous exercise, and is involved in energy output/maintenance in muscle tissue. Potential control of abuse is fraught with difficulties because of the normal endogenous level variations. Because creatine does not currently appear on any banned list, it may be used without any risk of penalty as of this date.

Sodium bicarbonate has been in use for enhancement of training and prolonged exercise levels (Webster et al., 1993). The mechanism of action is presumably the neutralization of excess lactate that builds in muscle tissue as exercise and strenuous activity is continued. There is little hope of ever controlling bicarbonate abuse, as large amounts exist in both the diet as well as in the body, and an analytical method that would isolate bicarbonate from the myriad of other inorganic ions naturally present in the body would be difficult at best. It is not a banned drug in any sports federations.

Table 1.5 Some Drugs Used by Athletes to Escape Detection

Androstendione	Polypeptide hormones: EPO, HCG, HGH, etc.
Bromantan	Mesocarb/Sydnocarb
Cafedrine	Norandrostendione
Clenbuterol	Oral-Turinabol Metabolite (Chlorodianabol Metabolite)
DHEA (Dehydroepiandrosterone)	Probenecid
DHT (Dihydrotestosterone)	Theodrenaline
Epitestosterone	

Table 1.6 Banned Drugs Used in Animals Raised for Food

Clenbuterol	Nandrolone
Clostebol	Trenbolone
Methenolone	Zeranol

Sydnocarb (Mesocarb) is a polar derivative of amphetamine, and it is classed as a psychostimulant (Breidbach, Sigmund, and Donike, 1995). Its use would confer an advantage in those sports where short-term stimulation would be useful. Because of its polar structure as well as its instability under some conditions of laboratory analysis, Mesocarb is poorly detected by some screening procedures. Recent papers demonstrate how to detect the drug by standard methods in order to enforce a ban on its use by athletes (Thieme et al., 1995; Deboer et al., 1995).

Table 1.5 summarizes some drugs used by athletes to escape detection. Some have been banned by name; others have not. The ability to legally prove abuse of some of these agents is extremely doubtful, even if an unequivocal confirmation test exists.

The drugs listed in table 1.6 have been found in urine samples taken from people who have consumed meat from animals treated with those same drugs. Thus, it is possible to have a "false-positive" drug test when individuals did not take a drug to enhance performance, but only consumed a meal; in fact, they did not even know that they had been exposed to the drug at all.

Future Directions in Drug Testing

New developments in drug testing may make the process cheaper, faster, and more reliable. On the other hand, it is also likely that new drugs will be developed that escape detection. The introduction of high-resolution mass spectrometry-mass spectrometry (MS-MS) analysis; liquid chromatography-MS-MS assays for unstable compounds and polypeptide hormones; and isotope ratio MS analysis for use in the TEPIT assay will make the testing process more expensive, slower, and more difficult. These latter instruments and associated assays are considerably more complicated, and will require more staff, further training, and greatly increased overhead costs in such a testing lab.

Confirmation assays are under development for HCG, GnRH, HGH, erythropoietin, and other abused natural products. The IOC had budgeted funds for a research project to develop a definitive test for HGH. In addition, there have been preliminary reports that a test for EPO is nearing completion. Some federations have been using the hemocrit blood test as an indicator of EPO abuse; e.g., above a certain value, the athlete is simply prohibited from competing, without any punitive action taken. The use of an indirect test such as the hemocrit for "proof" of drug use would not appear to be legally sound, at least in the United States. Although the mass spectrometric technology clearly exists for the development of the assay and valid detection of these products today, there is another major component to the detection of abuse of these products. Namely, what levels constitute abuse and what levels simply reflect "normal" fluctuations of these compounds that are present in all athletes. Thus, the moral, legal, and ethical issues of calling a drug test positive for any of these agents are extremely complex, and not easy to define. Under current guidelines, MS should be used for all confirmatory procedures, yet only RIA or other immunoassay methods currently are available for these peptide hormones.

Athletic federations may allow blood samples to be used for testing purposes. Although in some cases, blood (plasma) may contain higher concentrations of a drug than does urine, only limited amounts of blood may be taken (10–20 ml), whereas much larger amounts of urine are more easily obtainable. Thus, any potential benefit of blood as the testing matrix may be minimal. When esters of testosterone are abused, they cannot be detected intact in urine but can in plasma, which will constitute proof of T abuse. This is an important observation because T esters are not endogenous (produced in the body), so detection of an intact T ester constitutes proof of exogenous T supplementation. Thus, the controversy over the use of the TEPIT ratio will be avoided and the interpretation of the test result will become obvious (The first scientific proof that this technique is feasible appeared in de la Torre et al., 1995a,b). However, the use of blood is questionable, as the international athletic federations of the sports must still approve the use of blood.

Hair analysis may be used. The hair of a drug user does contain many of the drugs taken by that individual, and analysis of older sections of the hair can reliably indicate chronic use. Recent reviews of clinical analysis of hair samples (Deng et al., 1999; Gleixner and Meyer, 1997) show that testosterone and other steroids may be found in human hair, and stanozolol has recently been found in the hair of rats treated with stanozolol (Hold et al., 1996). Thus, additional research needs to be done to determine what steroids and other drugs are excreted into hair, as well as whether hair is a valid sample for athletic drug testing programs. Table 1.7

Table 1.7 Common Drugs Detected in Human Hair

1. Alprazolam	14. Ethylmorphine
2. Amitryptyline-Nortryptyline	15. Fentanyl-Sufentanyl
3. Androecgonine methyl ester (crack cocaine usage)	16. Fluitrazepam and 7-amino-flunitrazepam
4. Amphetamines	17. Haloperidol
5. 6-Acetyl-morphine (Heroin use)	18. Lorazepam
6. Cannabinoids	19. Morphine
7. Cocaine and metabolites	20. Methadone
8. Chloroquine and Desethylchloroquine	21. Meprobamate
9. Clenbuterol	22. Ofloxacine
10. Clozapine	23. Pentazocine
11. Carbamazepine	24. Phenobarbital
12. Dextropropoxyphene and Norpropoxyphene	25. PCP
13. Digozine	26. Stanozolol
	27. Testosterone

summarizes the drugs known to be excreted into human hair as of late 1997 (Deng et al., 1999).

In order for drug testing to become more effective as a deterrent and also to enhance health and promote fairness in competition, it has to become more widespread, and include unannounced (out-of-competition) testing. If athletes know that no one will escape detection for drug abuse and all competitors will face the same uniformly enforced sanctions for use of drugs, most abuse will cease. Athletes are still afraid of being at a disadvantage by not using certain performance-enhancing agents, because they believe that a majority of their competitors (in certain sports) do use performance-enhancing agents.

Sanctions against athletes must be more fairly and uniformly applied. This does not mean that an athlete should be punished in all cases in which his or her sample shows the presence of a drug, because circumstances do arise in which other factors determine whether or not true drug abuse has occurred. Such circumstances must always be based on scientific facts or level of uncertainty in the interpretation of the results, not on politics, quotas, or other irrelevant criteria. In addition to the actual test results, which are almost never in error, scientific facts that should decide a positive drug case include, but are not limited to, any evidence of sabotage, fluctuation of testosterone/epitestosterone levels (such as that resulting from female hormonal cycle variance (Engelke, Geyer, and Donike, 1995, Engelke, Flenker, and Donike, 1996), genetics, evidence of endocrine disease, sample history, conditions during preparation for testing, and the chain of custody. In addition, any positive case showing very low levels of a drug coupled with a normal steroid profile, indicating no chronic use, should not be called positive, because it has been shown that nandrolone metabolites may be generated from the use of some birth control medications (Reznik et al., 1987). The drug boldenone and its metabolites have been found in totally naive people who have never taken either boldenone or any steroid (Schänzer et al., 1995), and several anabolic steroid metabolites have been found in people who have consumed animals that were treated with the steroids as fattening agents during the raising of the animal (Debruyckere, de Sagher, and Peteghem, 1992, 1995; Kicman et al., 1994; Hemmersbach et al., 1995). In addition, pretest consumption of alcohol, incorrect storage of the urine sample, or use of certain specific deconjugation enzymes used during sample preparation (Geyer et al., 1996a) can artificially raise a TEPIT ratio and create a false-positive testosterone sample. It should always be borne in mind that a publicly announced drug testing positive probably will ruin the athlete's career, so that when there is *any* doubt about a result or its interpretation, a "positive test result" should be considered negative.

The monetary implications and political overtones associated with a positive drug found in an elite or famous athlete are too great to predict anything other than controversy and protracted legal challenges in many cases. Unannounced out-of-competition testing may improve any drug control program's effectiveness, but universal application of such an approach will be difficult to implement worldwide.

References

Aguilera, R., Becchi, M., Grenot, C., Casabianca, H., and Hatton, C.K. (1996a). Detection of testosterone misuse: comparison of two chromatographic sample preparation methods for gas chromatographic-combustion/isotope ratio mass spectrometric analysis. *Journal of Chromatography Biomedical Applications* 687(1): 53–54.

Aguilera, R., Becchi, M., Grenot, C., Casabianca, H., Hatton, C.K., Catlin, D.H., Starcevic, B., and Pope, H.G. (1996b). Improved method of detection of testosterone abuse by gas chromatography/combustion/isotope ratio mass spectrometry analysis of urinary steroids. *Journal of Mass Spectrometry* 31: 169–176.

Baba, S., Shinohara, Y., and Kasuya, Y. (1980). Differentiation between endogenous and exogenous testosterone in human plasma and urine after oral administration of deuterium-labeled testosterone by mass fragmentography. *Journal of Clinical Endocrinology and Metabolism* 50(5): 889–894.

Bamberger, M., and Yaeger, D. (1997). Bigger, stronger, faster. *Sports Illustrated*, 14 April, 62–70.

Barron, D., Barbosa, J., Pascual, J.A., and Segura, J. (1996). Direct determination of anabolic steroids in human urine by on-line solid-phase extraction/liquid chromatography/mass spectrometry. *Journal of Mass Spectrometry* 31: 309–319.

Beckett, A.H., Tucker, G.T., and Moffat, A.C. (1967). Routine detection and identification in urine of stimulants and other drugs, some of which may be used to modify performance in sport. *Journal of Pharmacy and Pharmacology* 19: 273–294.

Bertrand, M., Masse, R., and Dugal, R. (1978). GC-MS: Approach for the detection and characterization of anabolic steroids and their metabolites in biological fluids at major international sporting events. *Farmaceutische Tijdschrift Voor Belgie* 55(3): 85–101.

Bhasin, S., Storer, T.W., Berman, N., Callegari, C., Clevenger, B., Phillips, J., Bunnell, N., Tricker, R., Shirazi, A., and Casaburi, R. (1996). The effects of supraphysiologic doses of testosterone on muscle size and strength in normal men. *New England Journal of Medicine* 335(1): 1–7.

Bradley, C.A., and Sodeman, T.M. (1990). Human growth hormone; its use and abuse. *Clinics in Laboratory Medicine* 10(3): 473–477.

Breidbach, A., Sigmund, G., and Donike, M. (1995). Combination of screening procedures—mesocarb detection as an example. In Donike, M., Geyer, H., Gotzmann, A., and Mareck-Engelke, U., eds. *Proceedings of the 12th Cologne Workshop on Dope Analysis*, pp. 301–304. Cologne: Sport and Buch Strauss.

Brooks, R.V., Firth, R.G., and Sumner, N.A. (1975). Detection of anabolic steroids by radioimmunoassay. *British Journal of Sports Medicine* 9: 89–92.

Brooks, R.V., Jeremiah, G., Webb, W.A., and Wheeler, M. (1979). Detection of anabolic administration to athletes. *Journal of Steroid Biochemistry* 11: 913–917.

Carlström, K., Palonek, E., Garle, M., Oftebro, H., Stanghelle, J. and Björkhem, I. (1992). Detection of testosterone administration by increased ratio between serum concentrations of testosterone and 17α-hydroxyprogesterone. *Clinical Chemistry* 36: 1779–1784.

Casoni, I., Ricci, G., Ballarin, E., Borsetto, C., Grazzi, G., Gugliblmini, C., Manfredini, F., Mazzoni, M., Pattrracchini, M., Vitali, E.D.P., Rigolin, F., Bartalotta, S., Franze, G.P., Masoti, M., and Conconif (1993). Hematological indices of erythropoietin administration. *International Journal of Sports Medicine* 14: 307–311.

Catlin, D.H., Hatton, C.K., and Starcevic, S.H. (1997). Issues in detecting abuse of xenobiotic anabolic steroids and testosterone by analysis of athletes' urine. *Clinical Chemistry* 43(7): 1280–1288.

Catlin, D.H., Kammerer, R.C., Hatton, C.K., Sekera, M.H., and Merdink, J.L. (1987). Analytical chemistry at the games of the XXIIIrd Olympiad in Los Angeles, 1984. *Clinical Chemistry* 33(2): 319–327.

Chung, B.C., Choo, H.Y.P., Kim, J.W., Eom, K.D., Kwon, O.S., Suh, J., Yang, J.S., and Park, J.S. (1990). Analysis of anabolic steroids using GC/MS with selected ion monitoring. *Journal of Analytical Toxicology* 14: 91–95.

Conn, P.M., and Crowley, W.F. (1994). Gonadotropin-releasing hormone and its analogs. *Annual Reviews of Medicine* 45: 391–405.

Coutts, S.B., Kicman, A.T., Hurst, D.T., and Cowan, D.A. (1997). Intramuscular administration of 5α-dihydrotestosterone heptanoate: changes in urinary hormone profile. *Clinical Chemistry* 43(11): 2091–2098.

Cowan, D.A., Kicman, A.T., Walker, C.J., and Wheeler, M.J. (1991). Effect of administration of human chorionic gonadotropin on criteria used to assess testosterone administration in athletes. *Journal of Endocrinology* 131: 147–154.

Deboer, D., Ooijen, R.D.V., and Maes, R.A.A. (1995). Thermostable derivatives of mesocarb and its p-hydroxy-metabolite. In Donike, M., Geyer, H., Gotzmann, A., and Mareck-Engelke, U., eds. *Proceedings of the 12th Cologne Workshop on Dope Analysis*, pp. 305–316. Cologne: Sport and Buch Strauss.

Debruyckere, G., deSagher, R., and Peteghem, C.V. (1992). Clostebol positive urine after consumption of contaminated meat. *Clinical Chemistry* 38: 1869–1873.

Debruyckere, G., deSagher, R., and Peteghem, C.V. (1995). Detection of interferences in urinary anabolic steroid analysis. In Donike, M., Geyer, H., Gotzmann, A., and Mareck-Engelke, U., eds. *Proceedings of the 12th Cologne Workshop on Dope Analysis*, pp. 173–184. Cologne: Sport and Buch Strauss.

de la Torre, R., Segura, J., and Polettini, A. (1995a). Detection of testosterone esters in human plasma by GC/MS & GC/MS/MS. In Donike, M., Geyer, H., Gotzmann, A., and Mareck-Engelke, U., eds. *Proceedings of the 12th Cologne Workshop on Dope Analysis*, pp. 59–80. Cologne: Sport and Buch Strauss.

de la Torre, R., Segura, J., Polettini, A., and Montagna, M. (1995b). Detection of testosterone esters in human plasma. *Journal of Mass Spectrometry* 30: 1393–1404.

Dehennin, L. (1994). Detection of simultaneous self-administration of testosterone and epitestosterone in healthy men. *Clinical Chemistry* 40: 106–109.

Dehennin, L., and Matsumoto, A.M. (1993). Long-term administration of testosterone enanthate to normal men: alterations of the urinary profile of androgen metabolites potentially useful for detection of testosterone misuse in sport. *Journal of Steroid Biochemistry and Molecular Biology* 44: 179–189.

Deng, X.S., Kuroso, A., Pounder, D.J. (1999). Detection of anabolic steroids in head hair. *Journal of Forensic Science* 44(2): 343-346.

Doerge, D.R., Bajic, S., Blankenship, L.R., Preece, S.W., and Churchwell, M.I. (1995). Determination of ß-agonist residues in human plasma using liquid chromatography/atmospheric pressure chemical ionization mass spectrometry and tandem mass spectrometry. *Journal of Mass Spectrometry* 30: 911–916.

Donike, M. (1976). The detection of doping agents in blood. *British Journal of Sports Medicine* 10(3):147–154.

Donike, M., Bärwald, K.R., Kostermann, K., Schänzer, W., and Zimmermann, J. (1983). The detection of exogenous testosterone. In H. Heck, W. Hollmann, H. Liesen, and R. Rost, eds. *Sport: Leistung und Gesundheit*, pp. 293–298. Cologne: Deutscher Arzte-Verlag.

Donike, M., and Stratmann, D. (1974). Temperature programmed gas-chromatographic analysis of nitrogen containing drugs. Reproducibility of retention times and sample sizes by automatic injection (II). The screening procedure for volatile drugs at the 20th Olympic Games, Munich, 1972. *Chromatographia* 7(4): 182–189.

Donike, M., Ueki, M., Koroda, Y., Geyer, H., Nolteemsting, E., and Rauth, S. (1995). Detection of dihydrotestosterone (DHT) doping: alterations in the steroid profile and reference ranges for DHT and its 5α-metabolites. *Journal of Sports Medicine and Physical Fitness* 35: 235–250.

Ekblom, B. (1996). Blood doping and erythropoietin. *American Journal of Sports Medicine* 24(6): S-40–42.

Engelke, U.M., Flenker, U., and Donike, M. (1996). Stability of steroid profiles (5): the annual rhythm of urinary ratios and excretion rates of endogenous steroids in female and its menstrual dependency. In Donike, M., Geyer, H., Gotzmann, A., and Mareck-Engelke, U., eds. *Proceedings of the 13th Cologne Workshop on Dope Analysis*, pp. 177–190. Cologne: Sport and Buch Strauss.

Engelke, U.M., Geyer, H., and Donike, M. (1995). Stability of steroid profiles (4): ratios and excretion rates of endogenous steroids in female urines collected four times over 24 hours. In Donike, M., Geyer, H., Gotzmann, A. and Mareck-Engelke, U., eds., *Proceedings of the 12th Cologne Workshop on Dope Analysis*, pp. 135–156. Cologne: Sport and Buch Strauss.

Falk, O., Palonek, E., and Björkhem, I. (1988). Effect of ethanol on the ratio between testosterone and epitestosterone in urine. *Clinical Chemistry* 32: 1462–1464.

Franke, W.W. and Berendonk, B. (1997). Hormonal doping and androgenization of athletes: a secret program of the German Democratic Republic government. *Clinical Chemistry* 43(7): 1262–1279.

Garle, M., Ocka, R., Palonek, E., and Björkhem, I. (1996). Increased urinary testosterone/epitestosterone ratios found in Swedish athletes in connection with a national control program. Evaluation of 28 cases. *Journal of Chromatography Biomedical Applications* 687(1): 55–60.

Geyer, H., Schänzer, W., Mareck-Engelke, U., and Donike, M. (1996a). Factors influencing the steroid profile. In Donike, M., Geyer, H., Gotzmann, A., and Mareck-Engelke, U., eds. *Proceedings of the 13th Cologne Workshop on Dope Analysis*, pp. 95–114. Cologne: Sport and Buch Strauss.

Geyer, H., Schänzer, W., Schindler, U., and Donike, M. (1996b). Changes of the urinary steroid profile after sublingual application of dihydrotestosterone (DHT). In Donike, M., Geyer, H., Gotzmann, A., and Mareck-Engelke, U., eds. *Proceedings of the 13th Cologne Workshop on Dope Analysis*, pp. 215–230. Cologne: Sport and Buch Strauss.

Gleixner, A., and Meyer, H.H.D. (1997). Methods to detect anabolics in hair: Use for food hygiene and doping control. *American Laboratory*, December, 44–47.

Haning, R.V., Jr., Flood, C.A., Hackett, R.J., Loughlin, J.S., McClure, N., and Longcope, C. (1991). Metabolic clearance rate of dehydroepiandrosterone sulfate, its metabolism to testosterone, and its intrafollicular metabolism to dehydroepiandrosterone, androstenedione, testosterone, and dihydrotestosterone in vivo. *Journal of Clinical Endocrinology and Metabolism* 72(5): 1088–1095.

Haning, R.V., Jr., Hackett, R.J., Flood, C.A., Loughlin, J.S., Zhao, Q.Y., and Longcope, C. (1993). Plasma dehydroepiandrosterone sulfate serves as a prehormone for 48% of follicular fluid testosterone during treatment with Mentropins. *Journal of Clinical Endocrinology and Metabolism* 76(5): 1301–1307.

Heinonen, E.H. (1994). Pharmacokinetic aspects of l-deprenyl (selegiline) and its metabolites. *Clinical Pharmacology and Therapeutics* 56: 742–749.

Hemmersbach, P., Tomten, S., Nilsson, S., Oftebro, H., Havrevoll, O., Oen, B., and Birkeland, K. (1995). Illegal use of anabolic agents in animal fattening-consequences for doping analysis. In Donike, M., Geyer, H., Gotzmann, A., and Mareck-Engelke, U., eds. *Proceedings of the 12th Cologne Workshop on Dope Analysis*, pp. 185–192. Cologne: Sport and Buch Strauss.

Hoberman, J.M., and Yesalis, C.E. (1995). The history of synthetic testosterone. *Scientific American*, February, 60–65.

Hold, K.M., Wilkins, D.G., Crouch, D.J., Rollins, D.E., and Maes, R.A. (1996). Detection of stanozolol in hair by negative ion chemical ionization mass spectrometry. *Journal of Analytical Toxicology* 20(10): 345–349.

Jacobs, J.B., and Samuels, B. (1995). The drug testing project in international sports: Dilemmas in an expanding regulatory regime. *Hastings International and Comparative Law Review* 18(3): 557–589.

Kaboris, M., Platen, P., and Donike, M. (1996). Detection of human growth hormone urine of athletes. In Donike, M., Geyer, H., Gotzmann, A., and Mareck-Engelke, U., eds. *Proceedings of the 13th Cologne Workshop on Dope Analysis*, pp. 215–230. Cologne: Sport and Buch Strauss.

Kammerer, R.C. (1993). Drug testing and anabolic steroids. In Yesalis, C.E., ed. *Anabolic Steroids in Sport and Exercise,* pp. 283–308. Champaign, IL: Human Kinetics.

Kammerer, R.C. (in press). Drug testing and anabolic steroids. In Yesalis, C.E., ed. *Anabolic Steroids in Sport and Exercise*, 2nd ed. Champaign, IL: Human Kinetics.

Kammerer, R.C., Merdink, J.L., Jagels, M., Catlin, D.H., and Hui, K.K. (1990). Testing for fluoxymesterone (Halotestin) administration to man: Identification of urinary metabolites by gas chromatography-mass spectrometry. *Journal of Steroid Biochemistry* 36(6): 659–666.

Karila, T., Kosunen, V., Leinonen, A., Taehtelae, R., and Seppaelae, T. (1996). High doses of alcohol increase testosterone-to-epitestosterone ratio in females. *Journal of Chromatography Biomedical Applications* 687(1): 109–116.

Kicman, A.T., Brooks, R.V., Collyer, S.C., Cowan, D.A., Nanjee, M.N., Southan, G.J., and Wheeler, M.J. (1990). Criteria to indicate testosterone administration. *British Journal of Sports Medicine* 24: 253–264.

Kicman, A.T., Coutts, S.B., Walker, C.J., and Cowan, D.A. (1995). Proposed confirmatory procedure for detecting 5α-dihydrotestosterone doping in male athletes. *Clinical Chemistry* 41(11): 1617–1627.

Kicman, A.T., Cowan, D.A., Myhre, L., Nilsson, S., Oftebro, H., Havrevoll, O., Oen, B., and Birkeland, K. (1994). Effect on sports drug tests of ingesting meat from steroid (methenolone)-treated livestock. *Clinical Chemistry* 40: 2084–2087.

Laidler, P., Cowan, D.A., Hider, R.C., Keane, A., and Kicman, A.T. (1995). Tryptic mapping of human chorionic gonadotropin by matrix-assisted laser desorption/ ionization mass spectrometry. *Rapid Communications in Mass Spectrometry* 9: 1021–1026.

Leith, W. (1991). Cyclists don't die like this. *The Independent on Sunday*, July 14, 3–4.

Liu, C., and Bowers, L.D. (1995). Studies towards confirmation of HCG using HPLC/MS. In Donike, M., Geyer, H., Gotzmann, A., and Mareck-Engelke, U., eds. *Proceedings of the 12th Cologne Workshop on Dope Analysis*, pp. 235–242. Cologne: Sport and Buch Strauss.

Liu, C., and Bowers, L.D. (1996). Immunoaffinity trapping of urinary human chorionic gonadotropin and its high-performance liquid chromatographic-mass spectrometric confirmation. *Journal of Chromatography Biomedical Applications* 687(1): 213–220.

Maltin, C., Delday, M., Hay, S., Smith, F., Lobley, G., and Reeds, P. (1987). The effect of the anabolic agent, clenbuterol, on the overloaded rat skeletal muscle. *Bioscience Reports* 7: 143–148.

Meikle, A.W., Arver, S., Dobs, A.S., Sanders, S.W., Rajaram, L., and Mazar, N.A. (1996). Pharmacokinetics and metabolism of a permeation-enhanced testosterone transdermal system in hypogonadal men: influence of application site—a clinical research center study. *Journal of Clinical Endocrinology and Metabolism* 81:1832–1840.

Meikle, A.W., Mazar, N.A., Moellmer, J.F., Stringham, J.D., Tolman, K.G., Sanders, S.W., and Cdell, W.D. (1992). Enhanced transdermal delivery of testosterone across nonscrotal skin produces physiological concentrations of testosterone and its metabolites in hypogonadal men. *Journal of Clinical Endocrinology and Metabolism* 74(3): 623–628.

Norli, H., Esbensen, K., Westad, F., Birkeland, K.I., and Hemmersbach, P. (1995). Chemometric evaluation of urinary steroid profiles in doping control. *Journal of Steroid Biochemistry and Molecular Biology* 54(1-2): 83–88.

Oftebro, H. (1992). Evaluating an abnormal urinary steroid profile. *Lancet* 359: 941–942.

Oftebro, H., Jensen, J., Mowinckel, P., and Norli, H.R. (1994). Establishing a ketoconazole suppression test for verifying testosterone administration in the doping control of athletes. *Journal of Clinical Endocrinology and Metabolism* 78: 973–977.

Palonek, E., Gottlieb, C., Garle, M., Björkhem, I., and Carlström, K. (1995). Serum and urinary markers of exogenous testosterone administration. *Journal of Steroid Biochemistry and Molecular Biology* 55(1): 121–127.

Papadakis, M.A., Grady, D., Black, D., Tierney, M.J., Gooding, G.A.W., Schambelan, M., and Grunfeld, C. (1996). Growth hormone replacement in healthy older men improves body composition but not functional ability. *Annals of Internal Medicine* 124: 708–716.

Park, J.S., Park, S., Lho, D.S., Choo, H.P., Chung, B., Yoon, C., Min, H., and Choi, M.J. (1990). Drug testing at the 10th Asian Games and 24th Seoul Olympic Games. *Journal of Analytical Toxicology* 14: 66–72.

Raynaud, E., Audran, M., Brun, J.F., Fedou, C., Chanal, J.L., and Orsetti, A. (1992). False-positive cases in detection of testosterone doping. *Lancet* 340: 1468–1469.

Raynaud, E., Audran, M., Pages, J., Fedou, C., Brun, J.F., Chanal, J.L., and Orsetti, A. (1993). Determination of urinary testosterone and epitestosterone during pubertal development: a cross-sectional study in 141 normal male subjects. *Clinical Endocrinology* 38: 353–359.

Reznik, Y., Herrou, M., Dehennin, L., Lemaire, M., and Leymarie, P. (1987). Rising plasma levels of 19-nortestosterone throughout pregnancy: determination by radioimmunoassay and validation by gas chromatography-mass spectrometry. *Journal of Clinical Endocrinology and Metabolism* 64(5): 1086–1088.

Roche, T., and Davis, W. (1972). Evaluating growth promoters for beef cattle. *Farm and Food Research* 7: 146–148.

Rogozkin, V.A., Morozov, V.I., and Tchaikovsky, V.S. (1979). Rapid radioimmunoassay for anabolic steroids in urine. *Schweizerische Zeitschrift fur Sport Medizin* 27(4): 169–173.

Satchell, M. (1996). Raising "boxcars" out in the barn. *U.S. News and World Report*, 18 March, 40–41.

Schänzer, W. (1996). Metabolism of anabolic androgenic steroids. *Clinical Chemistry* 42(7): 1001–1020.

Schänzer, W., Delahaut, P., Geyer, H., Machnik, M., and Horning, S. (1996a). Long-term detection and identification of metandienone and stanazolol abuse in athletes by gas-chromatography-high-resolution mass spectrometry. *Journal of Chromatography Biomedical Applications* 687(1): 93–108.

Schänzer, W., Geyer, H., Gotzmann, A., Horning, S., Mareck-Engelke, U., Nitschke, R., Nolteemsting, E., and Donike, M. (1995). Endogenous production and excretion of boldenone (17α-hydroxyandrosta-1,4-dien-3-one), an androgenic anabolic steroid. In Donike, M., Geyer, H., Gotzmann, A., and Mareck-Engelke, U., eds. *Proceedings of the 12th Cologne Workshop on Dope Analysis*, pp. 211–212. Cologne: Sport and Buch Strauss.

Schänzer, W., Horning, S., Opfermann, G., and Donike, M. (1996b). GC/MS identification of long-term excreted metabolites of the anabolic steroid 4-chloro-1,2-dehydro-17α-methyltestosterone in human. *Journal of Steroid Biochemistry and Molecular Biology* 57(5/6): 363-376.

Segura, J., de la Torre, R., Pascual, J.A., Ventura, R., Farre, M., Ewin, R.R., and Cami, J. (1995). Antidoping control laboratory at the games of the XXV Olympiad Barcelona '92. In Donike, M., Geyer, H., Gotzmann, A., and Mareck-Engelke, U., eds. *Proceedings of the 12th Cologne Workshop on Dope Analysis*, pp. 413–430. Cologne: Sport and Buch Strauss.

Southan, G.J., Brooks, R.V., Cowan, D.A., Kicman, A.T., Unnadkat, N., and Walker, C.J. (1992). Possible indices for the detection of the administration of dihydrotestosterone to athletes. *Journal of Steroid Biochemistry and Molecular Biology* 42(1): 87–94.

Stenman, U.H., Kallio, L.U., Korhonen, J., and Alfthan, H. (1997). Immunoprocedures for detecting human chorionic gonadotropin: clinical aspects and doping control. *Clinical Chemistry* 43(7): 1293–1298.

Thieme, D., Grosse, J., Lang, L., and Mueller, R.K. (1995). Detection of mesocarb metabolite by LC-TS/MS. In Donike, M., Geyer, H., Gotzmann, A., and Mareck-Engelke, U., eds. *Proceedings of the 12th Cologne Workshop on Dope Analysis*, pp. 275–284. Cologne: Sport and Buch Strauss.

Thieme, D. J., Grosse, R., and Mueller, R.K. (1996). Application of high-resolution and tandem-MS to the identification of anabolic agents. In Donike, M., Geyer, H., Gotzmann, A., and Mareck-Engelke, U., eds. *Proceedings of the 13th Cologne Workshop on Dope Analysis*, pp. 285–297. Cologne: Sport and Buch Strauss.

Volek, J.S., and Kraemer, W.J. (1996). Creatine supplementation: Its effect on human muscular performance and body composition. *Journal of Strength and Conditioning Research* 10(3): 200–210.

Webster, M.J., Webster, M.N., Crawford, R.E., and Gladden, L.B. (1993). Effect of sodium bicarbonate ingestion on exhaustive resistance exercise performance. *Medicine and Science in Sports and Exercise* 25(8): 960–965.

Wide, L., Bengtsson, C., Berglund, B., and Ekblom, B. (1995). Detection in blood and urine of recombinant erythropoietin administered to healthy men. *Medicine and Science in Sports and Exercise* 27(11): 1569–1576.

2

CHAPTER

Doping Control Testing Policies and Procedures: A Critique

David L. Black, PhD, DABFT, DABCC
Aegis Sciences, Nashville, TN

Competitive amateur athletes are subjected to drug testing as a condition of participation, under various rules and procedures. Although all amateur athletic federations rules differ in specific policies regarding drug testing and in the application of these policies, common elements must be present to ensure accuracy and fairness. This chapter addresses the forensic issues in doping control of testing accuracy, athlete rights, burden of proof, and due process, and concludes with specific recommendations for reform.

Testing Accuracy

Doping control is a special application of forensic analytical toxicology, where the test results may result in adverse consequences to an individual's rights, privileges, or freedoms. Specifically, in elite sport an incorrect positive test report may result in loss of right to train or compete, loss of endorsements and income, or the premature termination of the athlete's career. A significant responsibility rests with the athletic organization to ensure that the doping control program is properly understood by the athletes and administrators, and that all procedures are followed by both the athlete and the athletic organization. Ultimately, the accuracy and fairness of the doping control policy is determined by the application of the drug testing program, which begins with the notification of the requirement to test the athlete and the collection of a sample.

These critical comments and the recommendations that follow them are based on experience in representing over 20 athletes in doping control cases. I have represented these athletes, serving as an expert on the issues of proper forensic analysis and test interpretation. In every case except one still pending at the time of this writing, the athlete was ultimately exonerated of the drug use accusation. These cases have been argued within various athletic federations, national governing bodies, and United States state and federal courts. One case was decided by the United States Supreme Court. Another case was successfully argued before the Court of Arbitration in Sport. Without exception, these cases have revealed inequities and injustice within the current drug testing and review hearing processes used in elite sport.

Forensic Analytical Toxicology

Historically, the International Olympic Committee (IOC) has certified laboratories to conduct the necessary testing to enforce IOC, national governing body, and federation doping control policies. The IOC-led program has relied on laboratory personnel to develop methods, validate methods, regulate, and issue certification for testing, to review and interpret test results, and testify to the accuracy of the process. The program has not recognized a forensic sample–handling requirement of the doping control program and has not required rigorous documentation of analytical processes, such as that required for proper forensic analysis. The forensic analytical process requires that complete chain of custody documentation is maintained regarding the original samples as well as all portions of the original samples actually tested. This documentation ensures the correct association of testing results to a

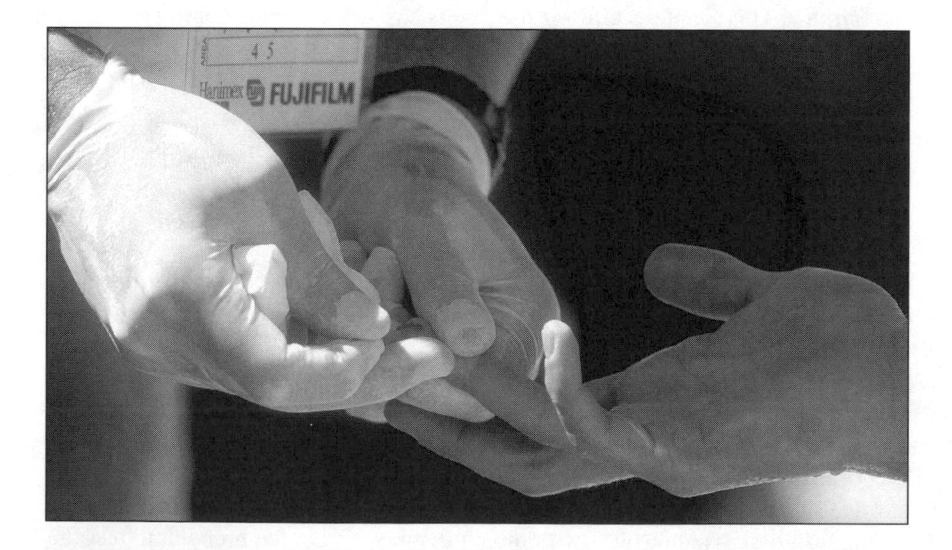

Australian Michael Klim providing a blood sample during the World Swimming Championships at Perth, Australia, 1998.
© Al Bello/Allsport

specific athlete. To ensure the accuracy and integrity of the process requires inspection and unbiased peer review of certified laboratories as well as their procedures, policies, and documentation of analysis. The current IOC laboratory certification program lacks impartial peer review and critical inspection of analytical and forensic sample handling procedures.

Urine, and other biological samples, collected to enforce current doping control programs must be treated as "evidence" throughout the collection, transportation, and analysis process. The information obtained from the testing process is "evidence" to be used to form the foundation of the accusation against an athlete. Typically no other evidence will exist, separate from the sample test results and associated data, to justify an accusation of drug use. The integrity of a doping control program is solely dependent on the sporting organization administering the program, and not on the athlete subject to the procedures and policies. Thus, confidence in any doping control program rests entirely on the completeness and accuracy of the drug testing program. A failure by the sport governing bodies to insist on completeness and accuracy—and impartial and unbiased inspection and certification of the laboratories—compromises the fairness of the program and ultimately compromises confidence in the program. The current practice of overlooking or ignoring laboratory errors of commission and omission has in many cases resulted in athletes being falsely accused of drug use. The IOC, national governing bodies, and athletic federations have abdicated their responsibilities by allowing the laboratory staff to function as fact gatherers, while at the same time wielding far too much influence over the people responsible for prosecuting and judging athletes accused of doping.

Notification and Sample Collection

When athletes are selected for drug testing, they should be notified, identified with a photograph, and then escorted at all times. An escort and constant supervision are necessary to protect against any opportunity for drug-using athletes to adulterate or manipulate the sample collection, thereby invalidating or complicating the test result. Subsequent to notification to be tested, athletes should be allowed only fluids from randomly selected sealed containers of water as necessary. Sealed containers protect the athletes from the actual, or claimed, unknowing ingestion of a banned substance.

Upon arrival at the collection area, athletes should be required to remove any jackets or bulky clothing, and wash their hands before providing the urine sample. They must each be allowed to choose randomly from a selection of sealed and sterile containers that will be used to collect the urine specimen.

The collector must ensure that the selected collection container remains with the athlete at all times until the process is completed. Collection of the urine sample must be conducted by a collector of the same sex, preferably with direct observation, or semi-direct observation if necessary, depending on the athletic organization policy.

The collector must immediately check the urine sample to ensure that the temperature range is 32-38°C (90-100°F), the specific gravity is equal to or greater than 1.005, and the pH is in the 4.0-8.0 range. These checks verify that the urine sample is normal. If the sample temperature, specific gravity, or pH is not acceptable, the abnormal sample collection should be completed, and then the athlete should be required to wait and provide a second sample. In the presence of the athlete, the laboratory staff should split the urine sample into two containers typically marked "A" and "B" and secure the containers with tamper-evident seals. The collector and athlete must complete sample custody and control forms that identify the athlete, the collector, the sample control numbers, any medications or supplements used by the athlete, and which have the signature of the athlete acknowledging correct sample identification. A copy of the custody and control form is provided to the athlete to document the collection event. The collector must initiate chain of custody documentation for the samples by recording receipt of the sample from the donor, as well as release of the samples to a courier for transport to the laboratory. Samples collected must remain in the custody and control of the collector at all times until release to the courier for transport.

Delay of transport beyond 12 hours requires the samples be refrigerated. Delay of transport beyond 24 hours requires the samples be frozen. Delivery of samples to the laboratory should be by commercial overnight courier providing delivery within three days of sample collection. Samples delivered more than three days after collection, and not received frozen by the laboratory, should not be accepted or analyzed by the laboratory because of uncertainty in sample storage conditions resulting in possible bacterial growth and contamination. Upon receipt at the laboratory, the original "A" and "B" split samples chain of custody should continue with documentation of release by courier, receipt by laboratory, and with the correct notation of date and time of receipt, as well as the name and signature of the receiving individual. Chain of custody of the original "A" and "B" split samples must continue in the laboratory with documentation of all handling and storage of the samples by date, time, individual, and purpose of handling.

Forensic Analysis

A number of other writers have reviewed the lists of banned substances, technical procedures and methods, and the technologies used for doping control. In summary, the urine sample collected from the athlete is transported to the laboratory and the sample is submitted to a series of screening tests. The screening tests are designed to determine whether the urine sample submitted is normal and whether the sample contains a banned drug (i.e., the screening test is positive). The primary purpose of the screening test is to identify the majority of samples that are negative, so that greater attention and additional testing can be given to the minority that are positive. The samples testing positive during the screening are subjected to a second confirmation test, usually gas chromatography or mass spectrometry, to specifically identify what drug is present and in what quantity. These technical aspects are the focus of most reports in contemporary testing programs, to the exclusion of the necessary forensic documentation and interpretation of results.

The forensic sample–handling and chain of custody documentation is an essential part of the analytical testing process and should be considered as important as the analytical methods or procedures in doping control programs. It is very important, from a forensic perspective, that the laboratory receiving the samples protects the sample storage or testing areas from unescorted access by visitors or unauthorized laboratory personnel. The security of the laboratory must be sufficient to document all individuals who have access to the samples, the records, and the test results.

Upon receipt by the laboratory, the original sample packaging and sample seals must be inspected to assess for breakage or tampering. The laboratory staff must document any unusual condition of the shipping package. Original samples must be stored refrigerated to protect the samples against bacterial or fungal growth. Chain of custody documentation must be completed contemporaneously with each handling and accessing of the original samples. The staff should inspect the "A" sample seals for breaking or tampering before opening to remove an aliquot, or portion, for screening analysis. Any evidence of breakage or tampering of the original "A" bottle seal must be documented and may require rejection of the sample for analysis. The "A" sample containers should be opened only one at a time, with aliquots assigned to a screening batch of multiple aliquots. Each sample portion should be tested for pH and specific gravity to verify that the sample is consistent with a normal random urine. Each screening batch must consist of a calibrator, a negative quality control sample, a positive quality control sample, and a set of "A" sample aliquots. Laboratory personnel must provide chain of custody documentation of all handling and processing of the batch of "A" aliquots, recording the location and actual purpose of each handling of the aliquots.

Upon completion of analysis, the laboratory must critically review the forensic and analytical records to ensure that the analysis is complete and accurate. Screening samples testing negative must be reported as negative, and screening samples testing positive must be scheduled for confirmatory analysis. To conduct the confirmation test, the original "A" sample is opened and a fresh aliquot is removed for analysis. The confirmation batch must consist of a calibrator for the drug to be confirmed as present, a negative quality control, a positive quality control containing the targeted drug, and the "A" sample aliquot(s).

After completing the "A" confirmation analysis, the laboratory should critically review the forensic and analytical records for completeness and accuracy. Confirmation samples testing negative must be reported as negative, and samples testing positive are normally reported as positive. Special interpretive consideration must be given for any report concerning altered or elevated testosterone/epitestosterone (T/E) ratio, caffeine, ephedrine, pseudoephedrine, or elevated epitestosterone. The interpretation of altered T/E ratios is complex due to an incomplete understanding of epitestosterone production in the human, diurnal variation of steroid production in the male and female, female birth control medication use, and the many cases of athletes with normal urine testosterone concentrations but suppressed epitestosterone concentrations, leading to an alleged positive T/E ratio greater than six. Caffeine interpretation is difficult due to the prevalence of caffeine in food and beverages and the influence of hydration on urine caffeine concentrations. Ephedrine and pseudoephedrine are also difficult to interpret due to the prevalence of these chemicals in over-the-counter cold products, diet aids, and supplements. These products also interfere with the testing for the presence of amphetamines and may contribute to a false conclusion of amphetamine abuse. Elevated epitestosterone is a poorly understood analytical finding, especially since this product is not a pharmaceutical product generally available and is also believed to be an anti-androgenic compound. The laboratory then issues positive reports to the appropriate athletic organization, and the athlete is notified.

The athlete is provided an opportunity to be present at the opening and testing of the "B" split sample (counter analysis) in the same laboratory that conducted the "A" split sample analysis. The athlete also may have a legal representative or analytical expert present to view the opening and testing of the "B" sample. If the athlete chooses not to attend in person or have a representative or expert present, the laboratory typically will select a surrogate witness to verify that the seal is intact on the "B" split sample and for comparison of color consistency with the "A" split sample.

Following verification that the seal is intact, the "B" sample is opened and an aliquot processed to reconfirm the finding in the "A" split sample. The "B" sample aliquot should be tested by pH and specific gravity to verify that the sample is consistent with the "A" split sample; in addition, the color and transparency of the "A" and "B" sample should be similar. The "B" split sample reconfirmation batch must consist of a calibrator for the drug to be confirmed as present, a negative quality control, a positive quality control containing the targeted drug, and the "B" sample aliquot(s). When the "B" reconfirmation analysis is completed, the forensic and analytical records must be critically reviewed before issuing a report. Reconfirmation "B" samples testing negative or with results either qualitatively or quantitatively significantly different than the "A" split sample results must be reported as negative, and samples testing positive must be reported as positive. Before issuing a final positive report for the reconfirmation of the "B" split sample, all the forensic and analytical documentation for both the "A" and "B" split sample analysis should be critically reviewed to ensure completeness and accuracy.

The chain of custody documentation must be complete and allow for an uninterrupted documentation of the original sample collection by the subject athlete to the final "A" and "B" analytical results. Any breaks in the chain of custody require the sample be reported as negative, since the results cannot be associated with the subject athlete. Any minor deviations from normal analytical methods or procedure must be documented by memoranda verifying that such changes do not alter the final analytical conclusion.

Athlete Rights

All rhetoric aside, current doping control policies and practices presume that an athlete is guilty until proven innocent following a positive drug test report. This is perhaps the single most harmful policy characterizing current doping control programs. The consequence of this policy is to relieve the laboratories and athlete organization of their institutional responsibilities to adhere to their procedures and to administer their programs with accuracy and fairness. The stigma, cost, and psychological effect on the accused athlete are profound. The stigma resulting from the accusation removes any opportunity for fairness or unbiased review within the hearing process. The accused athlete is confronted with immediate significant expense in having to retain an attorney and an expert to represent his or her interests and attempt to prove the athlete's innocence. The immediate loss of moral support by their federations often leaves athletes psychologically unable to effectively participate in developing a defense. The athlete is immediately deemed to have diminished rights within the review and hearing process within the athlete's own federation or governing body. The athlete and the athlete's retained representatives are further disadvantaged by the necessity of dealing with complex forensic analytical issues and also with complex and confusing procedural issues.

Burden of Proof

The current doping control procedures and policies result in an accusation of banned substance abuse based on a single urine specimen collection and analysis. All the evidence forming the accusation against the athlete remains in the possession of the accuser.

The accused athlete, while currently treated as guilty until proven innocent, must have an attorney and a technical expert make an appeal to obtain the evidence forming the accusation. The IOC-accredited laboratories controlling the analytical data and information are often slow to provide all the forensic handling and analytical documentation. Although athletes can request a standard litigation support packet, in the author's experience the information provided is always incomplete, resulting in both delay of process and the need for repeated appeals for documentation. In addition, it is now United States Olympic Committee (USOC) policy that accused athletes must pay for the litigation support packet. This means that athletes must pay for a copy of the very evidence forming the basis of the accusation and the data necessary to be used to help understand the accusation and argue their innocence.

The current doping control programs are further complicated by the issue of testing for use of testosterone or use of a drug that results in an increase in the amount of testosterone. The analytical requirements of identifying a synthetic chemical or drug not normally found in the human body are extremely challenging. High standards of analytical performance must be achieved to ensure against false test findings or false accusations of use of banned synthetic drugs. However, the testing to identify testosterone administration must rise to a higher standard, since the presence of testosterone is normal in both male and female athletes.

The current procedures and interpretation of test data to identify an elevated T/E, which requires indirect evidence of testosterone use, are grossly inadequate. The testing process, and testing interpretation, cannot account for all the variables that may influence the testosterone or epitestosterone concentrations in urine. Historically, persuasive arguments were made by IOC experts that a T/E ratio greater than 6:1 provided evidence beyond a reasonable doubt that testosterone had been used. Subsequently it has been acknowledged that some individuals naturally have T/E ratios greater than 6:1. The original IOC hypothesis that an elevated T/E ratio would document, and result only from, an excess of testosterone, has not been proven in practice. Most T/E ratios greater than 6 are in fact a consequence of a normal testosterone urine concentration and a suppressed epitestosterone urine concentration.

Epitestosterone is a natural steroid poorly studied or understood within the field of endocrinology. Normal biological factors influencing the production of epitestosterone in humans, and thus the T/E ratio, are not understood. It is well documented that hormone and steroid production in males and females fluctuates over time and that disease, diet, and supplements will alter natural concentrations. The issue is more complicated in female athletes, with hormone and steroid production more variable than in the male. The T/E ratio in females is complicated further through the use of birth control medications, which specifically contain steroids to influence the natural female hormone and steroid production.

An additional complication affecting female athletes and their use of birth control medications is the generation of urine metabolites that suggest the use of banned nandrolone (19-nortestosterone; deca-durabolin). Female athletes have been falsely accused of nandrolone use based on positive urine test results for nandrolone metabolites.

These complicated test interpretation issues have been exposed over time as athletes, accused of banned substance use, have developed arguments in their defense. The evolution of a better understanding of how these factors affect test results has come at the expense of athletes subjected to poorly formed doping program procedures and policies. The doping programs have typically rushed to employ sophisticated technology and instrumentation without the benefit of understanding the full consequences of the information produced. In developing a strict liability program, procedures have not been put into place to require evidence and test interpretation that satisfy the requirement of "beyond a reasonable doubt." The need to develop a "beyond a reasonable doubt" standard has been impaired by the "guilty until proven innocent" doctrine.

Due Process

In order to ensure accuracy in drug testing laboratories and fair treatment of athletes, athletic federations have a responsibility to follow clear procedures and policies.

Athletic Federation Policy

As a consequence of the "guilty until proven innocent" policy embedded in today's testing programs, the athlete's federation is most likely unwilling to support the athlete financially during the appeal process. This is a critically important issue because the athlete is placed in a position of having to petition the athletic federation for the evidence forming the basis of the accusation from the laboratory. The athlete requires advice and guidance regarding federation or national governing body policy to understand appeal procedures and deadlines.

Analysis of the "B" Split Sample

The "B" split sample analysis is scheduled for reconfirmation at the laboratory reporting on the "A" split sample positive results. Because of the international nature of amateur athletics, the procedure may require an immediate significant expense to the athlete, who must attend the reconfirmation testing or arrange for a representative to be present. The short-term expense to an athlete who needs to retain legal counsel, obtain expert consulting, and travel to the "B" split sample analysis can easily exceed $10,000 (US).

Litigation Support Packet

Immediately following the completion of the "B" split sample reconfirmation analysis, the athlete and legal representatives must appeal for the litigation support packet. The litigation support packet should be forthcoming and at no cost to the athlete. The litigation support packet should contain all of the analytical and forensic sample handling documentation for both the "A" and "B" split samples analysis. The documentation should include, at a minimum, the following:

- documentation of original "A" and "B" sample collection and transport to the laboratory;
- receipt of the samples at the laboratory;
- analytical data for "A" sample integrity checks (pH, specific gravity);
- analytical data for "A" sample screening;
- analytical data for "A" sample confirmation;
- analytical data for "B" sample integrity checks (pH, specific gravity);
- analytical data for "B" sample reconfirmation;
- chain of custody for "A" and "B" split samples documenting all handling, storage conditions, and location, as well as the opening of container and the aliquots removed;
- chain of custody for all "A" and "B" sample aliquots used for screening and confirmation analysis;
- sequence tables and batch forms identifying all samples and sequence of samples in the batches analyzed;
- quality control results identifying both expected and measured results;
- copies of the analytical procedure used for identifying the drug present;
- narrative statement describing sample handling and processing, and the documentation procedure for errors; and

- narrative statement describing quality control procedures and the documentation procedure for errors.

A complete litigation support packet should contain between 50 and 150 pages of documentation, depending on the drug identified and the procedures used. The litigation packet should be certified and all pages numbered sequentially to identify the complete package of data.

Timely Hearings

Hearings should take place in a timely manner. Ideally one or more members of a hearing panel should possess the technical expertise required to comprehend the forensic toxicology issues certain to be raised in the hearing. Unfortunately, panels are not always made up of experts, nor are they always timely. Furthermore, when experts are present, they all too often have a close relationship to an IOC-accredited laboratory or a sports federation. In other words, they do not participate as truly independent experts.

Recommendations for Policy Reform

A change in policy to shift the burden of proof to the IOC laboratory and the athletic organization would result in a paradigm shift, creating the opportunity for avoiding many of the false accusations of drug use by athletes. This change alone could go a long way in restoring credibility to the IOC doping control program. Shifting the focus from the athlete's need to prove innocence to the laboratory's need to provide proof of guilt would change attitudes throughout the process and better protect innocent athletes. The laboratory requirement must be to adhere to all policies and procedures that ensure a complete and accurate forensic report. A change in attitude challenging the laboratory to ensure completeness and accuracy will result in greater attention to laboratory protocol and errors.

Hearings

Because of the highly technical nature of issues presented in drug-related cases, a forensic toxicology expert should sit on the hearing panel or be appointed as an advisor to the panel. The expert should be independent from the IOC-certified laboratories and the athletic federation. The expert should function essentially as *amicus curiae,* or neutral consultant, to the panel and not be present as an advocate for the athletic federation or athlete.

Hearings should also occur within a reasonable period of time following the completion of the "B" split sample reconfirmation. The athlete and athlete representatives should be allowed a reasonable period of time to prepare arguments, but the career life span of many athletes is so short as to demand timely case hearing.

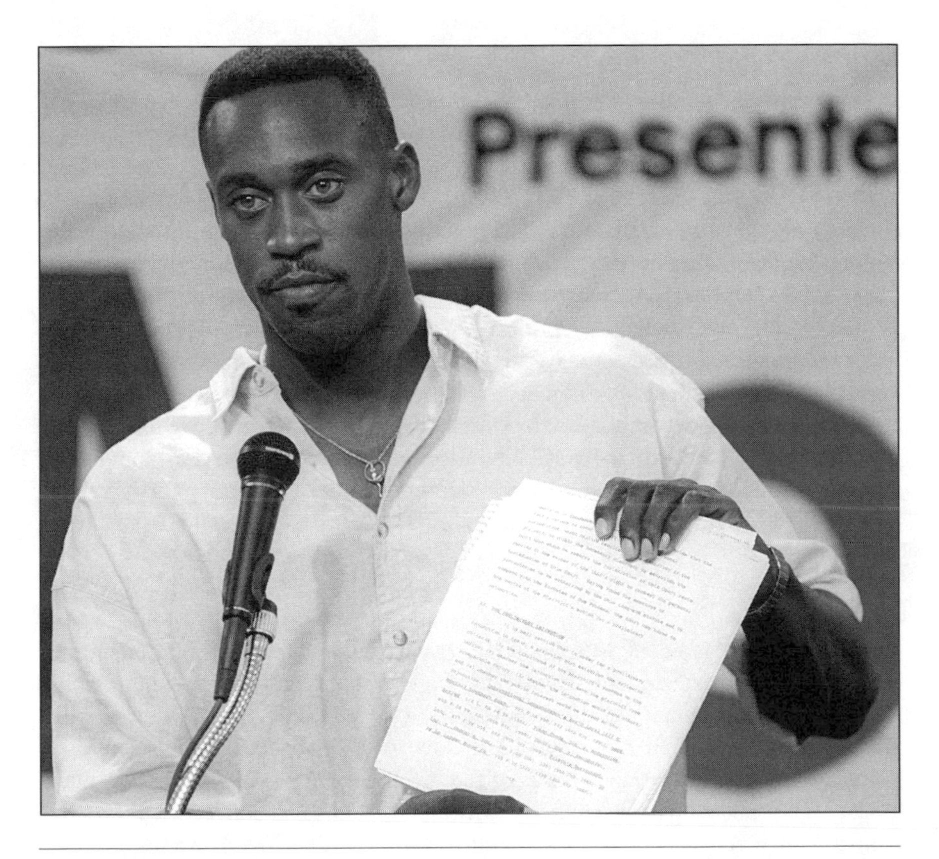

Butch Reynolds of the United States argues against his two-year drug ban at a 1992 news conference. An American court ruled in Reynold's favor, but the IAAF refused to lift its ban.
© Mike Powell/Allsport

Second Opinion Analysis

To further protect the rights of athletes, and to shift the burden of proof to the laboratory, the appeal of a "B" test should result in reconfirmation analysis in a second certified laboratory. The "B" split sample should be shipped with chain of custody documentation with a specific request to reconfirm the results of the "A" split sample. The current practice of allowing the "B" split sample to be reconfirmed in the same laboratory that issued the original positive finding does not allow for a second independent analysis and opinion to be provided. This policy would further ensure that the "A" split sample analysis laboratory would follow proper procedure and assemble complete documentation for the "A" sample screening and confirmation testing. A "second analytical opinion" procedure must allow for timely analysis of the "B" sample and must provide specific policies regarding conflicts in sample integrity checks or positive test results.

Litigation Support Packet

The current procedure is for IOC laboratory directors to review the "A" split sample data and to report a conclusion of a positive test result directly to the athletic organization. There is currently no separate review process to evaluate the "evidence" of the positive finding (i.e., the litigation support packet) and to consider alternative explanations for a positive finding before notification of the athlete. Implementing an independent review board, verifying both the accuracy of the analytical data and completeness of the chain of custody documentation, would be a simple method of protecting athletes against flawed analysis. An independent review board could decide that the litigation support packet is insufficient to form the foundation of an accusation, or might insist on investigations of errors of omission or commission before accusing the athlete of drug use. Such a procedure could ensure that IOC laboratories follow all necessary laboratory analytical policies and could ultimately correct the current disparity between IOC facilities.

T/E Ratio

The T/E ratio test should be suspended until a greater understanding of the natural production of epitestosterone is understood and a better analytical method identifying the use of synthetic testosterone can be developed. The T/E ratio should absolutely not be applied to female athletes, because of the current lack of scientific knowledge of natural variance limits of female androgen production. In the future a drug, or suspected performance enhancement chemical practice, should not be banned until a consistent evaluation method has been developed and subjected to independent peer review. "Natural" products should not be placed on the banned drug or practices list until a proper interpretation of the test data has been developed through a peer review process.

Recommendations for Laboratory Procedure Reform

The following changes in procedure would ensure that laboratory testing is accurate, impartial, and timely.

Laboratory Accreditation

The certification of doping control laboratories should be administered through a third-party organization or independent certifying agency. Laboratories should be challenged with survey samples to assess their technical capabilities and inspected to verify the forensic handling and control of samples tested. Inspection procedures should also evaluate and verify facility security, written procedures, quality control, quality assurance, instrument maintenance, and qualifications of personnel. In order to ensure impartial decisions, the inspectors and the certification process must be completely independent from the athletic organization personnel responsible for administering hearings and reviews.

Method Validation

A standard procedure for analytical method validation must be developed. Forensic laboratories must assess their methods to determine limits of detection, limits of quantitation, linear range, and precision of analysis. Objective criteria applying to all data generated must describe quality control acceptance and rejection criteria, and objective Gas Chromatography-Mass Spectrometry data acceptance criteria. Minimum reporting thresholds for confirmation analysis should be established to create consistency among laboratories and consistency in treatment of athletes. Standardization of data assessment and reporting procedures is necessary to ensure consistent performance among laboratories and to establish performance standards for the many laboratories.

Alternative Matrix

Research should be funded through the IOC and federations to investigate alternative matrix analysis. Current testing of urine only is limiting in several ways. Androgenic anabolic steroids are banned drugs used by athletes during training, but discontinued before competition in order to "pass" the urine test. A number of products and techniques are employed by athletes to flush the drugs from their system before competition, or chemicals are used to interfere with the test performance to create a "false-negative" report. However, analysis of hair can document drug use weeks and months before the competitive event, depending on the length of the hair. Although several reports in the peer-reviewed literature have documented the ability to isolate and identify androgenic anabolic steroids from hair, these methods require additional validation. The hair used in such testing does not have to be crown hair, but may be any body hair. Hair testing would create an opportunity to "look back" over the training period to identify androgenic anabolic steroid use, and would provide an excellent sample type for random, out-of-competition testing.

Testing urine at the time of competition is complicated by the potential use of a performance-enhancing drug several days before an event. Arguments may be presented that the drug in the urine at the time of the event is residual from prior use, and not evidence of an effort to enhance performance at the competitive event. In addition, many of the banned drugs are pharmaceutical products used legally by physicians to treat disease; the administration of medication by a physician to treat acute illness has been a continuing point of argument in alleged doping cases.

Saliva samples could document the use of a banned drug within a period of hours before a competitive event, and thus indicate use with intent of performance enhancement. Because saliva is an ultrafiltrate of the blood, the drug in saliva is an indirect indicator of the blood concentration of drug. Saliva represents a better sample choice than blood, since saliva may be obtained without a needle stick and without the potentially controversial invasive practices associated with taking blood. Research needs to be conducted to validate the procedure; however, saliva methods have been reported in the peer-reviewed literature that document detection of many of the drug classes banned. Saliva represents an excellent sample matrix that could be used to identify drug use at the time of competition.

Conclusions

The purpose of doping control is to reduce and ultimately eliminate the use of banned substances in sport. This is a worthy goal, but it should not be pursued at the financial and psychological expense of athletes who have committed no offense. The present system of doping control too often violates the rights of athletes. Sport governing bodies that conduct drug testing must adhere to strict standards of collection, documentation, and interpretation of data. Their failure to do so will result in doping control programs that are neither fair nor, in the final analysis, effective.

Bibliography

Black, David L., ed. 1995. *Drug Testing in Sports.* Niles, IL: Preston Publications.

Bowers, L.D. 1997. Analytical advances in detection of performance-enhancing compounds. *Clinical Chemistry* 43(7): 1299-1304.

Catlin, D.H., Hatton, C.K., and Starcevic, S.H. 1997. Issues in detecting abuse of xenobiotic anabolic steroids and testosterone by analysis of athletes' urine. *Clinical Chemistry* 43(7): 1280-1288.

Committee on the Judiciary, U.S. Senate, Report to the Chairman. *Drug Misuse: Anabolic Steroids and Human Growth Hormone.* 1989. Washington, DC: United States General Accounting Office.

Dubin, Charles L., Commissioner. 1990. *Commission of Inquiry into the Use of Drugs and Banned Practices Intended to Increase Athletic Performance.* Ottawa, Canada: Canadian Government Publishing Center.

International Amateur Athletic Federation. 1994. *Procedural Guidelines for Doping Control.* Barcelona, Spain: International Amateur Athletic Foundation.

International Olympic Committee. 1995. *IOC Medical Code.* Lausanne, Switzerland: International Olympic Committee.

Wadler, G.I., and Hainline, B. 1989. *Drugs and the Athlete*. Philadelphia: F.A. Davis.

Yesalis, C.E. 1993. *Anabolic Steroids in Sport and Exercise.* Champaign, IL: Human Kinetics Publishers.

3

CHAPTER

Difficulties in Estimating the Prevalence of Drug Use Among Athletes

Charles E. Yesalis III, ScD
Pennsylvania State University, University Park, PA
Andrea N. Kopstein, PhD
National Institute on Drug Abuse, Rockville, MD
Michael S. Bahrke, PhD
Human Kinetics, Champaign, IL

Sport is an integral part of American culture, as it is in many other cultures around the world. It has multiple purposes, including personal fulfillment, enjoyment, and entertainment—all of which have resulted in sport becoming a multibillion-dollar global business. "To the victor go the spoils," and with large amounts of money and adulation at stake, some competitors will cheat to obtain these objectives. One method of cheating is to use performance-enhancing drugs.

The use of drugs to enhance physical performance has been a facet of athletic competition since the beginning of recorded history (Prokop, 1970; Strauss and Curry, 1987). The legendary Berserkers of Norse mythology used bufotenin for stimulating effects, whereas West Africans used Cola accuminita and Cola nitida during running competitions in ancient times (Prokop, 1970; Boje, 1939). The gladiators in the Roman Coliseum used stimulants to overcome fatigue and injury, and the ancient Greeks ate hallucinogenic mushrooms as well as sesame seeds with the goal of enhancing performance (Wadler and Hainline, 1989). For centuries South American Indians have chewed coca leaves to increase endurance (Boje, 1939; Karpovich, 1941).

During the 19th century, performance-enhancing drug use among athletes was commonplace. Swimmers, distance runners, sprinters, and cyclists used drugs such as caffeine, alcohol, nitroglycerine, digitalis, cocaine, strychnine, ether, opium, and heroin in attempts to gain a competitive edge over their opponents (Boje, 1939; Hoberman, 1992; Prokop, 1970). Indeed, the first fatality attributed to a performance-enhancing drug was that of an English cyclist who overdosed on tri-methyl during a race between Bordeaux and Paris in 1886 (Prokop, 1970). In 1939, in a paper entitled "Doping," Boje stated,

> There can be no doubt that stimulants are today widely used by athletes participating in competitions; the record-breaking craze and the desire to satisfy an exacting public play a more and more prominent role, and take higher rank than the health of the competitors itself. (439-440)

Today, athletes employ a wide variety of drugs to enhance performance, including anabolic steroids, human growth hormone, insulin-like growth factor, erythropoietin, thyroid hormone, insulin, human chorionic gonadotropin, gonadotropin-releasing hormone, clenbuterol, L-dopa, clonidine, dehydroepiandrosterone, ephedrine, gamma hydroxy butyrate, and amphetamines. Currently, over 100 substances are banned by the International Olympic Committee, including over 17 individual anabolic steroids and related compounds (*International Olympic Committee Medical Code*, 1995).

Our concerns over drug use in sport are generally founded in one or more of the following moral and ethical issues: (1) The athlete may suffer physical or psychological harm as a result of drug use. (2) The use of drugs by one athlete may coerce other athletes to use drugs to maintain parity. (3) The use of drugs in sport is unnatural in that any resulting success is due to external factors. (4) The athlete who uses drugs has an unfair advantage over athletes who do not use them (Yesalis, 1993).

Given these concerns, it is important to be able to accurately assess the magnitude of drug use in sport. If we underestimate drug use (i.e., false negatives), it is very likely that these concerns will, at least in part, be realized. If we overestimate drug use (i.e., false positives), we could injure the reputations of individuals, teams, or even nations.

Until the mid-1970s, all that was known regarding the incidence of performance-enhancing drug use in sport was based on anecdotes, testimonials, and rumors reported by journalists and others (Gilbert, 1969a,b,c; Scott, 1971; Wade, 1972; Wright, 1978). High levels of steroid use were reported in weightlifting, powerlifting, bodybuilding, professional football, and the throwing events in track and field; even use by high school athletes was reported as early as 1959 (Frazier, 1973; Gilbert, 1969a,b,c). Although investigative journalism still serves as an indicator of the level of drug use in sport, other sources of information also are available. These include government records and investigations as well as the results of systematic surveys and drug testing associated with athletic competition.

This chapter discusses the difficulties faced in accurately estimating the prevalence of drug use among athletes by examining the four major methods generally employed in estimating use: investigative journalism, government investigation, drug testing, and surveys, with particular attention given to the veracity of responses to survey questions.

Investigative Journalism

Journalists, using primarily the personal observations, accounts, or opinions of self-selected informants, both anonymous and attributed, have detailed during the past four decades a sustained epidemic of drug use in sport at the professional, Olympic, collegiate, and even the high school levels (Bamberger and Yaeger, 1997; Fish, 1993a; Gilbert, 1969a,b,c; Janofsky, 1988; Johnson, 1985; Kelley, 1991; Keteyian, 1989; Litsky, 1993; Rosellini, 1992; Scott, 1971, Todd, 1983; Wade, 1972; Zimmerman, 1986). The writings and testimonials of former athletes and others in, or around, sport generally have confirmed that doping in sport is a serious problem (Alzado, 1991; Courson, 1991; Francis, 1990; Hoberman, 1992; Huizenga, 1994; Klecko and Fields, 1989; Mix, 1987; Voy, 1991).

Although using investigative methods to assess the incidence of performance-enhancing drug use in sport is often less expensive and time-consuming than the other methods, it is fraught with methodological limitations. Individuals who use or have used drugs and who serve as informants may project their behavior onto others in an attempt to rationalize their drug use—as they may say, "Everybody does it." Consequently, an overestimate of the level of drug use may result. Conversely, athletes, coaches, team physicians, and others involved in competition may either refuse to cooperate with journalists or deny drug use to protect themselves, teammates, their school, or the reputation of their sport. In fact, the Dubin Commission (1990; see discussion later in this chapter) referred to a "conspiracy of silence" and a "pact of ignorance" among those in sport regarding discussion of the issue of drug use. Testimonials on drug use in sport are generally only given by former athletes, because current athletes fear possible retribution from coaches, teammates, or sport federation officials. Even former athletes may be reticent to discuss drug use because they could be ostracized by the news media, as well as by their fans and former teammates. In turn, this could affect their livelihood by resulting in the loss of paid speaking engagements, endorsements, autograph signings, and induction into halls of fame. Each of these disincentives could result in an underestimate of drug use in sport.

Similarly, sport federation officials, when interviewed, have often tended to either deny that a major doping problem exists within sport or have at least downplayed its magnitude (*Chicago-Sun Times,* 1994; *Milwaukee Sentinel,* 1993; *Sports Medicine Digest,* 1996). When pushed, sport officials have stated "We've had problems in the past, but now things are different" (*Champaign News Gazette,* 1995; *Chicago Tribune,* 1992, *USA Today,* 1998b; Yesalis, 1996).

Another potential problem within investigative journalism is the scope of the investigation and its effect on the generalizability of the findings. Often reports will focus on a few athletes, teams, or sports. Even if the findings are valid, can they be legitimately generalized beyond the scope of the investigation? It is most likely that they cannot.

Government Investigations

During the past three decades, the U.S. Congress has held several hearings on performance-enhancing drug use in sport (U.S. Congress, 1988, 1989a, 1989b, 1990). During these hearings, current and former athletes, and some coaches and sport federation officials, with few exceptions, have supported the notion that there is a significant doping problem. However, from a methodological perspective, once again, the volunteered opinions and observations of a relatively small sample of individuals, selected in a nonrandom manner, were used to estimate the extent of doping in a relatively small number of sports at various levels of competition.

Spawned by the Ben Johnson doping incident in the 1988 Seoul Olympic Games, the Dubin Commission (1990) in Canada investigated the extent of drug use in Olympic sport. Although the proceedings employed a more aggressive legal format, including cross-examination of witnesses under oath, it fell well short of the

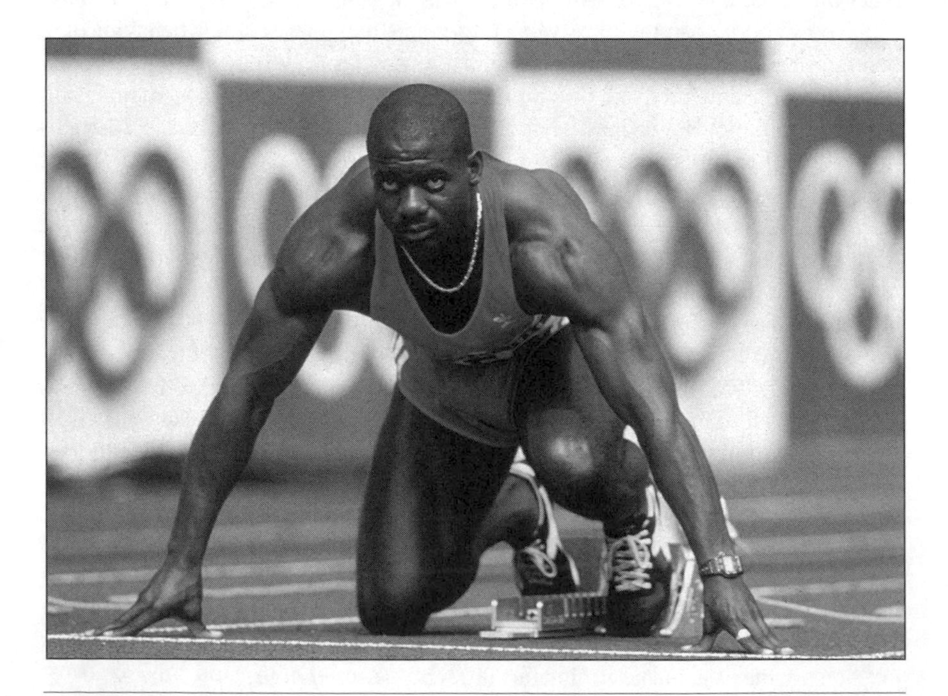

Canadian sprinter Ben Johnson at the start of the men's 100-meter final at the 1988 Seoul Olympic Games. Johnson finished first, but was disqualified when the post-race drug test revealed he had used stanozolol, an anabolic steroid.

adversarial format of a trial, and relied heavily on the veracity and recall of selected witnesses. Nevertheless, after 91 days of testimony from a parade of witnesses, the Commission concluded:

> Unfortunately, the noble sentiments and lofty ideals proclaimed in the Olympic Charter are a far cry from the reality of international competition. This reality has not until recently been widely known, but the conspiracy of silence has now been broken and the truth revealed. Truth is not always pleasant. (516)

Franke and Berendonk's (1997) analysis of a large cache of captured Stasi, or secret police, files from the former German Democratic Republic paints a chilling picture of sustained collusion among high-level government, sports medicine, drug testing, sport federation, and East German Olympic officials to systematically dope East German athletes. Even though the face validity of these data is seemingly great, at least 15 of those accused by the authors of collaborating in this doping conspiracy have sought relief in the German courts (Franke, 1998). However, to date, all have lost. In fact, these Stasi files have served as primary evidence for a wide-scale criminal prosecution of the individuals involved (*Des Moines Register,* 1997; Franke, 1998; *USA Today*, 1997).

Although the internal validity of Franke and Berendonk's conclusions appears quite strong, the external validity (generalizability) is brought into question in that all the data involve one, now defunct, country. Notwithstanding, the temptation to draw parallels with the former Soviet Union's and the current Communist China's sport systems is great.

Drug Testing

During the past 10 years, less than 3 percent of Olympic and National Football League athletes who were tested were shown to be positive for banned substances (Catlin and Murray, 1996). These results appear to be at great odds with most of the conclusions of investigations conducted by journalists and the government organizations discussed previously. This is likely a result of the fact that drug testing as a method of estimating the level of performance-enhancing drug use is seriously flawed in that testing can often be circumvented by the user, increasing the probability of a false negative. In the case of testing only at competitive events, athletes usually can determine when to discontinue use of training drugs (such as anabolic steroids) prior to testing in order to allow the metabolites of the drugs to clear the body and, thus, avoid a positive test (Kammerer, 1993; Yesalis and Cowart, 1998). When faced with unannounced, out-of-competition testing, drug-using athletes have available a number of strategies to successfully circumvent the testing process (Kammerer, 1993; Longman, 1995; Yesalis, 1996; Yesalis and Cowart, 1998). For example, athletes can titrate their dose by using transdermal patches or skin creams containing testosterone, and, combined with the results of self-testing from private laboratories, remain below the maximum allowable testosterone/epitestosterone ratio of 6:1 (Kammerer, 1993; Longman, 1995; Yesalis and Cowart, 1998).

Another factor allowing drug-using athletes to escape detection is the lack of effective tests for certain performance-enhancing drugs. At present, there is no effective test to detect the presence of exogenous human growth hormone, which is used by power, strength, and sprint athletes for its anabolic (muscle-building) effects. According to a *Sports Illustrated* article (Bamberger and Yaeger, 1997) on doping in sport, some athletes jokingly referred to the Atlanta Olympics as the "Growth Hormone Games." A related anabolic hormone, insulin-like growth factor, is also available to athletes, and as with human growth hormone, there is no effective test for detecting its use. There is also no viable test as yet for erythropoietin, which is used by some athletes to increase their number of red blood cells, thus improving the oxygen-carrying capacity of their blood and ultimately the athlete's endurance performance (Kammerer, 1993; *USA Today*, 1998b). Significant numbers of high school, collegiate, and Olympic athletes have probably used creatine, a substance found naturally in the body that has been demonstrated to enhance performance (Volek and Kraemer, 1996). Because it is a food supplement, it does not appear on the list of banned drugs. However, a person would need to eat more than 10 to 20 pounds of meat daily to equal the standard loading dose now being taken by athletes: easy for a tiger, tough for a human! Is this a performance-enhancing substance? The data obtained in controlled studies appear to indicate that it is.

Surveys

The vast majority of survey research on the use of performance-enhancing drugs has focused on anabolic steroid use among adolescents. Although there has been an ongoing series of cross-sectional surveys of National Collegiate Athletic Association athletes (Anderson et al., 1991, 1993; Anderson and McKeag, 1985; *NCAA News*, 1997), only a handful of surveys have explored this issue among professional and Olympic athletes (Pearson, 1994; Pearson and Hansen, 1990; Yesalis et al., 1996).

Survey research is dependent on self-reported data about the attitudes, motivations, beliefs, and behaviors known only to the respondent. A frequent concern about survey research, especially surveys dealing with illegal, controversial, or socially stigmatized behaviors, is the veracity of responses given by the participants. Illicit drug use, including the use of anabolic steroids and many other performance-enhancing drugs, which are also illegal and socially stigmatized, is no different. Thus, the extent to which athlete respondents honestly report their drug use is unknown.

Background

This focus on the validity of self-report is not new. In Hyman's 1944 article titled, "Do They Tell the Truth?" he evaluated how willing people were to admit they cashed war bonds, a socially unacceptable behavior at the time. Hyman found that many people who were documented as having redeemed war bonds subsequently denied their behavior (Harrell, 1985).

In the 1950 Denver Validity Study, Parry and Crossley studied rates of distortion and compared the accuracy of reporting of socially neutral and socially desirable behaviors. The study included questions about the respondents' age, their charitable contributions, possession of a driver's license, ownership of a library card, possession of a telephone, and other factors. Records from the library, the Community Chest, and other pertinent organizations were used to check the accuracy of reporting. Questions asking for information that could be easily verified had accuracy rates of 90 percent or higher when compared to the external criteria. Researchers found evidence of exaggerated responses related to socially desirable behaviors. Of the respondents reporting they contributed to the Community Chest, 34 percent reported contributions that could not be confirmed by Community Chest records. Errors in the other direction, such as failing to report a socially desirable behavior such as donating to the Community Chest, were consistently very small (under 5 percent). The latter type of distortion was probably a function of memory lapse or other sources of unreliability. Socially neutral behaviors such as owning a library card were exaggerated by only 9 percent of the sample (Harrell, 1985).

Social Desirability

According to social desirability theory (Crowne and Marlowe, 1960; Edwards, 1957), distortion of self-reports occurs as a function of the perceived social acceptability of the behavior in question. Survey respondents may under-report their drug use to conceal their behaviors from the interviewer, the general public, sponsors of the survey, and other members of their households in order to present themselves, or perhaps their sport, in a way they feel is more socially acceptable. Conversely, respondents who view substance use positively may exaggerate reported use in order to impress others or to live up to a self-image they perceive in a positive light (Schuman and Presser, 1981).

The likelihood of over-reporting socially desirable behavior and under-reporting socially undesirable behavior has not diminished with time. Cannell and Fowler researched socially undesirable behavior in 1963 in a study that compared self-reported information on hospitalizations with hospital records. Socially undesirable hospitalizations (i.e., threatening or embarrassing conditions) were denied by respondents at a much higher rate than hospitalizations for other types of disorders (Harrell, 1985). In 1979, Bradburn et al. examined an assortment of behaviors. For the socially positive behavior of voting in a recent primary, rates of exaggeration were as high as 48 percent. On the other hand, drunken driving was denied by 54 percent of the respondents whose driving record indicated otherwise (Harrell, 1985).

Validity of self-report appears in many instances to be a function of personal norms and self-expectations. For example, because of the virilizing qualities of anabolic steroids (Kochakian, 1976), women might be more secretive about their anabolic steroid use than men or even adolescents.

Factors other than social desirability also threaten the validity of self-reporting. Respondents may be reluctant to disclose behaviors that have specific legal and social consequences. Most drugs that have been shown to enhance physical performance are used in violation of the rules of sport federations (Wadler and Hainline, 1989) and state and federal laws (Yesalis et al., 1997).

Drug use may be reported inaccurately because of variations in memory related to past drug consumption among respondents. Moreover, rare behaviors are often recalled but routine behaviors cannot always be recalled to immediate memory (Bradburn et al., 1987). Respondents may have difficulty accurately recalling the number of times they used cigarettes or alcohol in an interval as long as a year. In the experience of the authors, athletes have a strong recollection regarding whether or not they have ever used a particular type of performance-enhancing drug. However, limitations of memory do come into play when respondents are asked to recall the specific name of a drug (generic/ brand name), dosage, number of episodes of use (cycles), time frames for drug use, etc.

Respondents may vary in their comprehension of the question being asked in a particular survey, and some respondents may have reading difficulties that preclude an accurate response. The complexity of the scales for reporting frequencies and amounts of drug use can also be a source of confusion and variation.

Mode of administration affects the reporting of sensitive topics, and it is important to have a good understanding of how privacy or lack of privacy during an interview affects the veracity of reporting. Literature on substance use survey questions indicates that when surveys are self-administered, levels of reporting are increased, compared to administration of the same questions by an interviewer. Respondents of all ages are generally reluctant to admit that they have engaged in illegal and/or embarrassing activities to an interviewer (Tourangeau and Smith, 1996; Tourangeau et al., 1997). In addition to self-administration, privacy is one explanation for the much higher rates of drug use reported in school-based surveys like the Monitoring the Future Study and the Youth Risk Behavior Survey as compared to the National Household Survey on Drug Abuse (Gfroerer et al. 1997). The National Household Survey on Drug Abuse does provide a self-administered answer sheet for substance use, but adults are allowed to stay in the room when the respondent is 12 to 17 years of age.

Individual Variation

Studies that have examined the validity of self-report have consistently found that some people are more likely than others to provide inaccurate information. In 1944, Hyman found that certain subgroups of the population were more likely to deny war bond redemption. Persons with higher incomes were more likely than those with low incomes to distort their responses. Following analysis of data from the Denver Validity Study, Cahalan (1968) reported distorted responses differed by gender, age, and socioeconomic status. Women were less likely than men to exaggerate their contributions to the Community Chest. Cahalan found that younger people were more likely than older ones to exaggerate socially desirable behaviors such as charitable contributions and voting. When Weiss looked at self-reported voter registration and voting among African-American welfare mothers in 1968, she found differences by age, education, and social status. Older women with more education were more likely to exaggerate information related to voting. Weiss felt this was because they valued voting and wanted to present a more positive picture of themselves.

Although drug use may vary substantially among different populations such as high school, college, Olympic, and professional athletes, accuracy of their self-report may also vary among these groups. Arguably, adolescents may be more forthcoming regarding their illicit performance-enhancing drug use because they have less to lose than college, elite, or professional athletes whose scholarships or livelihoods depend on their participation and success in sport. The fear of guilt by association and its potential to adversely affect the athlete's place in sport history may result in a hesitancy to volunteer or be truthful.

Type of Drug

Findings from a series of methodological studies conducted in conjunction with the National Household Survey on Drug Abuse indicate that the more stigmatized the drug, the more likely the respondent will deny using it. This finding has been replicated in a number of other studies. Marijuana use is reported more validly than cocaine (Harrison, 1992, 1995; Fendrich and Xu, 1994; Mieczkowski et al., 1991a). Among an arrestee population, Harrison found that respondents were most willing to report marijuana followed by opiates, amphetamines, and then cocaine (Harrison, 1992).

Although the use of traditional "street" drugs may constitute misdemeanor violations of state and federal laws, it is the violation of sport rules that could have, at least from the perspective of the athlete, a greater impact on the athlete's life, including the loss of a scholarship, income, and other incentives. Thus, in sport, some drugs may be more stigmatized than others. For example, it can be argued that athletes might acknowledge marijuana use before they would admit anabolic steroid use, because marijuana use, although stigmatized, is, unfortunately, not a rare behavior, and society does not view this drug as enhancing athletic performance. Perhaps this explains, in part, the International Court of Arbitration for Sport overturning Canadian snowboarder Ross Rebagliati's positive drug test for marijuana at the Nagano Olympic Games and the reinstatement of his gold medal (*USA Today,* 1998b).

Accuracy

There is a wide array of inferential evidence for the validity of self-reported drug use. As contained in a report of the U.S. General Accounting Office (GAO: 46, 1993), examples of such evidence include the considerable proportion of respondents that *do admit* to illegal drug use; the general completion of survey items concerning sensitive behaviors; the statistical demonstrations of predictable relationships between drug use and items concerning drug use, attitudes, and delinquent activities; the similar prevalence rates obtained through an assortment of surveys; and the failure of people to report the use of a fictitious drug (which is included on most substance use surveys).

The large numbers of people who admit to drug use are readily demonstrated by the data available from the national surveys on this topic. In 1997, the Monitoring the Future Study revealed that more than half (54.3 percent) of seniors in high school had used some sort of illicit drug at least once in their lives (Johnston et al., 1997). In the 1996 National Household Survey on Drug Abuse, 6.1 percent of the respondents reported current use (current use refers to using at least once in the 30 days before the survey) of an illicit drug. This figure corresponds to an estimated 13 million Americans age 12 and older.

However, accuracy of reporting among adolescents, at least as it applies to anabolic steroid use, is somewhat suspect given the results of a 1988 study of high school athletes. Among the participants, 39 percent of male athletes and 56 percent of female athletes denied that they had even *heard of* using anabolic steroids to aid performance. This unawareness is noteworthy given that the study took place during a decade marked by significant media attention to drug use among athletes.

The reliability of surveys used in determining the prevalence of drug use among adolescents has been tested by DuRant et al. (1993, 1994). Although DuRant et al. (1994) have noted that self-report measurements on substance use by ninth-grade students provide a reliable method of determining drug use, they found self-reported lifetime anabolic steroid use had significantly decreased (5.4 percent to 4.8 percent) for males, and significantly increased for females (1.5 percent to 2.9 percent), when they readmin-istered their questionnaire four months later. Unfortunately, because the two questionnaires were administered anonymously, the two surveys could not be paired.

In an anonymous, self-administered survey of elite (adult) powerlifters, only 33 percent reported having ever used anabolic steroids (Yesalis et al., 1988); this in a sport in which many believe the use of these drugs is virtually universal (Starr, 1981; Todd, 1987; Wright, 1982). When a coinvestigator, whom the study participants knew, again questioned (via telephone) some of the athletes about their steroid use, 55 percent admitted prior use. Thus it is possible that the level of trust the subjects felt with the interviewer was a more important factor to them than anonymity.

In 1990, an attempt was made to survey 1,600 National Football League players via mail by the NFL Players Association (Courson, 1991). However, only 120 players (7.5 percent) were willing to participate. This extremely low response rate is notable because the survey was sponsored by the players' own professional association and the anonymity of respondents was guaranteed. Nevertheless, of those who did participate, 28 percent of all respondents and 67 percent of offensive linemen reported prior use of anabolic steroids. Only 3 percent of the participants reported steroid use in the past 12 months. When the participants were asked what percent of their fellow NFL players they believed had ever used anabolic steroids, the mean response was 32 percent; the estimate of use among fellow players for the past 12 months was 19 percent. This indirect survey technique (i.e., in which respondents estimate their competitors' anabolic steroid use level) relies to some extent on hearsay as well as the opportunity to project one's own behavior onto others, and the resulting estimates of use probably represent an upper bound or overestimation of use (Tricker et al., 1989; Yesalis et al., 1990). This indirect survey method is probably less threatening to the athlete in that it does not require the respondent to divulge information about himself or herself or about specific teammates; this method likely results in a higher level of participation in the study. Undoubtedly a certain amount of projection also takes place (Semeonoff, 1976). That is, the respondent protects himself or herself from anxiety by projecting or externalizing inappropriate behaviors to others, as if by projecting these behaviors (in this case anabolic steroid use) to someone else, one denies or rationalizes their existence within oneself. Also, anxiety related to one's own inappropriate behavior may be diluted if the behavior can be projected toward others in an effort to characterize the activity as less atypical or more mainstream. Thus, the true level of anabolic steroid use among athletes probably lies somewhere between the lower-bound estimates from self-reports and the upper-bound estimates obtained from the projective response techniques.

Apparently, only one study has examined the validity of self-report in identifying anabolic steroid use among athletes. To determine the validity of self-report in the detection of steroid use among weightlifters, Ferenchick (1996) compared self-report with assay results of simultaneous urine samples from 48 male weightlifters. The sensitivity of self-report in the detection of steroid use was 74 percent (a value that increased to 90 percent when lifetime use was considered) and specificity was 82 percent. Also, 22 of 23 participants in the study who declared current steroid use had at least one undeclared steroid identified in their urine. (However, this may not be unusual, since several studies [Debruyckere et al., 1992; Kicman et al., 1994] have found steroid-positive urine following the dietary consumption of meat contaminated with anabolic steroids.) In addition, 15 participants reported at least one drug that was not detected in the urine. (Again, this may not be unusual given the lack of purity and questionable content of black market drugs [Coleman et al., 1991; Fish, 1993a, 1993b; Musshoff et al., 1997; Walters et al., 1990], which may constitute as much as 50-80 percent of the anabolic steroids used by athletes [Office of Diversion Control, 1994]). Furthermore, 3 of 17 declared nonusers had objective evidence of steroids in their urine. All of this led Ferenchick to conclude that the validity of self-report may be inadequate to differentiate reliably between steroid users and nonusers. Whether these conclusions are applicable to elite athletes is questionable; it can be argued that, because they tend to have more money, elite athletes have greater access to pharmaceutical-grade steroids prescribed by physicians.

Time Frame

Another issue deserving comment is that some studies have focused their attention on anabolic steroid use during the past month or 12 months (Anderson et al., 1991;

Anderson et al., 1993; Anderson and McKeag, 1985; *NCAA News*, 1997) rather than focusing on any past use of these drugs. Anabolic steroids are not necessarily temporary performance enhancers; they are capable of providing the athlete with increased muscle mass and strength, much of which can be maintained for a number of years through training alone. One might then argue that once a strength athlete uses anabolic steroids, he is never really the same person. Consequently, is there a difference between a college football player who does not currently use steroids but used them in high school to gain enough weight to win a scholarship and a college player who used the drugs during the summer season to retain his starting position in the fall?

Non-Responders

A review of studies of the use of anabolic steroids across various levels of competition showed response rates ranging from 7.5 to 99.5 percent (not all studies reported response rates) (Yesalis and Bahrke, 1995; Courson, 1991). There is no information on individuals who chose not to volunteer information, but it is reasonable to hypothesize, based on the preceding discussion, that a disproportionate number of those who did not participate were anabolic steroid users, which would result in an under-reporting bias.

Credibility

For some time there has been a lack of trust and communication between members of the athletic community and the scientific and medical communities regarding anabolic steroids and other performance-enhancing drugs. In part, this is a function of a poor understanding by clinicians and researchers of the motivations of athletes, and vice versa. The medical community has lost much credibility as a result of repeated denials that anabolic steroids significantly enhance performance (American College of Sports Medicine [ACSM], 1977; Elashoff et al., 1991). For the past three decades, some physicians and scientists have dogmatically reported that any weight an athlete gains while taking steroids is mainly the result of fluid retention and that any strength gain is largely psychological (a placebo effect). Along the same line, some members of the sports medicine community have, with the best of intentions, adopted an overly aggressive educational strategy and have used strong, but often unfounded, pronouncements regarding the adverse health effects of anabolic steroids. Athletes, on the other hand, simply have not witnessed long-time steroid users "dropping like flies." This credibility gap has been exacerbated by the apparent contradiction between these warnings of dire health consequences and new clinical applications of these drugs such as the 10-center worldwide trial sponsored by the World Health Organization to test the efficacy of anabolic steroids as a male contraceptive (World Health Organization Task Force on Methods for the Regulation of Male Fertility, 1996) as well as multicenter trials to assess the effects of testosterone supplementation in older men (*Endocrine News,* 1996). The doses used in these studies equal or exceed those used by endurance and sprint athletes, among others (Yesalis, 1993).

Recommendations

An approach for determining the validity of self-reported drug use is to evaluate responses that should be consistent over time. Lifetime use of a substance can logically never decline. Therefore, one can look at the rates of recanting of earlier lifetime use. For anabolic steroid use, one can look at the lifetime use reported in the Monitoring the Future Study by cohorts of students. An example is the eighth graders who were surveyed in 1991. These same students were tenth graders in the 1993 survey and seniors in the 1995 survey. See table 3.1.

Validation of self-report requires comparing study results to some method that is more accurate. Research on the use of self-report methods has shown them to be valid for documenting recreational drug use, especially for adolescents (McClary and Lubin, 1985; Smart and Blair, 1978). When the recreational drug use rates from self-report studies have been compared with external methods of documenting drug use (e.g., reports by others, or blood and urine samples), the self-report use rates have been similar to or only slightly lower than the rates derived by the other methods (Ausel et al., 1976; Bonito et al., 1976; Deaux and Callaghen, 1984; Petzel et al., 1973; Stacy et al., 1985). Unfortunately, because of the shortcomings of testing for drugs in sport, discussed previously, the applicability of this validation strategy is somewhat limited.

Finally, researchers need to concentrate on making self-reported data better. To help maximize accurate reporting, the Committee on Privacy and Confidentiality of the American Statistical Association (1429 Duke Street, Alexandria, Virginia, 22314-3402) recommends that sponsors of surveys should

1. assure participants that the information provided will be kept confidential,
2. ensure participants' responses will be used only for statistical purposes, and
3. provide participants with information so they can make an informed decision about whether or not to participate (informed consent).

Table 3.1 Lifetime Use of Anabolic Steroids by Cohort

Cohort	8th grade	10th grade	12th grade
1991 8th graders	1.9	1.7	2.3
1992 8th graders	1.7	1.8	1.9
1993 8th graders	1.6	2.0	2.4
1994 8th graders	2.0	2.0	(not available until 1998)

Additional strategies for reducing concealment or under-reporting also include

1. establishing rapport with the respondent by choosing skillful interviewers and enlisting respondent support by giving them the objectives of the study,
2. concentrating more on recent events because there are definite limits to the type and amount of detailed information that respondents can recall, and
3. careful questionnaire construction and fieldwork procedures to evaluate potential response bias associated with method of inquiry. This usually requires pretesting the questionnaire.

Summary

It is important for us to be able to accurately assess the prevalence of drug use in sport, primarily to protect the health of athletes and maintain a "level playing field." Unfortunately, the four major methods (investigative journalism, government investigation, drug testing, and surveys of athletes) used in determining the prevalence of drug use among athletes suffer from significant methodological weaknesses, often precluding accurate assessment. In particular, the responses of athletes to the questions of journalists, drug use surveys, or even government investigations may be influenced by the athlete's desire to respond to the questions in a socially desirable manner, memory lapse, the illegal nature of the substances being surveyed, and a general distrust of those doing the questioning, among others. Drug testing, at the very least, is hamstrung by significant limitations in technology. All these limitations would likely result in a significant under-reporting bias. Future investigations and research will need to address these shortcomings if a more accurate estimate of drug use among athletes is to be obtained.

Note

Significant portions of the text are taken from C. Yesalis, 2000, *Anabolic Steroids in Sport and Exercise*, 2nd ed. (Champaign, IL: Human Kinetics).

References

Alzado, L. 1991, July 8. I'm sick and I'm scared. *Sports Illustrated*, 20-27.

American College of Sports Medicine. 1977. Position statement on the use and abuse of anabolic-androgenic steroids in sports. *Medicine and Science in Sports and Exercise* 9: 11-13.

Anderson, W.A., Albrecht, M.A., McKeag, D.B., Hough, D.O., and McGrew, C.A. 1991. A national survey of alcohol and drug use by college athletes. *The Physician and Sportsmedicine* 19: 91-104.

Anderson, W., Albrecht, M., and McKeag, D. 1993. Second replication of a national study of the substance use/abuse habits of college student-athletes. Final report. *NCAA News*.

Anderson, W., and McKeag, D. 1985. *The Substance Use and Abuse Habits of College Student-Athletes* (Research Paper No. 2). Mission, KS: National Collegiate Athletic Association.

Ausel, S., Mandell, W., Mathias, L., et al. 1976. Reliability and validity of self-reported illegal activities and drug use collected from narcotic addicts. *International Journal of the Addictions* 11: 325-336.

Bamberger, M., and Yaeger, D. 1997, April 14. Over the edge. *Sports Illustrated* 86: 60-70.

Boje, O. 1939. Doping. *Bulletin of the Health Organization of the League of Nations* 8: 439-469.

Bonito, A., Nucro, D., and Schaffer, J. 1976. The veridicality of addicts' self-reports in social research. *International Journal of the Addictions* 11: 719-724.

Bradburn, N., Sudman, S., et al. 1979. *Improving Interview Methods and Questionnaire Design*. Washington, DC: Jossey-Bass.

Bradburn, N., Rips, L. and Shevell, S. 1987. Answering autobiographical questions: The impact of memory and inference on surveys. *Science* 236: 157-161.

Cahalan, D. 1968. Correlates of respondent accuracy in the Denver validity survey. *Public Opinion Quarterly* 32: 607-621.

Cannell, C., and Fowler, F. 1963. Comparison of a self-enumerative procedure and a personal interview: A validity study 27: 250-264.

Catlin, D., and Murray, T. 1996. Performance-enhancing drugs, fair competition, and Olympic sport. *Journal of the American Medical Association* 276: 231-237.

Champaign News Gazette. 1995, April 9. USOC officials cite test failures.

Chicago Sun-Times. 1994, January 27. ITF disputes Becker charges.

Chicago Tribune (1992, July 22) Drugs still mystery Olympic ingredient, 1,7.

Colman, P., A'Hearn, E., Taylor, R., and Le, S. 1991. Anabolic steroids—analysis of dosage forms from selected case studies from the Los Angeles County Sheriff's Scientific Services Bureau. *Journal of Forensic Sciences* 36: 1079-1088.

Courson, S. 1991. *False Glory*. Stamford, CT: Longmeadow Press.

Crowne, D., and Marlowe, D. 1960. A new scale of social desirability independent of psychopathology. *Journal of Counseling Psychology* 24: 349-354.

Deaux, E., and Callaghen, J. 1984. Estimating statewide health risk behavior: A comparison of telephone and key information survey approaches. *Evaluation Review* 8: 467-492.

Debruyckere, G., de Sagher, R., and Van Peteghem, C. 1992. Clostebol-positive urine after consumption of contaminated meat. *Clinical Chemistry* 38: 1869-1873.

Des Moines Register. 1997, October 5. Athletes live with steroids' toll.

Dubin, C. 1990. *Commission of Inquiry into the Use of Drugs and Banned Practices Intended to Increase Athletic Performance* (Catalogue No. CP32-56/1990E,

ISBN 0-660-13610-4). Ottawa, ON: Canadian Government Publishing Center.

DuRant, R., Rickert, V., Ashworth, C., Newman, C., and Slavens, G. 1993. Use of multiple drugs among adolescents who use anabolic steroids. *New England Journal of Medicine* 328: 922-926.

DuRant R., Ashworth, C., Newman, C., and Rickert, V. 1994. Stability of the relationships between anabolic steroid use and multiple substance use among adolescents. *Journal of Adolescent Health* 15: 111-116.

Edwards, A. 1957. *The Social Desirability Variable in Personality Assessment and Research*. New York: Dryden.

Elashoff, J., Jacknow, A., Shain, S., and Braunstein, G. 1991. Effects of anabolic-androgenic steroids on muscular strength. *Annals of Internal Medicine* 115: 387-393.

Endocrine News. 1996, February. Testosterone replacement therapy: May improve life for aging males 21: 1-7.

Fendrich, M., and Xu, Y.C. 1994. The validity of drug-use reports from juvenile arrestees. *International Journal of Addiction* 29: 971-985.

Ferenchick, G. 1996. Validity of self-report in identifying anabolic steroid use among weightlifters. *Journal of General Internal Medicine* 11: 554-556.

Fish, M. 1993a. Experts suspect “a whole country” may be cheating. *The Atlanta Journal/Constitution*, E3.

Fish, M. 1993b. Steroids: Riskier than ever. *Atlantic Journal/Constitution*, D1.

Francis, C. 1990. *Speed Trap*. New York: St. Martin’s Press.

Franke, W. 1998, February 9-14. Hormonal doping of athletes: The German Democratic Republic’s secret program. In *Drugs and Athletes: A Multidisciplinary Symposium*. American Academy of Forensic Sciences, San Francisco.

Franke, W., and Berendonk, B. 1997. Hormonal doping and androgenization of athletes: A secret program of the German Democratic Republic government. *Clinical Chemistry* 43: 1262-1279.

Frazier, S. 1973. Androgens and athletes. *American Journal of Diseases of Children* 125: 479-480.

General Accounting Office (GAO). 1993. *Drug Use Measurement Strengths, Limitations, and Recommendations for Improvement*. Report GAO-PEMD 93-18. Washington, DC, Superintendent of Documents, U.S. Government Printing Office.

Gilbert, B. 1969a, June 23. Drugs in sport: Part 1. Problems in a turned-on world. *Sports Illustrated*, 64-72.

Gilbert, B. 1969b, June 30. Drugs in sport: Part 2. Something extra on the ball. *Sports Illustrated*, 30-42.

Gilbert, B. 1969c, July 7. Drugs in sport: Part 3. High time to make some rules. *Sports Illustrated*, 30-35.

Gfroerer, J., Wright, D., and Kopstein, A. 1997. Prevalence of youth substance use: The impact of methodological differences between two national surveys. *Drug and Alcohol Dependence* 47: 19-30.

Harrell, A. 1985. Validation of self-report: The research record. In B.A. Rouse, N.J. Kozel, L.G. Richards, eds., *Self-Report Methods of Estimating Drug Use: Meeting Current Challenges to Validity*, NIDA Research Monograph 57, National Institute on Drug Abuse, Department of Health and Human Services, pp. 12-21.

Harrison, L. 1992. Trends in illicit drug use in the USA: Conflicting results from national surveys. *International Journal of Addiction* 27: 817-847.

Harrison, L. 1997. The validity of self-reported drug use in survey research: An overview and critique of research methods. In L. Harrison and A. Hughes, eds., *The Validity of Self-Reported Drug Use: Improving the Accuracy of Survey Estimates*, NIDA Research Monograph 167, National Institute on Drug Abuse, National Institutes of Health, NIH Pub. No 97-4147, Department of Health and Human Services, pp. 17-36.

Hoberman, J. 1992. The early development of sports medicine in Germany. In J. Berryman and R. Park, eds., *Sport and Exercise Science: Essays in the History of Sports Medicine*. Champaign, IL: University of Illinois Press.

Huizenga, R. 1994. *You're OK It's Just a Bruise*. New York: St. Martin's Press.

Hyman, H. 1944. Do they tell the truth? *Public Opinion Quarterly* 8: 557-559.

International Olympic Committee Medical Code. 1995. Lausanne, Switzerland: IOC; ISBN 92-9149-003-2.

Janofsky, M. 1988, November 17. System accused of failing test posed by drugs. *New York Times.*

Johnson, W. 1985, May 13. Steroids: a problem of huge dimensions. *Sports Illustrated.*

Johnston, L., O'Malley, P., and Bachman, J. In press. *National Survey Results on Drug Use from the Monitoring the Future Study, 1975-1997. Vol. I, Secondary School Students*. National Institute on Drug Abuse, National Institutes of Health, U.S. Dept. of Health and Human Services.

Kammerer, R.C., 1993. Drug testing and anabolic steroids. In C. Yesalis, ed., *Anabolic Steroids in Sport and Exercise*. Champaign, IL: Human Kinetics.

Karpovich, P.V. 1941. Ergogenic aids in work and sports. *Research Quarterly*, 12 (Suppl.): 432-450.

Kelley, S. 1991, July 10. This chapter of Alzado's story is sad. *Seattle Times*.

Keteyian, A. 1989. *Big Red Confidential: Inside Nebraska Football.* New York: Contemporary Books.

Kicman, A., Cowan, D., Myhre, L., Nilsson, S., Tomten, S., and Oftebro, H. 1994. Effect of sports drug tests of ingesting meat from steroid (methenolone)-treated livestock. *Clinical Chemistry* 40: 2084-2087.

Klecko, J., and Fields, J. 1989. *Nose to nose: Survival in the trenches in the NFL.* New York: Morrow.

Kochakian, C., ed. 1976. *Anabolic-Androgenic Steroids*. New York: Springer-Verlag.

Litsky, F. 1993, Friday, January 15. D.E.A. says more players at risk. *New York Times,* B9.

Longman, J. 1995, April 9. U.S.O.C. experts call drug testing a failure. *New York Times,* 11.

McClary, S., and Lubin, B. (1985). Effects of type of examiner, sex, and year in school on self-report of drug use by high school students. *Journal of Drug Education* 15: 49-55.

Mix, R. 1987, October 19. So little gain for the pain. *Sports Illustrated.*

Mieczkowski, T. 1990. The accuracy of self-reported drug use: An evaluation and analysis of new data. In R. Weisheit, ed., *Drugs and Crime and the Criminal Justice System*, Cincinnati: Anderson Publishing Company.

Milwaukee Sentinel. 1993, July 12. NFL drug users find invisible assistance.

Musshoff, F., Daldrup, T., and Ritsch, M. 1997. Anabole steroide auf dem deutschen Schwarzmarkt. *Archiv für Kriminologie* 1916: 152-158.

NCAA News. 1997, September 15. Survey shows steroid use on decline, 1.

Office of Diversion Control. 1994. *Report of the International Conference on the Abuse and Trafficking of Anabolic Steroids*. Washington, DC: United States Drug Enforcement Administration Conference Report.

Parry, H., and Crossley, H. 1950. Validity of response to survey questions. *Public Opinion Quarterly* 14: 61-80.

Pearson, B. 1994, February 7. Olympic survey: Olympians of winters past. *USA Today*, C5.

Pearson, B., and Hansen, B. 1990, February 5. Survey of US Olympians. *USA Today*, C10.

Petzel, T., Johnson, J., and McKillip, J. 1973. Response bias in drug surveys. *Journal of Consulting and Clinical Psychology* 40: 437-439.

Prokop, L. 1970. The struggle against doping and its history. *Journal of Sports Medicine and Physical Fitness* 10(1): 45-48.

Rosellini, L. 1992, February 17. The sports factories. *U.S. News & World Report,* 48-59.

Schuman, H., and Presser, S. 1981. *Questions and Answers in Attitude Surveys. Experiments on Question Form, Wording and Context*. New York: Academic Press.

Scott, J. 1971, October 17. It's not how you play the game, but what pill you take. *New York Times Magazine*.

Semeonoff, B. 1976. *Projective Techniques*. London: Wiley.

Smart, R., and Blair, N. 1978. Test-retest reliability and validity information for a high school drug use questionnaire. *Drug and Alcohol Dependence* 3: 265-271.

Sports Medicine Digest. 1996, September. Drug testing results in Atlanta confound expectations, 103.

Stacy, A., Widaman, K., and Hays, R. 1985. Validity of self-reports of alcohol and other drug use. A multitrait-multimethod assessment. *Journal of Personality and Social Psychology* 49: 219-232.

Starr, B. 1981. *Defying Gravity: How to Win at Weightlifting*. Wichita Falls, TX: Five Starr Productions.

Strauss, R., and Curry, T. 1987. Magic, science and drugs. In R.H. Strauss, ed., *Drugs and Performance in Sports*. Philadelphia: Saunders.

Todd, T. 1983, August. The steroid predicament. *Sports Illustrated*, 66-77.

Todd, T. 1987. Anabolic steroids: The gremlins of sport. *Journal of Sport History* 14: 87-107.

Tourangeau, R., and Smith, T. 1996. Asking sensitive questions. *Public Opinion Quarterly* 60: 275-304.

Tourangeau, R., Smith, T., and Rasinski, K. 1997. Motivation to report sensitive behaviors on surveys: Evidence from a bogus pipeline experiment. *Journal of Applied Social Psychology* 27: 209-222.

Tricker, R., O'Neill, M., and Cook, D. 1989. The incidence of anabolic steroid use among competitive bodybuilders. *Journal of Drug Education* 19: 313-325.

USA Today. 1997, October 15. Coaches Charged, 3C.

USA Today. 1998a, February 4. Drug wars, 10C.

USA Today. 1998b, February 20. IOC mum on latest positive drug test, 13E.

USA Today. (1998c, March 19). In the swim world, 7C.

U.S. Congress. Subcommittee on Crime of the U.S. House Committee on the Judiciary. 1988, July 27. *Hearing on H.R. 3216. Legislation to amend the controlled substance act to make the anabolic steroid methandrostenolone a Schedule I Controlled Substance*.

U.S. Congress. Subcommittee on Crime of the U.S. House Committee on the Judiciary. 1989a, March 23. *Hearing on H.R. 995. The Anabolic Steroid Restriction Act of 1989.*

U.S. Congress. Committee on the Judiciary of the U.S. Senate. 1989b, April 3. *Hearing on Steroid Abuse in America*.

U.S. Congress. Subcommittee on Crime of the U.S. House Committee on the Judiciary. 1990, March 22. *The Abuse of Steroids in Amateur and Professional Athletics.*

Volek, J., and Kraemer, W. 1996. Creatine supplementation: Its effect on human muscular performance and body composition. *Journal of Strength & Conditioning Research* 10: 200-210.

Voy, R. 1990. *Drugs, Sport, and Politics*. Champaign, IL: Leisure Press.

Wade, N. 1972. Anabolic steroids: Doctors denounce them, but athletes aren't listening. *Science* 176: 1399-1403.

Wadler, G., and Hainline, B. 1989. Drugs and the athlete. Philadelphia: Davis.

Walters, M., Ayers, R., and Brown, D. 1990. Analysis of illegally distributed steroid products by liquid chromatography with identity confirmation by mass spectrometry or infrared spectrophotometry. *Journal of the Association of Official Analytical Chemists* 73: 904-926.

Weiss, C. 1968. Validity of welfare mothers: Interview responses. *Public Opinion Quarterly* 32: 622-633.

World Health Organization Task Force on Methods for the Regulation of Male Fertility. 1996. Contraceptive efficacy of testosterone-induced azospermia and oligozoospermia in normal men. *Fertility and Sterility* 65: 821-829.

Wright, J. 1978. *Anabolic steroids and sports*. Natick, MA: Sports Science Consultants.

Wright, J. 1982. *Anabolic steroids and sports II.* Natick, MA: Sports Science Consultants.

Yesalis, C. 1993. *Anabolic Steroids in Sport and Exercise*. Champaign, IL: Human Kinetics.

Yesalis, C. 1996, August 1. No medals for drug testing. *New York Times,* A27.

Yesalis, C., Herrick, R., Buckley, W., et al. 1988. Self-reported use of anabolic-androgenic steroids by elite powerlifters. *Physician and Sportsmedicine* 16: 91-100.

Yesalis, C.E., Buckley, W.A., Anderson, W.A., Wang, M.O., Norwig, J.A., Ott, G., Puffer, J.C., and Strauss, R.H. 1990. Athletes' projections of anabolic steroid use. *Clinical Sports Medicine* 2, 155-171.

Yesalis C. and Bahrke, M. 1995. Anabolic-androgenic steroids: Current issues. *Sports Medicine* 19: 326-340.

Yesalis, C., Bahrke, M., and Ortner, C. 1996). Steroidi Anabolizzanti Mascolinizzanti: Dal si dice al quanto: uno sguardo alla situazione internazionale. *Sport & Medicina* 5: 27-35.

Yesalis, C., Barsukiewicz, C., Kopstein, A., and Bahrke, M. 1997. Trends in anabolic-androgenic steroid use among adolescents. *Archives of Pediatric and Adolescent Medicine* 151: 1197-1206.

Yesalis, C., and Cowart, V. 1998. *The Steroids Game,* Champaign, IL: Human Kinetics.

Zimmerman, P. (1986, November 10). The agony must end. *Sports Illustrated*, 17-21.

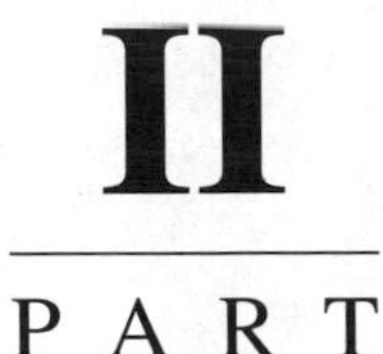

PART

The History, Ethics, and Social Context of Doping

4

CHAPTER

Significant Events in the History of Drug Testing and the Olympic Movement: 1960–1999

Jan Todd, PhD, and Terry Todd, PhD
The University of Texas at Austin

When we were asked to write a comprehensive history of drug testing and the Olympic movement for this book, it sounded like a relatively simple task. However, we quickly realized that we faced two significant research problems. The first was to find a way to tell the story of drug testing and the Olympic movement without all the internal International Olympic Committee (IOC) documents. Although the Avery Brundage Collection yielded a number of early minutes and Medical Commission reports, and although the minutes of the IOC General Sessions are now available, the IOC Executive Committee minutes and its Medical Commission minutes are closed to the public for a period of 30 years after they are published. As Dr. Robert K. Barney of the University of Western Ontario's Olympic Studies Centre explained, they were "embargoed." Because the IOC is essentially a private corporation, it is not legally required to make these kinds of documents available to the public.[1] Even so, we have done our best to track the official IOC actions and decisions, using what IOC documents were available to us. We have relied on secondary sources such as newspapers and magazines to fill in the many gaps left in the IOC record.

Our second research problem was the sheer magnitude of this undertaking. After exhausting the available Olympic sources, we began working our way through the last 39 years of the *New York Times*, the *Los Angeles Times*, and the *Washington Post*. We soon had more than 300 articles related to this topic, yet we knew we still did not have the full story. So, we went online, typed "drug testing and Olympics" in just one internet search engine, and discovered—to our horror—that 7,023,268 possible sources of information awaited our review. We were staggered, but once we righted ourselves we began to think about the project in a different way. We began with the idea of creating a traditional, narrowly focused essay. However, after confronting the enormous number of books and articles available on this topic we decided that a road map for others to follow might be a more useful scholarly contribution.

What follows is an annotated timeline of the significant events and decisions related to drug testing and the Olympic Games. In this timeline we have attempted to trace the significant doping scandals of the last 30 years; we have included information about the IOC's drug testing policies; and when possible we have cited the books and scholarly journal articles we believe will be of use to others exploring this territory. In addition, we have attempted to highlight some of the important journalistic treatments of doping that awakened the public to this growing problem. Although the documentation we have compiled is extensive, it is not exhaustive. We did not consider it necessary to list every Olympic athlete who has ever tested positive during the past 39 years, nor have we included every possible print source for the events and decisions included in this timeline. We have simply tried to point readers to good starting points for their own research.

We should also note that, like many histories, this timeline is biased in a number of ways. First, it is based almost exclusively on sources available in the English language. Second, the timeline covers the activities of the United States Olympic Committee (USOC) to a much greater extent than it does any other national Olympic committee or international sports federation in the Olympic movement. And third, although we have tried to be objective in the preparation of this document, our personal long-time opposition to the use of anabolic steroids and other ergogenic drugs in competitive sport situations is no doubt apparent. History is not merely what we remember but also a reflection of who remembers it. In this instance, the fact that we are Americans with a deep commitment to the anti-drug movement in sport has colored the chronology that follows.

1960–1969

1960—At the 57th Session of the IOC, held in San Francisco, the use of amphetamine sulfate or "pep pills" is discussed by the assembly. Delegate Bo Eklund suggests that the IOC engage in scientific research about its potential dangers to sport.[2]

1960—Dr. John Ziegler, a physician from Olney, Maryland, begins giving methandrostenelone, an anabolic steroid manufactured by Ciba Pharmaceutical Company and sold under the trade name of Dianabol, to three U.S. weightlifters: Tony Garcy, Bill March, and Lou Riecke. All three were good lifters, but not the best in the country. Very quickly, all three made astonishing progress, gaining muscle mass as well as strength. All three became national champions and March and Riecke both set world records. At first, it was believed that their use of a new training technique—isometric contraction—had created the changes, but soon the secret was out, and anabolic steroids began to spread from sport to sport in the United States and beyond.[3]

1960 August 8—The father of Olympic swimmer Sylvia Russka charges that "pep pills" were found in the women's dressing room at the 1960 Olympic Trials for swimming and diving in Detroit. Weikko Russka of Berkeley, Sylvia's father and the Berkeley YMCA coach, said three teams were guilty—Santa Clara, Multnomah (Portland), and the Los Angeles Athletic Club. Santa Clara and Multnomah won every event, and broke the American record in each event as well.

1960—At the Rome Olympic Games, Danish cyclist Knut Jensen collapses during the road race, suffers a fractured skull, and dies. In the investigation of Jensen's death, it is revealed that he had taken Ronicol, a blood circulation stimulant. Jensen's is the first death in Olympic competition since 1912.[4]

1961 June 21—The IOC sets up its first Medical Committee. There are four members: Arthur Porritt of New Zealand, Ryotaro Azuma of Japan, Joaquim Ferreira Santos of Brazil, and Josef Gruss of Czechoslovakia. The committee is asked by Avery Brundage to investigate the doping situation and make recommendations to the IOC about how to proceed. However, no recommendations come from the Medical Committee until the Tokyo meeting in 1964. Prince Alexandre de Merode, of Belgium, is added later as a replacement for the deceased Ferreira Santos. The prince makes his first public appearance as a representative of the Medical Committee in 1965 in Madrid.[5] According to the IOC Web site on 5 May 1998, however, the IOC Medical "Commission" did not begin until the appointment of Prince Alexandre de Merode as its chairman and its first meeting was on the 26th and 27th of September, 1967.[6]

1963 January—The European Council on Doping and the Biological Preparation of the Athlete Taking Part in Competitive Sports, an IOC subcommittee, meets to discuss the doping problem in international sport. This group, chaired by Colonel Marceau Crespin of France, is composed of doctors, pharmacists, biologists, jurists, athletes, coaches, and journalists. At the end of the proceedings, the group adopts several motions, the most significant of which is the council's request for the IOC to establish an international commission whose purpose would be to (1) educate officials and athletes about the dangers of doping, (2) study the behavior of athletes involved in doping, and (3) appoint a permanent board charged with keeping track of doping methods and keeping a list of proscribed drugs and activities. The council further argues in favor of drug testing for artificial stimulants, tranquilizers, drugs that modify the blood pressure or respiratory action, and hormones.[7]

1964—At the 63rd Congress of the IOC in Tokyo, delegates unanimously vote to condemn doping by athletes. It is further agreed that the IOC will (1) formally condemn the use of drugs, (2) sanction each person or national organizing committee who uses or promotes the use of drugs, (3) ask athletes to sign a pledge on non-drug use as part of their application process, and (4) ask national organizing committees to inform athletes that they are subject to examination and testing.[8]

1965—France and Belgium pass anti-sports-doping laws.[9]

1966 March 3—The IOC meets in Rome. Sir Arthur Porritt of New Zealand, head of the IOC Medical Committee, presents his committee's report on the doping problem and asks for support for several recommendations. Porritt and his committee note that "only a long-term education policy stressing the physical and moral aspects" of the drug problem would ever stop athletes from doping. As short-term measures, however, he suggests (1) beginning such an education program, (2) asking all athletes to sign a pledge testifying that they have not used drugs during their training, (3) asking all international sport organizations to adopt rules banning drug use, (4) asking for an official condemnation of doping by the IOC, (5) asking that the IOC be given powers to sanction both individuals and sport organizations believed to be involved with doping, and (6) and making arrangements for the medical examination of competitors at the Olympic Games.[10]

1966 September 5—The Congress of the International Amateur Athletic Federation (IAAF) announces that track-and-field competitions in future Olympic Games and European Championships will be subject to spot checks for drugging. Athletes are to be chosen at random, as was done in the soccer World Cup in England.[11]

1967 May 9—At the IOC meeting in Tehran, Iran, the committee votes to adopt a drug- and sex-testing policy. New IOC regulations require (1) that all Olympic athletes must sign a pledge swearing that they will not use drugs to improve performance, (2) that athletes must submit to medical examinations to ascertain their sex, and (3) that the IOC will set up a medical center at the Mexico City Games where doctors can check "for the use of dope and other stimulants."

Doping is defined by the IOC as "the use of substances or techniques in any form or quantity alien or unnatural to the body with the exclusive aim of obtaining an artificial or unfair increase of performance in competition."[12] Specifically mentioned on the new IOC list of banned substances are alcohol, pep pills, cocaine, vasodilators, opiates (opium, morphine, heroin, pethidine, and metathadin), and hashish. IOC Secretary General J.W. Westerhoff says at a press conference announcing the decision, "It will be impossible for athletes to refuse to submit to medical checks."[13]

1967—British cyclist Tommy Simpson dies from amphetamine-related complications during the Tour de France.[14]

1968 October 7-11—At the IOC Congress, Prince de Merode introduces the members of the Medical Commission and explains the procedures he and his team have put into place for the testing of athletes for amphetamines use and to determine athletes' sex at the 1968 Games. IOC President Avery Brundage then clarifies the IOC position on drug testing, explaining that although organized by the IOC, the "actual responsibility (for the testing and its legal repercussions) should remain with the international federations, who therefore must give a written agreement." Following de Merode's report, and this point of clarification by Brundage, the following statement is read to the assembly:

> The representatives of 22 European national Olympic committees and of 16 international federations assembled in Versailles on 8th September 1968 to

> convey to the IOC Medical Commission their congratulations of the excellent work which has been accomplished in Grenoble for the control of sex and anti-doping. They firmly hope that the IOC will give full powers to this commission to carry on the tests at the Olympic Games in Mexico City in October 1968, in full collaboration with the international federations.

The recommendation of the federations is adopted.[15]

1968 October 12—The Olympic Games open in Mexico City. Drug testing protocol for the Games: The Olympic Medical Committee will select a sport at random each morning of the Games. From the list of competitors in that sport they will then test ten competitors, again chosen at random. In team sports, at least two members of each team are to be tested. Urine tests are done before competition. If traces of drugs are found, the athlete cannot compete.[16]

An American weightlifter asked by reporters about the new ban on amphetamines replies, "What ban? Everyone used a new one from West Germany. They couldn't pick it up in the test they were using. When they get a test for that one we'll find something else. It's like cops and robbers."[17]

1968—At the Olympic Games, Dr. Tom Waddell, a U.S. decathlete who placed sixth in the Games, told the *New York Times* that he estimated a third of the men on the U.S. track-and-field team were using anabolic steroids at the pre-Olympic training camp held at Lake Tahoe.[18]

1968 October 24—Soccer player Jean-Louis Quadri collapses during a game in Grenoble, France, and is dead on arrival at the hospital. His autopsy reveals that he was heavily medicated with amphetamines at the time.[19]

1968 November 3—Cyclist Yves Mottin wins a regional bicycle competition and then succumbs to complications from excessive amphetamine use. He dies two days later in a hospital in Grenoble, France.[20]

1969—*British Journal of Sports Medicine* publishes a special issue entitled "Doping in Sport."[21]

1969—Dr. H. Kay Dooley, member of the USOC medical team at the Lake Tahoe training camp set up before the 1968 Olympic Games, tells a reporter, "I don't think it's possible for a man to compete internationally without using anabolic steroids. All the weight men on the Olympic team had to take steroids. Otherwise they would not have been in the running." When questioned about his involvement with the drugs, Dooley answers, "I did not give steroids at Tahoe, but I did not inquire what the boys were doing on their own. I did not want to be forced into a position of having to report them for the use of a banned drug. A physician involved in sports must keep the respect and confidence of the athletes with whom he is working."[22]

1969 January 25-26—IOC Medical Commission meets in Lausanne, Switzerland. Major agenda items for discussion include (1) refining the procedures for the blood testing of modern pentathletes for alcohol, and (2) discussing the use of "hormonoid" substances. The discussion of hormones is prompted by a letter from the Union Cycliste Internationale (UCI) protesting the Medical Commission's "apathy" related to the Dutch masseur whom the UCI sent home after learning that he had administered an anabolic steroid without prescription. The UCI wished to know why the IOC had not removed from the Games the athlete who had received the steroid since these drugs were officially banned at that time. In the IOC Medical Commission minutes, it appears that a major portion of the discussion on this matter centered on the fact that the UCI had dared to question the authority of the IOC. The minutes read: "A very important point was also emphasized which was clearly stated *as soon as* our anti-doping fight was instituted; under no circumstances would we accept denouncements."[23]

1969 June—*Sports Illustrated* author Bil Gilbert publishes the first segment of a three-part exposé entitled "Drugs in Sport." Gilbert takes the IOC to task for not implementing a more effective drug testing program, arguing that delaying the decision to ban drugs from sports is helping to promote their use. In a publisher's note Gilbert speculates that "the doctor and the chemist may soon be as important to an athlete as a coach." Gilbert adds that a friend in the pharmaceutical industry "explained how all the money has thus far gone into therapeutic drugs. Yet he has no doubt that soon they'll be working on additives and that a drug can be found that will, say, help someone run a mile ten seconds faster than he normally could."[24]

1969 June 6-10—At the IOC meeting in Warsaw, Prince de Merode, president of the IOC Medical Commission, explains that the commission has adopted a test for the presence of alcohol in the blood of athletes in the modern pentathlon.[25]

1970–1979

1970 November—At the Weightlifting World Championships in Columbus, Ohio, after all three medalists in each of the first three bodyweight categories test positive for stimulants, the International Weightlifting Federation (IWF) decides to cancel the testing and reinstate the former winners. The reason given is that the fourth, fifth, and sixth place finishers were not tested.[26]

1971—American weightlifter Ken Patera breaks the code of silence surrounding the use of anabolic steroids by athletes. He tells reporters he is anxious to meet Russian superheavyweight Vassili Alexeev in competition at the 1972 Olympic Games. In their previous contest, which Alexeev barely won, Patera did not feel they were on equal footing. "Last year," said Patera, "the only difference between me and him was that I couldn't afford his pharmacy bill. Now I can. When I hit Munich next year, I'll weigh in about 340, maybe 350. Then we'll see which are better—his steroids or mine."[27]

In a 1983 interview, Patera told Terry Todd that he "didn't hear a peep out of anyone from the U.S. Olympic Committee," after his comments were published in *The Los Angeles Times*.[28]

1972—At the Sapparo Winter Olympic Games, the IOC tests 211 athletes. One hockey player is found positive for the stimulant ephedrine.[29]

1972 August 21-24—In his report to the IOC on behalf of the Medical Commission, Prince de Merode praises the medical facilities in Munich, adding that

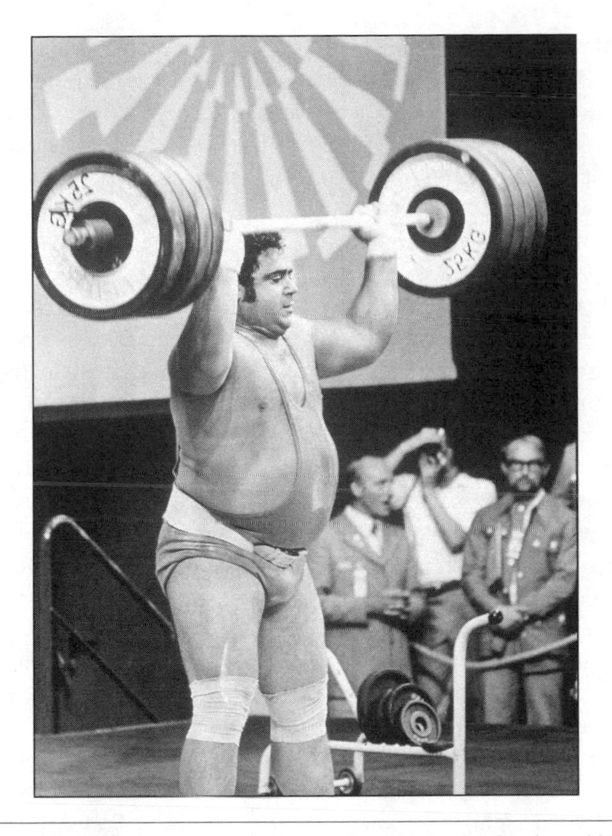

Super heavyweight Vassili Alexeev of the Soviet Union. Alexeev dominated his weight division through most of the 1970s.

500 females have already passed the sex control test. Of special interest, however, is the part of de Merode's report in which he explains that the Commission has decided not to enforce "Rule 26" at the Sapporo Games for "technical reasons." Rule 26 states, "the team of an athlete who has been shown to have used dope is excluded if the team can benefit from this usage." De Merode then goes on to suggest an amendment to Rule 26 that would allow it to be enforced only "after consulting the international federations concerned."[30]

1972—Sixteen-year-old swimmer Rick DeMont of California wins the gold medal in the 400-meter freestyle at the Munich Olympic Games. DeMont then turns up positive for ephedrine, which he maintains came from an asthma medicine. He has listed the drug on the assigned form. The IOC disqualifies him and removes his medal.[31]

1972—Track-and-field team member Jay Sylvester unofficially polls all male track-and-field contestants at the Munich Olympic Games. He finds that 68 percent have used some form of anabolic steroid in their training.[32]

1973—U.S. Senate subcommittee holds hearings on drugs and athletics. Hammer-thrower Harold Connolly, the gold medalist in 1956, argues that an athlete should do anything, short of killing himself, to succeed.[33]

1973 February 9—The IOC refuses to return Rick DeMont's medal. C.H. Buck, outgoing head of the USOC requested the return at a meeting with the IOC in Lausanne, Switzerland. "The IOC was firm that it had to follow the ruling of its medical committee and we have reached the end of the rope on that point," Buck says.[34]

1973 February 14—The American Academy of Allergists unanimously adopts a resolution upholding the use of ephedrine for athletes with asthma.[35]

1973 October—Dr. Roger Bannister, head of the British Sports Council, announces that British scientists have developed tests for anabolic steroids. Two articles appear in the *British Journal of Sports Medicine.* The first describes using radioimmunoassay, and the second article describes a testing process using gas chromatography and mass spectrometry. The IOC decides to adopt both procedures in order to guarantee accuracy.[36]

1973 October 5-7—In his Medical Commission report to the IOC, Commission chair Prince de Merode announces that the list of banned substances will henceforth be "closed" six months before the beginning of the Olympic Games in order to give athletes time to come into compliance. In addition, de Merode announces that in the future, the second, and confirming test, will be automatically performed in order to speed up the testing process.[37]

1974—Scottish weightlifting coach, David P. Webster, concerned about the growing use of drugs in sport, publishes a pamphlet entitled *The Truth About Drugs* for distribution throughout the weightlifting community. Webster writes, "I find it distressing that national and international officials will not make a very strong stand in this matter. . . For example, why are anabolic steroids not included in the IOC Medical Commission list of doping substances? The list produced for its meeting in Munich on 19th May 1971 did not contain anabolic steroids. The fact that at the time it was difficult to trace the drug should not in my opinion have prevented the inclusion on such a list. Surely the definition of doping is sufficient to make the use of steroids illegal."[38] Webster's pamphlet contains an excellent bibliography of early references to steroid use in both the scientific and popular journals.

1974 February—At the British Commonwealth Games in Auckland, New Zealand, the new British drug tests are used on a trial basis for the first time. Nine of the 55 samples tested contain steroids. No sanctions are imposed.[39]

1974 April—Following the annual meeting of the IOC Medical Commission in Innsbruck, Austria, it is announced that testing for anabolic steroids will take place at the 1976 Olympic Games in Montreal. (No screen for testosterone will be used.) Medical Commission members also work at that meeting on the language for Rule 26(a), which sets out the procedures for dope testing and suggests punishments for offenders.[40]

1974 October 21-24—In his report to the IOC, de Merode explains the new tests for anabolic steroids and reports that after consulting with medical specialists he and his commission are confident that "steroids could be detected, provided the last dose was taken within three weeks before the test." Anyone taking steroids outside that window of time will not be caught. The prince also notes that Montreal has been chosen as the first testing site for anabolic steroids rather than the Winter Games in Innsbruck because it was believed that more summer athletes were likely to use the drugs.

The other major business at this IOC Congress is the adoption of Rule 26(a), the legislation setting up the IOC's anti-drug program. Prince de Merode's Medical Commission drafted this legislation at their April meeting, and he objects in his report to the IOC assembly that the language of the rule has changed since it left the hands of his committee. However, despite his objections, the wording stands as proposed by the IOC Executive and is ratified by the assembly, becoming Annex 12: Rule 26(a)—Medical. It reads:

1. Doping is forbidden. The IOC will prepare a list of prohibited drugs.
2. All Olympic competitors are liable to medical control and examination, in conformity with the rules of the Medical Commission.
3. Any Olympic competitor refusing to take a doping test or who is found guilty of doping shall be eliminated. If the Olympic competitor belongs to a team, the match or competition in question shall be forfeited by that team. After the explanations of the team have been considered and the case discussed with the International Federation concerned, a team in which one or more members have been found guilty of doping may be disqualified from the Olympic Games. In sports in which a team may no longer compete after a member has been disqualified, the remaining members may compete on an individual basis in agreement with the IOC.
4. Olympic competitors in sports restricted to women must comply with the prescribed tests for femininity.
5. A medal may be withdrawn by order of the Executive Board on a proposal of the Medical Commission.
6. A Medical Commission may be set up to implement these rules. Members of the commission may not act as team doctors.
7. The above regulations shall in no way affect further sanctions by the international federations.[41]

1975—At the European Cup for track and field, the steroid test is "officially" administered for the first time. Two athletes who test positive for steroids are disqualified from the competition and are subsequently sanctioned by the IAAF.[42]

1976—At the Innsbruck Winter Games, 356 samples are analyzed with only two positives. One is for ephedrine in Nordic skiing, the other is for codeine in ice hockey. No steroid screens are performed at these games.[43]

1976—At the Olympic Track and Field Trials in Eugene, Oregon, 23 athletes fail the doping control.[44]

1976 February 2–3—The IOC meets in Innsbruck. Prince de Merode proposes, and the IOC approves, a motion that doping and femininity controls should be initiated at all regional games of the IOC.[45]

1976 May 21–23—At the annual meeting of the IOC, Prince de Merode reports on the progress of the doping procedures for the forthcoming Olympic Games in Montreal. He expresses great satisfaction with the facilities, and announces again that in addition to amphetamines, athletes will be tested for anabolic steroids (before the games), ephedrine, and—for fencers and modern pentathletes only—alcohol. In addition, Prince de Merode proposes that all national governing bodies for sport should establish a medical department. He reports, "Modern top competition is unimaginable without doctors. The lives and health of our sportsmen are at stake." De Merode further praises the new links being made between research scientists and the IOC. "The medical commission has realized the imperative existence of a link between scientific research and itself. It has thus decided to appoint a certain number of advisers, chosen from eminent experts in scientific research."[46]

1976—Frank Shorter places second in the marathon at the Montreal Olympic Games and is asked by reporters if he will compete at Moscow in 1980. "Yeah," Shorter says, "if I can find some good doctors."[47]

1976—At the Montreal Olympic Games, Lasse Viren of Finland wins gold medals in the 5,000 and 10,000-meter races amid speculation that he is blood doping.[48]

1976—At the Montreal Olympic Games, East Germany's women swimmers become the subject of controversy with their big shoulders and deep voices. One East German coach reportedly tells a reporter who asks about possible steroid use and comments about the women's deep voices, "We have come here to swim, not sing."[49]

1976 July 25—At the Montreal Olympic Games, weightlifter Dragomir Ciroslan (22 years old) is disqualified after placing fifth in his weight class. Ciroslan is the Romanian record holder in the middleweight class. He is the first weightlifter to be disqualified under the random drug testing system. (As of November 1, 1999, Ciroslan was serving as U.S. Olympic Weightlifting Team coach in Colorado Springs, Colorado).[50]

1976 July 30—At the Montreal Olympic Games, weightlifters Mark Cameron, of Middletown, RI (heavyweight class) and Petř Pavlašek of Czechoslovakia (super heavyweight class, sixth place) are disqualified for anabolic steroid use. Women's discus competitor Danuta Rosani of Poland is also disqualified. All three are caught in the random steroid tests. The USOC issues a statement saying they are "shocked and appalled" at the disqualification of Cameron. Phillip O. Krumm, USOC president, criticizes the IOC Medical Commission for announcing the decision without informing the USOC. The USOC says Cameron will not be dropped from the team and will be permitted to remain in the Olympic village. According to Dr. John B. Anderson, head of the U.S. medical delegation to Montreal, "Cameron was disqualified on a test before the competition. He knew his test would be positive but he was playing a game. He felt the statistics were on his side and he took the calculated risk that he wouldn't be one of the athletes tested. He lost."[51]

1976—By the end of the Montreal Olympic Games, 275 tests have been run and a total of eight athletes are found positive for steroids. A second American weightlifter, Phil Grippaldi, is suspended. In total, seven weightlifters and one female field event specialist test positive.[52]

1976 August—The USOC approves the formation of a panel of experts to study the medical and scientific aspects of sport. Dr. Irving Dardik, cardiovascular surgeon from Tenafly, New Jersey, is named head. Dardik was on the USOC medical staff at Montreal and says the medical committee will do research, help athletes, and "look into areas considered taboo," including anabolic steroids and other drugs. Dr. John Anderson, another member of the new medical committee says, "It's become a medical Olympics. Twenty-five percent of our time in Montreal was spent on trying to explain to athletes all the details of the tests and the drugs that they could and couldn't take. It's gone too far." Dardik further claims that the testing done in Montreal was inconsistent. Some of the tests were conducted by the various sport organizations. Mac Wilkins, Olympic discus champion, for instance, was tested twice at the Games, on the day he arrived and the day after his event, but the IOC did not officially test him even though he won.[53]

1976 September—*Physician and Sportsmedicine* publishes a report on the drug testing at the 1976 Summer Olympic Games.[54]

1977—The American College of Sports Medicine publishes its official position paper on steroid use. The paper concludes that there is no evidence that steroids increase muscle mass or strength.[55] Many elite athletes ridicule this conclusion.

1977 January—Dr. John Anderson, head of the U.S. medical delegation at Innsbruck and at Montreal, charges that the IOC is not paying enough attention to drug problems. "The majority of the IOC members are looking at the trees, not the whole picture," he states in a *New York Times* interview. The *Times* interview was prompted by an article in *Frontiers* magazine, a periodical published by the Academy of Natural Sciences in Philadelphia. In that article, Anderson urged that sex testing be abolished and also raised a number of questions about the IOC testing protocols. "It was rumored in Montreal that the female gymnasts from certain eastern bloc nations received testosterone injections at a certain stage of growth in order to prematurely close the epiphyseal lines of the long bones," he explained, thus creating "a small, short, muscular agile female who probably had a very definite advantage over her competitors." More pessimistically, Anderson wrote, "I think in 1980 it will become evident to the world in general and the athletes in particular, that man has gone a bit too far in manipulating individuals, and it would seem to this observer that 1984 will come and go without the Olympic Games."[56]

1977 January 28—Dr. Irving Dardik meets with Colonel Don Miller, USOC executive director, to discuss the first phase of budgetary requirements to establish a sports medicine program at the USOC training center in Squaw Valley, California. Drug testing is one reason for the establishment of the program.[57]

1977 June 11—At Baden-Baden, West Germany, Dieter Count Landsberg-Velen, vice president of the West German Sports Federation, announces that the federation has approved a ban on the use of muscle-building steroids in international competition. Using drugs, Landsberg-Velen declares, is "a violation of human dignity."[58]

1977 June 15–18—In his report to the IOC in Prague, Prince de Merode discusses the need for IOC-approved drug testing laboratories to be located throughout the world. He suggests that the IOC begin officially recognizing those labs capable of doing IOC-type testing and that it work to encourage other laboratories to upgrade and become certified.[59]

1977 August—The European Cup for track and field takes place in Helsinki, Finland. Three Finns, a Norwegian, and an East German test positive. The Finnish athletes are discus thrower Markku Tuokko, javelin thrower Steppo Hovinen, and high jumper Asko Pesonen. Ilona Slupianek, shot putter, is the East German athlete and the first woman to fail an Olympic-type drug test. The Norwegian athlete is Knut Hjeltnes, discus. Hjeltnes was previously banned for a positive test in Oslo in July at a pre-Cup event.[60]

1977 November 9—The IAAF "indefinitely" bans the five athletes found positive at the European Cup. John Holt, IAAF general secretary, says that the bans might be reduced under "mitigating circumstances."[61]

1977 November 20—Following appeals, the IAAF reduces the suspensions to one year, thus allowing all five athletes to be eligible to participate in the European Championships in Prague in 1978.[62]

1978—Dr. James E. Wright publishes *Anabolic Steroids and Sports*, which will be widely circulated in the weightlifting and bodybuilding communities.[63]

1978—Viktor Kuznetsov is disqualified at the World Swimming Championships after testing positive for anabolic steroids. He won the bronze medal in the 100-meter backstroke.[64]

1978 October—At the European Track and Field Championships, five athletes are disqualified, including pentathlon gold medalist Nadechda Tkacenko of the USSR. Yevgeny Mironov, USSR, who earned a silver medal in men's shot put, is also disqualified.[65]

1978 November—The USOC Medical Committee meets in Colorado Springs and recommends that drug testing procedures be implemented at all national championships. Until now, there has not been a comprehensive doping program in the United States.[66]

1979—During the course of the year, the IAAF bans seven women track athletes for positive drug tests: three Romanians, two Bulgarians, and two Soviets. A report in *Sports Illustrated* notes, "Now even athletes with slight builds, such as middle-distance runners, believe steroids provide explosive power."[67]

1979 January—Renate Neufeld (Spassov) defects to West Germany and tells of the horrors of living in the state-run sport school. The 20-year-old East German claims she was given steroids as "vitamins." According to Neufeld, "The trainer told me the pills would make me stronger and faster and that there were no side effects."[68]

1979 January—Drs. Arnold Beckett and D.A. Cowan, the leaders of Britain's drug testing movement, publish "Misuse of Drugs in Sport" in the *British Journal of Sports Medicine*.[69]

1979 November—Jerry Kirshenbaum publishes "Steroids: The Growing Menace," in *Sports Illustrated*.[70]

1979 December 6—At a pre-Olympic conference in New York City, Dr. Robert Dugal and Dr. Michael Bertrand, who are in charge of drug tests at Lake Placid, announce that the new test is more precise and that procedures will change. A minimum of 400 urine samples will be collected. Random tests will be used and all medal winners tested. The drug test team consists of 40 people, 25 of whom are chemists or biochemists. Twelve new gas chromatographs, three computers, and four mass spectrometers will be used to conduct the tests. There are now 300 drugs on the IOC banned list.[71]

1980–1989

1980—Although no official drug positives are found during the course of the Moscow Olympic Games, IOC drug testing expert Manfred Donike unofficially screens urine samples for exogenous testosterone. According to Donike's new test (which involves measuring the ratio of testosterone to epitestosterone in the urine) 20 percent of all athletes tested—males and females—would have failed his new testosterone screen if it were officially administered. To register a positive on Donike's experimental test, the athlete has to be over the 6:1 (testosterone to epitestosterone) ratio. The 20 percent figure included sixteen gold medalists. Donike uses these unofficial test results to convince the IOC to add his testosterone screen to their testing protocols.[72]

1980—Ilona Slupianek, banned for steroid use in 1977 at the European Cup, wins the gold medal in the shot put at the Moscow Olympic Games. Following her victory, a panel of track and field experts selects Slupianek as "Sportswoman of the Year."[73]

1980—Budget allocation for Lake Placid's testing program is $1.4 million.[74]

1980 February 10-3—At the IOC meeting in Lake Placid, New York, Prince de Merode is asked what the Medical Commission is doing about the "blood injections" or blood doping. According to *IOC Minutes* the prince reports that "This practice was not thought to be very widespread or of much assistance to an athlete."[75]

1980 June—A lengthy article in the *Physician and Sportsmedicine* charges that 20 years after initiating a drug testing program, the IOC's doping problems only continue to grow.[76]

1981 January—U.S. discus thrower Ben Plunknett and Australian Gael Mulhall test positive for anabolic steroids at the Pacific Conference Games in New Zealand. Plunknett, who set world records in the discus at later meets in Modesto, California and Stockholm, Sweden, is stripped of his record and placed on suspension by the IAAF when the test results are completed. As a *Time* article puts it, "He will, however, retain a less desirable record: first person to lose a world record because of steroid use."[77]

1981 September 28—Sebastian Coe, spokesperson for a group of 30 Olympic athletes who attended the IOC congress in Baden-Baden, asks for a lifetime ban on all competitors who use drugs barred by international rules. "We also call for a lifetime ban on coaches and the so-called doctors who administer this evil."[78]

1982—Dr. Robert Kerr, infamous for prescribing anabolic steroids and other drugs for Olympic athletes, publishes *The Practical Use of Anabolic Steroids With Athletes*. Kerr equates drug use with plastic surgery such as breast implants, writing: "It really doesn't matter, the important factor is that they (the athletes) are going to take them anyway. If they are taking them anyway, then at least I can play a role in guiding them in the right direction. . . . If I should stop performing this work right now, who would my few thousand . . . patients go to for help, understanding and guidance?"[79]

1982—Powerlifter Frederick C. Hatfield publishes *Anabolic Steroids: What Kind and How Many*. Hatfield's cookbook for steroid-enhanced performance suggests that steroid users have a different ethic than other athletes. "Many who hold to this ethic," writes Hatfield, "recognize that science is ever advancing in technology and knowledge. New ethic athletes are pioneers . . . implicit in their philosophy is the notion that no amount of legislation has ever been able to halt the progress of science . . . (Drug use is unethical) by your moral code, but not by OURS!"[80]

1982—Santa Monica bodybuilder Dan Duchaine privately publishes *The Underground Steroid Handbook*. Over the next decade, Duchaine will emerge as one of the leading authorities on how to administer anabolic steroids and other drugs to athletes. In the introduction, Duchaine writes, "We know this book will make us a lot of enemies just because we address the topic of steroid use in a realistic manner. Right off, let's state our position on a few things. We like steroids. We use them."[81]

1982 July—An article in *Physician and Sportsmedicine* announces that caffeine and exogenous testosterone are being added to the IOC's banned substances list. In both cases a positive test for these two drugs will be based on the level or percentage of the drug in the body.[82]

1983 February 7—After returning from meetings with the Los Angeles Organizing Committee, IOC president Juan Antonio Samaranch tells reporter Robert Pariente in answer to a question regarding the efficacy of the IOC testing program, ". . . we must make sure that our tests are beyond reproach or challenge. We cannot risk creating a scandal. . . . There are, no doubt, those who cheat, and we know it; . . . the really guilty people are not necessarily the athletes, who are often young and 'innocent'; it is those who encourage them to take drugs."[83]

1983 April 28—The IOC announces that it will reconsider the use of tests for testosterone and caffeine following an announcement by the Los Angeles Olympic Organizing Committee (LAOOC) that it will not test for testosterone and caffeine unless scientific proof is presented showing that the tests were valid.[84]

1983 June—In an interview in *Flex* magazine, Dr. Robert Kerr, a physician who admits to helping athletes with their drug programs, suggests that human growth hormone can create "greatly enhanced gains, beyond what you would expect to achieve using anabolic steroids." Kerr, clearly in favor of the drug, also claims that he has seen increases in muscle mass of as much as 40 pounds in a six-week period, but with a reduction of body fat at the same time.[85]

1983 August 1—*Sports Illustrated* publishes Terry Todd's lengthy article, "The Steroid Predicament." Publication of this article, just two weeks before the problems at the 1983 Pan American Games, contributes to the media frenzy on the question of drugs and sports by providing journalists with a detailed look at the issues involved.[86]

1983—At the Pan American Games in Caracas, Venezuela, officials use the testosterone/epitestosterone screen for the first time. American weightlifter Jeff Michaels is caught and suspended through 14 August 1985.

Over the course of the Pan American Games, 15 athletes, representing 10 nations, are found positive. Included in that number are 11 weightlifters, 1 cyclist, 1 fencer, 1 sprinter, and 1 shot putter. In addition, 12 members of the U.S. track-and-field team pack their bags and fly home after the weightlifting positives are announced, rather than risk the drug testing procedure. The 1983 Pan American Games are, by far, the largest drug scandal in the history of doping control to that time.[87]

1983 August 24—The USOC announces that in the future there will be mandatory, random testing at any meet where American athletes qualify for spots on international teams.[88] USOC president William Simon goes on to say that the USOC assumes the responsibility for drug testing all athletes, which will likely mean clashes with some national governing bodies.

However, during the buildup to the Los Angeles Games, the USOC announces no positive test results, an apparent attempt to avoid bad publicity. Following the completion of the 1984 Olympic Games, when pressed by reporters, the USOC reveals that 86 tests administered during the pre-Olympic season were positive. However, no athletes were denied a chance to compete in the Olympic Games, except for two track-and-field athletes who were denied spots on the U.S. team, and no sanctions were levied against those athletes found to be positive.[89]

1983 August 27—A front page article in the *New York Times* reveals that USOC officials allowed athletes who have failed precompetition drug screens to compete in the Pan American Games. According to USOC president William Simon, approximately 10 athletes approached the USOC before the Caracas competition and asked to be pretested to see if they could pass the IOC drug screen. Simon acknowledges that as many as eight of the tests contained traces of anabolic steroids but no penalty was imposed because the tests were voluntary.[90]

1983 December 4—*Los Angeles Times* staff writers Elliott Almond, Julie Cart, and Randy Harvey join forces for an exposé on the activities of Dr. Robert Kerr, who has been providing Olympic athletes with both anabolic steroids and human growth hormone. "If anabolic steroids are the unofficial drug of the Olympics, Dr. Robert Kerr is the Games' unofficial doctor," they write. "The controversial sports medicine specialist estimates that he has 4,000 patients, among them Olympic athletes from 19 countries as well as professional football, baseball, and basketball players."[91]

1984—Canadian physician and drug use expert Dr. Mauro Di Pasquale publishes *Drug Use and Detection in Amateur Sports*.[92] Following the publication of this book, Di Pasquale begins publishing regular "Updates" for those interested in keeping informed on the changing array of steroids and hormones available for athletes. The first "Update" appears in 1986.[93]

1984—S. Chinery publishes *In Quest of Size,* an advice book on the latest pharmacologic agents available to bodybuilders and weightlifters who want to increase strength and muscle mass.[94]

1984—Osteopath, some-time bodybuilder, and anti-steroid crusader Bob Goldman publishes *Death in the Locker Room*, the first book-length examination of the history and cultural impact of steroid use. Written from Goldman's evangelical perspective, the error-plagued book is widely discussed by the media, and it triggers a growing awareness of the dangers of steroid use for both athletes and the future of sports.[95]

1984—At the Calgary Winter Games, for the first time, the IOC includes beta-blockers (which lower the pulse rate) and diuretics in its testing protocols.[96]

1984 February—Olympic hammer thrower Harold Connolly, an opponent of the IOC's drug testing program, writes "Fair Play Through Drug Tests?" for *Muscle and Fitness* magazine.[97]

1984 May 8—Jeff Michaels of Chicago files suit in U.S. District Court seeking a temporary restraining order lifting his suspension from weightlifting following the 1983 Pan Am Games. He also seeks $1 million in damages.[98]

1984 May 19—The IWF Medical Committee meets to review Michaels's case in Ligano Sabbiardo, Italy. After reviewing the file, they tell him that his two-year IWF suspension must stand. The United States Weightlifting Federation supports him in his request for leniency. Michaels, holder of 40 American records and ranked sixth in the world, took a precompetition test in Caracas, so he felt he was safe. He is caught because his testosterone to epitestosterone ratio is over the 6-to-1 limit. Michaels charges that discrepancies in the testing procedure created an error. He denies ever taking the drugs.[99]

1984 June—In Federal Appeals Court, Judge Milton Shadur lifts American weightlifter Jeff Michaels's suspension from international competition on the grounds that Michaels was denied a proper hearing.[100]

1984 July 1—Dr. Paul Ward of Huntington Beach, California, coordinator of an elite track-and-field program for throwers of the shotput, hammer, and discus, admits that he is dispensing information to help athletes beat IOC drug tests. "This is a way to get as much information as possible to the athletes," says Ward, adding, "If they want to (use drugs) then you have to give them the right facts." Ward further states, "No one seems to have the guts to discuss this drug issue. Well, it's going on and you can't ignore it. The USOC and TAC [The Athletics Congress] take the posture of the ostrich. They stand there with their heads in the sand and their rears in the air. That's where their brains are."

Ward's main source of information on drug use is ex-powerlifter Richard Anthony "Tony" Fitton, who gave advice to Ward and the athletes about which drugs to take, in what dosages, and how to mask the results. In an interview, Fitton told a reporter, "I'm totally sympathetic with the athletes who are trying to find out about drug testing. I can recommend the products to them, and if they take them in the amounts I advise, they will have a top performance in the Olympic Games and I will guarantee that they will not test positive." Ward admits that he frequently gave athletes Fitton's telephone number. Fitton is the author of a privately published booklet sold to athletes at contests entitled, *Drug Testing . . . So What!! How To Beat the Test.* The message on Fitton's 1984 Christmas Card (which featured naked women) was "Have a Hormonious Holiday."[101]

1984 July 13—A nationwide investigation into the steroid black market results in warrants being issued for a physician, three pharmacists, and a gym owner in Hartford, Connecticut. One of the pharmacists, George Butler, had sold 400,000 doses of synthetic hormone to Tony Fitton, who consulted with Dr. Paul Ward of TAC's elite athlete program.[102]

1984 July 13—The deadline for the submission of names of the weightlifting team members for the 1984 Olympic Games is July 14. On Friday, July 13, Judge Milton Shadur issues a preliminary injunction ordering the USOC to name 13 lifters, including Michaels, asserting that such an order would force the IOC to consider Michaels's case. USOC attorneys immediately seek a stay of that court order.[103]

1984 July 14—In the Jeff Michaels case, the U.S. Court of Appeals for the Seventh Circuit denies the USOC's request for a stay. Court sets the date of July 23 for the formal hearing. The USOC is thus forced to name Jeff Michaels to the U.S. Weightlifting Federation team later the same day as the thirteenth man. However, the IOC then rules that despite the court injunction, Michaels will not be allowed to compete. Although he returns to competition some years later, he never again regains his early prominence.[104]

1984 July 16—Dr. Robert Kerr is profiled in *People* magazine. Kerr, an outspoken proponent of both anabolic steroids and human growth hormone tells *People* that human growth hormone is the "fad anabolic drug" of the 1984 Olympic Games.[105]

1984 July 22—In Boulder, Colorado, five officials of the U.S. Cycling Federation meet to discuss Alexi Grewal's suspension from cycling. Grewal tested positive for ephedrine at the Coors International Classic. He says he took the drug by mistake in an asthma medication. Grewal is suspended from cycling for 30 days, which means he cannot compete in the Olympic Games if his penalty stands. Grewal had been officially named to the U.S. cycling team by qualifying in a series of trials.[106]

1984 July 23—After a meeting from 6 P.M. on Sunday evening to 4 A.M. on Monday, the U.S. Cycling board agrees to allow Grewal to race in the Olympic Games. The cycling administrators decide to throw out Grewal's suspension because the tests "did not go far enough to determine the drug involved."[107]

1984 July 23—Tony Daly, orthopedist and sports medicine specialist from Inglewood, CA, and a member of the LAOOC's Medical Team, gives an interview attesting to the infallibility of the IOC's new testing procedures. "It's more sensitive than the equipment used last summer in the Pan American Games in Caracas," says Daly. Daly also explains that about 1,500 drug tests are planned for the 1984 Summer Olympic Games. The first four finishers in each division will be automatically tested with others chosen at random. The IOC will use eight mass spectrometers and gas chromatographs at Los Angeles, allowing officials to announce results within 24 hours. Daly also announces that levels have been set for testosterone and caffeine and that athletes over these allowable levels will be considered positive.[108]

1984 July 29—The Canadian Weightlifting Federation sends home two weightlifters before their competitions in the Los Angeles Games. Lifters Terry Hadlow and Luc Chagnon were given precompetition tests on July 16 at a training camp in Quebec. Both were positive for methyltestosterone.[109]

1984 July—Allan J. Ryan, editor of *Physician and Sportsmedicine*, examines the history of drug testing and discusses the American College of Sports Medicine's new position stance in an article entitled "Drug Problem Building since 1952 Olympics."[110]

1984 August 2—The IOC bans a member of the Japanese training staff from the Games. Volleyball player Mikiyasi Tanaka was found positive for ephedra. However, the Japanese delegation claimed that Tanaka's masseur—Yoshitaka Yahagi—had given the player an herbal cold remedy that contained the drug. No action was taken against the player. Yahagi, the masseur, was sent home and also banned from participation in the next Olympic Games.[111]

1984 August 5—Manfred Donike, member of the IOC Medical Committee, announces that unofficial tests have revealed the use of beta-blockers by most competitors in the Olympic pentathlon. Donike explains that the drug will go on the banned list for the 1988 games.[112]

1984 August 5—Thomas Johansson of Sweden, silver medalist in the superheavyweight class of Greco-Roman wrestling, is the first medalist to be found positive for steroids at the 1984 Olympic Games. Johannson admits to taking primobolan to gain weight after surgery for a broken nose.[113]

1984 August 9—California physician and steroid proponent Robert Kerr tells reporters that he has personal knowledge of more than 12 medalists who have beaten the IOC tests by stopping their drugs at the appropriate time. "As far as the athletes I deal with, all of them have performed well, and I would like to brag about how many gold medals and silver medals my patients have won in the last week, but I can't," says Kerr. Kerr claims that some athletes told him they continued taking drugs up to two weeks before the Games. He also admits that a number of his patients used human growth hormone in their training.

Dr. Tony Daly, Olympic Committee medical director says in the IOC's defense, "He can claim anything he wants to, but I know our system is foolproof and it's working. If the steroids are in the system . . . we're going to find them." He added, "Our system can find one part per billion, so they'd have to be long since gone, which means they're not doing them any good."[114]

1984 October—In an article for *Sports Illustrated,* Terry Todd examines the dilemmas posed by human growth hormone and warns readers that the soon-to-be-released biosynthetic version of the drug will cause increased use among athletes.[115]

1984 August—Marti Vaino of Finland is stripped of the silver medal he won in the 10,000 meters when he tests positive for anabolic steroids. In a later interview on Finnish television, Vaino claims, "I have gotten a confession from people whom I have trusted. They thought I should be helped against being overtrained, and they gave me testosterone and anabolic steroids without me knowing it."[116]

1984—The American College of Sports Medicine changes its position on steroid use and announces, "The gains in muscular strength achieved through high intensity exercise and proper diet can be increased by the use of anabolic-androgenic steroids in some individuals."[117]

1984 August 16—*Foreign Report*, a magazine published in London by the *Economist,* reports that over the previous 25 years a total of 59 Soviet athletes have died from drug-related causes.[118] (This article received subsequent criticism for having been politically motivated and poorly documented.)

1985—Dr. William N. Taylor publishes *Hormonal Manipulation: A New Era of Monstrous Athletes*.[119]

1985—Canadian weightlifters, returning from the 1985 World Championships in Moscow, are stopped at the Montreal airport and found to be in possession of tens of thousands of doses of anabolic steroids they purchased for resale in North America.[120]

1985—Customs officials stop Soviet weightlifters Anatoly Pisarenko and Alexander Kurlovich, the two top superheavyweight lifters in the world, at Montreal airport. Agents discover more than $10,000 worth of steroids in their luggage.[121] After being arrested, Pisarenko and Kurlovich are released, but their drugs are confiscated. The Soviet Weight Lifting Federation bans them for life, but then reinstates Kurlovich in time for him to win the gold medal in 1988.

1985 January—Dr. Tom Dickinson, part of the U.S. cycling team's medical support staff in Los Angeles, reveals that at least three and possibly as many as seven American cyclists used blood doping before racing in the 1984 Olympic Games. Maintaining that blood-doping was not banned at this time by the IOC, Pat McDonough, silver medalist in the team-pursuit competition tells reporters, "Nothing illegal was done. . . . In the Olympics, you know that everyone is getting the best medical help. So, if it's not illegal, you get it too."[122]

1985 January 18—The U.S. Cycling Federation officially bans blood doping and imposes sanctions on the three officials involved in administering the doping at the 1984 Games. However, U.S. Cycling Federation president David Prouty also announces that no cyclists will lose medals and that "no athletes will be held or considered responsible for the incident."[123]

1985 February—*Track and Field News* reports that following the embarrassment of the drug positives at the 1983 Pan American Games the USOC conducted a large number of both "informal" and "formal" tests in order to determine the level of use among American athletes before the 1984 Games. According to the report, 1332 athletes were formally tested (meaning that athletes faced sanctions if found positive), 611 were tested informally (without sanctions in place), and an additional 311 were tested at the specific request of allied athletic groups. It was found that 33 athletes were positive for stimulants and 53 were positive for anabolic steroids or testosterone. This included 10 positive tests at the 1984 Olympic Trials.[124]

1985 March—In a signed editorial in the *New England Journal of Medicine*, Dr. Harvey G. Klein, an expert in blood transfusions who works at the National Institute of Health, urges the USOC and IOC to add blood doping or blood packing to its proscribed list. Klein cites as part of his rationale the fact that several cyclists at the 1984 Games became ill after transfusions and that at least six members of the U.S. team used transfusions.[125]

1985 March—In an article in *Physician and Sports Medicine,* G. Legwold examines the legal aspects of implementing a blood doping policy for athletics.[126]

1985 March 24—Kenneth Clark, director of Sports Medicine for the USOC, announces that the USOC plans to get tougher on drug testing. Clark says that the USOC is now working on a new drug testing policy that will call for (1) testing at all national championships, (2) a one-year suspension for a first offense, and (3) a four-year suspension for a second offense. Dr. Irving Dardik and Dr. Robert Voy work with him. Their proposals will be submitted to the USOC in April for ratification. If approved, the 40 national governing bodies that make up the USOC must also ratify it before it goes into effect.[127]

1985 April 10—Richard Anthony (Tony) Fitton, steroid smuggler and former adviser to Dr. Paul Ward's elite athlete program, fails to appear in court to face sentencing on drug trafficking charges. This is Fitton's second offense for smuggling. He was also arrested in 1982, in Atlanta, and given a suspended sentence.[128]

1985 May 6—Peter V. Ueberroth, the commissioner of baseball, announces a new drug testing program for major league baseball. "We will include everyone from the owners on down," said Ueberroth before noting that the players themselves will not be tested until the players' union agrees to the program.[129]

1985 June 6—In his report to the IOC at their meeting in Berlin, Prince de Merode announces that (1) there are now 14 accredited IOC laboratories, (2) beta blockers will be added to the banned substances list, and (3) the Medical Commission has decided to ban blood doping, even though a test is not yet available to detect the procedure.[130]

1985 June 24—The USOC announces that it has set aside funds for a comprehensive doping program to ensure that athletes competing for spots on the 1998 Olympic team are drug-free. The new program calls for testing of all medal winners and others at random in Olympic qualifying events. It also calls for the testing of athletes in residence in Colorado Springs.[131]

1985 August—H.L. Nash examines the ban on blood doping for *Physician and Sports Medicine.*[132]

1985 September 6—Otto Jelinek, Canada's minister of sport, announces stiffer penalties for athletes found positive for drugs. He also announces a stepped-up program of random testing that would lead to the loss of government support for those caught. The move comes after Michael Vlau, a weightlifter, was suspended for life because of repeated drug use.[133]

1985 October—Genentech, a pharmaceutical company based in California, announces that it has received FDA approval to begin the manufacture of biosynthetic human growth hormone. The new drug will be marketed under the name Protropin.[134] Before this time, human growth hormone was only available from human cadavers, making it both scarce and expensive. The biosynthetic version marketed by Genentech and, later, by the Eli Lilly Company, will sell for substantially less.[135]

1986—Tom Donohoe and Neil Johnson publish *Foul Play: Drug Abuse in Sports*.[136]

1986 January—In a provocative article in *New Studies in Athletics,* published in London, H.G. Klein explores why the IOC, which outlawed blood doping 10 years earlier, has not put measures into place to stop the practice.[137]

1986 March—The U.S. Food and Drug Administration tightens its regulations regarding "approved" medical uses for anabolic steroids. The regulatory agency rules that methandrostenalone (sold by the trade name Dianabol) and methandriol may no longer be manufactured because of a lack of proof of medical need.[138]

1986 July—Canada's minister of sport, Otto Jelinek, cuts off government funding for six cyclists found positive for steroids. In a later interview, Jelinek says he is aware that his actions have "ruined their athletic careers," but feels it is necessary to stand firm against drug use.[139]

1986 August 27—At the Eighth Annual Sports Summit held in New York City, USOC president Robert Helmick calls for a national policy on drug testing. Helmick wants to unify the testing policies of the USOC, the National Football League, The National Collegiate Athletic Association, the National Basketball Association, and other sports organizations. Helmick also reports that since the USOC began regularly testing athletes in 1983, approximately 3,500 U.S. athletes have been tested and that 3,000 more will be tested by the end of 1986.

Canada's minister of sport, Otto Jelinek, also speaking at the meeting, criticizes Helmick for not suggesting uniformity in penalties as well as in policy. Jelinek states, "I am appreciative of his comments on uniformity in testing and random sampling. What concerns me still, is that he hasn't approached publicly the issue of uniformity in penalizing. We developed our policy in Canada: banning offenders for life."[140]

1986 October 12-17—IOC Medical Commission informs the IOC that Dr. Don Catlin, head of the IOC lab in Los Angeles, has assisted the Commission in revising its list of banned substances. Added to the list for the first time are diuretic drugs, which are used both to help lose weight and to increase urine production and thus mask the presence of other banned substances. The Medical Commission also notes that there are now 18 IOC-accredited laboratories.[141]

1987—Jonathan Harris publishes *Drugged Athletes: The Crisis in American Sports.*[142]

1987—Richard H. Strauss publishes *Drugs and Performance in Sports.*[143]

1987—Canadian scientist J.G. Macintyre surveys the scientific literature on the safety and efficacy of human growth hormone use by athletes for the scientific journal, *Sports Medicine.* Macintyre notes that although the scientific literature does not suggest that human growth hormone will increase performance, a number of people in the bodybuilding and weightlifting communities claim it is a miracle drug. One proponent of human growth hormone use, cited by Macintyre (Dan Duchaine, author of the *Underground Steroid Handbook*) states, "Wow, is this great stuff! It is the best drug for permanent muscle gains. . . . People who use it can expect to gain 30 to 40 lbs. of muscle in 10 weeks . . . we LOVE the stuff."[144] Macintyre concludes, "The lack of scientific support for its efficacy in sports and the potential hazards of its use will not deter the athlete who is determined to win at all costs . . . growth hormone use may become a problem of tremendous magnitude."[145]

1987 May—In his report to the IOC at their annual meeting in Istanbul, Prince de Merode reports that Dr. Manfred Donike has examined all the doping tests done in IOC labs during 1986 for a statistical analysis of the trends in doping. Donike found that two-thirds of all drug-positives were for anabolic steroids and two-thirds of the steroid-positives were for nandralone.[146]

1987—At the Pan American Games in Indianapolis, for the first time, drug testers discover probenecid in the tests of many athletes. Probenecid is a gout medication used by athletes to mask steroids. In January of 1988, probenecid will be added to the IOC list of banned substances.[147, 148]

1987 January—Dr. Don Catlin is quoted, in an article in the *Journal of the American Medical Association*, as saying, "Some sports may want to do testing, but they also don't want to have too many positive tests. Well, that can be arranged, but my position is that we will work with any group willing to follow certain basic guidelines we think are necessary to defend the credibility of the testing."[149]

1987 February—Nordic combined skier Kerry Lynch wins the silver medal at the 1987 World Championships. Later, in December of the same year, Lynch confesses that he used blood doping before the competition and is subsequently stripped of his medal and banned for two years. The director of nordic skiing, Jim Page, admits that he approved the blood doping and made arrangements to fly a physician to Switzerland to reinject red blood cells that were previously taken from Lynch. Page receives a lifetime ban for his participation. However, that ban is lifted in 1990 and in 1992 Page is named the USOC's Assistant Executive Director of Sport. In this new position, Page oversees the work of USOC drug control director Dr. Wade Exum. Lynch is later named an assistant coach of the U.S. Nordic Combined World Cup Team.[150]

1987 March—Michael Sawka, a researcher at the Army Research Institute of Environmental Medicine, reports that a clinical study of the effectiveness of blood doping found that transfusing athletes with additional red blood cells derived from two units of the athletes' own blood increases the subjects' aerobic potential between 4 percent and 18 percent.[151]

1987 April 10—Birgit Dressel, 26-year-old heptathlete from Germany, dies of complications from anabolic steroid use. The story of her death, and the unbearable agony she suffered in her last days, is chronicled in *Der Spiegel* following a criminal inquiry. At the center of the controversy surrounding her death is Armin Klumper, Dressel's doctor and the so-called "highest guru of German sports doctors," who took credit for her move from thirty-third to sixth in the world rankings.[152]

1987 May—David Jenkins, member of the 1972 British Olympic team and winner of a silver medal in the mile relay; Pat Jacobs, former strength coach for the University of Miami; Mike McDonald, world record–holding powerlifter; Dan Duchaine, author of *The Underground Steroid Handbook*; and 30 other local distributors located throughout the United States, are indicted for conspiracy to sell anabolic steroids, smuggling, and tax fraud. The 110-count indictment is the largest undercover investigation into the black marketing of anabolic steroids up to this time. Phil Halpern, the San Diego–based district attorney in charge of the investigation, estimates that this particular steroid ring sold more than $4 million worth of ergogenic drugs in the previous calendar year.[153]

1987 May 19—*Miami Herald* investigative reporter Angie Cannon explores the connections between steroid use and law enforcement in "Steroid-Using Police Cause Brutality Fears." Inspired by Harrison Pope and David Katz's study of the psychological effects of steroids, Cannon quotes former steroid-using policeman Freddy Gasca, who observed that users "get upset and angry. You won't take anything from anybody. . . . A street patrolman on steroids will get into more fights, more incidents than one who's not."[154] Later that year, *60 Minutes* aired a show about police and steroids that indicated the problem was widespread.

1987 August—In Rome, at the World Championships in Athletics, Ben Johnson sets a new world record at 100 meters while winning first place. Rumors of steroid use circulate.[155]

1987 August 30—The *Pittsburgh Press* begins a four-part series examining the problem of anabolic steroid use. Series author Bill Utterback focuses on the increasing number of deaths and medical problems associated with steroid use. Writes Utterback, "For two decades doctors have warned against the dangers of steroids. They talked about heart problems. They talked about liver problems. They talked about cancer. . . . Now the anti-steroid warnings are illustrated by clogged arteries, ruptured vessels, lifeless limbs, cancerous growths and softball-sized tumors. Real people are having real, life-threatening problems. The doctors were right."[156]

1987 September 10—Carl Lewis tells reporters in Brussels that the USOC and IOC need to hire an independent company to do their drug testing. This company should test for drugs that improve performance and for masking agents. Lewis believes this independent company should also have authority to release the names of athletes without first sending them to the IAAF or IOC.[157]

1988—Janet Mohun and Aziz Khan publish *Drugs, Steroids and Sports.*[158]

1988—Michael J. Asken publishes *Dying to Win: The Athlete's Guide to Safe and Unsafe Drugs in Sports.*[159]

1988—The IAAF publishes the proceedings of its second IAAF Medical Congress, held in Canberra, Australia, in 1977. Included in the proceedings are papers on both doping and sex tests for female competitors.[160]

1988—Peptide hormones are added to the IOC list of banned drugs. These include human growth hormone and ACTH, a synthetic hormone that stimulates the adrenal gland. The IOC announces a $2 million project to find a test for human growth hormone by the 2000 Olympic Games. (As of November 1999, no such test was yet approved.)[161]

1988—At the Women's World Weightlifting Championships, the Chinese team dominate the event, winning every one of the nine bodyweight divisions. Some months later, a member of the International Weightlifting Federation tells a CBS journalist (Terry Todd) that when the drug testing for those championships was completed, all nine winners tested positive for anabolic steroids. The International Weightlifting Federation official says the federation believes that if this information becomes public knowledge it will support the views of such IOC officials as Vice President Richard Pound, who has recommended that weightlifting be dropped from the Olympic program because of its ongoing drug problems. This worry leads the International Weightlifting Federation to contact the Chinese Weightlifting Federation via back channels and inform them that although the positives will not be made public, none of the Chinese lifters can be brought to the 1989 World Championships. In those championships, none of the 1988 winners appear, but once again a Chinese lifter wins every class. What lends credence to the story of the International Weightlifting official is that each one of the 1989 winners lifted exactly the same weights as did the winners in 1988. The snatches were the same, the clean and jerks were the same, and, of course, the totals were the same. Anyone experienced in lifting would argue that this was not the result of a coincidence.[162]

1988 February 22—Polish hockey player Jaroslaw Mirowecki is banned for testosterone use in the Calgary Olympic Winter Games. He was chosen at random. He and his coaches claim he was given the testosterone in a drink.[163]

1988 February—In *Maclean's* magazine's Winter Olympic special edition, C. Wood examines the problems of drug testing for the organizers of the Olympic Winter Games in Calgary.[164]

1988 February 9-11—The Medical Commission reports to the IOC in Calgary that it is working on a new code of ethics for drug testing labs that would, among other things, strictly forbid their doing pre-Olympic tests. Several reports of this nature surfaced before the Winter Games in Calgary. In addition, several new drugs are added to the list of banned substances including human chorionic gonadotropin, which causes the body to produce higher levels of testosterone.[165]

1988 April—Psychologists Harrison G. Pope and David L. Katz publish an article in the *American Journal of Psychology* in which they report, after surveying more than 40 steroid-using athletes, "Many reported prominent affective syndromes, and five reported five psychotic symptoms in association with steroid use."[166] Pope's study is widely publicized in the media, which become especially enamored of the term coined to describe this new disorder—"roid rage."[167]

1988 June—IOC sponsors the "First Permanent World Conference on Anti-Doping in Sport" in Ottawa, Canada. During the three-day conference, representatives of 28 countries examine drug testing issues and work to create an "international anti-doping charter." Among their proposals, which will be presented to the IOC Executive for implementation, is a request for random, out-of-competition testing.[168]

1988 July 13—Dr. James C. Puffer, U.S. team physician to Seoul, gives an interview to the *New York Times*. According to Puffer, several new tests will be added for the Seoul Olympic Games. The new tests will look for the use of phosphate loading to enhance oxygen-carrying capacity and bicarbonate loading to reduce lactic acid buildup.[169]

1988 July 29—1984 gold medalist Karl-Heinz Radschinsky is dropped from the West German weightlifting squad when the IOC declares they are opposed to his competing in Seoul. Radschinsky was convicted for selling anabolic steroids two years previously.[170]

1988 August 13—Mike Moran, USOC spokesperson, explains that between 6 and 10 track-and-field athletes who failed drug tests at the Olympic Trials in Indianapolis in July will be allowed to compete in the Olympic Games because the drug use was either "predeclared" or "inadvertent." All positives were for over-the-counter stimulants from herbal teas or cold medications.[171]

1988—At the Seoul Olympic Games, marijuana is screened for the first time. It is not officially banned by the IOC, but "some member nations are curious about the number of athletes who use it." In addition, it is estimated that the drug testing laboratory in Seoul will process about 200 samples a day. Drug testing equipment for Seoul costs $3 million. Again, officials will test the top four finishers in each division as well as athletes chosen at random following their competitions.[172]

1988 September 13—In Seoul, Korea, the 94th IOC Congress adopts a resolution addressing the issue of drug trafficking. The new rule gives the IOC the power to impose penalties for dealing or supplying drugs to athletes, up to and including life exclusion from the Games. The rule is prompted by a case in which a Soviet speed skater was allowed to compete at the Calgary Games after being caught passing steroids to a Norwegian cross-country skier.[173]

1988 September 14—Dr. Robert Voy, chief medical officer of the USOC, tells reporters that he is convinced athletes have found a new masking agent. "The cheaters are winning," says Voy. "They know how to beat the tests and what I'm hearing from a lot of people is that they have a fantastic new blocking agent that our labs cannot pick up." Later in the article, Voy says, "I have got to believe what the athletes are telling me. They tell me our drug testing program is a joke. Until we begin some kind of unannounced testing, essentially surprising the athletes, what we're doing is a waste."[174]

1988 September 17—A three-member arbitration panel upholds the USOC's right to deny Angel Meyers a place on the U.S. Olympic swimming team. In the hearing, Meyers continues to maintain that her birth control pills have created a false positive.[175] She returns in 1992 and wins the gold medal in the 4 × 100-meter relay in the Barcelona Games.

1988 September 17—Robert Helmick announces that the USOC's decision to ban Angel Meyers will stand. Meyers has qualified in five events at the U.S. swimming championships.[176]

1988 September 25—The Bulgarian weightlifting team pulls out of the Seoul Games and sends its team home after two of its gold medalists are found positive for diuretics. The IOC also disqualifies a Spanish weightlifter, Fernando Mariaca, for amphetamines administered by a team physician. Three other lifters are suspended before competition begins.[177]

1988 September 27—The IOC announces that Ben Johnson, gold medalist at 100 meters, is positive and will be stripped of his medal. Later in the morning, the IAAF announces that Johnson will be banned for two years. The Canadian government then announces that he will be banned for life from receiving any kind of government financial support. Two tests have shown that Johnson used stanozolol, an anabolic steroid. Richard Pound, an IOC vice president from Canada, states, "This is a disaster for Ben, a disaster for the Games, and a disaster for track and field. But let's turn this around to make the slate clean and show the world that we do mean business."

Johnson and his coach, Charlie Francis, tell IOC officials that he is innocent and must have been given something in a drink. Prince de Merode, head of the IOC Medical Commission rules out that possibility, saying that the tests also indicate a chronic suppression of Johnson's adrenal function.

In an interview, Juan Antonio Samaranch says, "We are showing that the system works. We are showing that my words are not only words, they are facts. We are winning the battle against doping."[178]

1988 September 27—The Canadian Track and Field Association announces that it will begin random, monthly testing. Canadian testing policy has been to test two out of the three top finishers in track-and-field competitions. At the Olympic Trials, Johnson was lucky and was not tested.[179]

1988 September 27—Dr. Jamie Astaphan, Ben Johnson's physician, appears on *Nightline* and denies that he has ever given Johnson steroids.[180]

1988 September 28—Canada announces it will investigate the Ben Johnson affair. Ben Johnson's doctor, Jamie Astaphan, is at the center of the controversy. The Ontario College of Physicians and Surgeons also announces it will investigate Astaphan.[181]

1988 September 29—Hungarian weightlifter Andor Szanyl is disqualified for stanozolol. He was the silver medalist in the 220-pound class. Following this announcement, Hungary pulls its team from the Games and sends them home. Szanyl was the 1985 world champion. Another Hungarian, Kalman Csengari, finishes fourth in the 75-kilo class, and then tests positive for testosterone.[182]

1988 September 30—Richard Pound, vice president of the IOC, announces that he will recommend dropping weightlifting from future Olympic Games. This is announced after a fifth weightlifter is found positive in Seoul. Three of the five are medal winners.[183]

1988 October—*Doping Express*, a book by journalist Anne Lise Hammer, is published in Norway. In that book, UCLA professor and Olympic drug testing expert Don Catlin says, "Certain federations are suppressing results, some out of stupidity, but not the IAAF. They know what they do."[184]

1988 October 3—As the Seoul Olympic Games end, U.S. and Soviet sports officials announce a new joint effort to eradicate drugs in sport. Robert Helmick says they hope to achieve "comprehensive year-round testing during training and competition." However, in the United States there are potential legal barriers to such a plan. A major problem is that individual sports are controlled by their own national governing bodies. The USOC is actually only in control of the Olympic Trials and team selection for the Games. For these reasons and because the Soviet Union dissolves soon thereafter, this joint effort never comes to fruition.[185]

1988 October 5—The Canadian government appoints a senior judge to investigate the use of drugs in Canadian sport with special focus on the Ben Johnson scandal. Charles W. Dubin is named to the post; he is an associate chief justice of the Supreme Court of Ontario.[186]

1988 October 18—Angel Meyers is suspended from competition through 1989 by the U.S. Swimming Board of Review. Meyers tested positive at the national championships where she set several world records, won her division, and qualified for the Olympic Games. The Board also rules that she will have to undergo "not less than three" random drug tests each year through 1992.[187]

1988 October 24—Canadian Track and Field Association indefinitely suspends Charlie Francis, Ben Johnson's coach. The Canadian association also ratifies the IAAF's two-year ban on Johnson.[188]

1988 November 16—U.S. Representative Charles B. Rangel of New York announces that he has sent letters to the heads of the NBA, NFL, and other professional sport organizations suggesting that they impose an immediate and lifetime ban on pro athletes who use drugs. "No ifs, no ands, no buts," says Rangel. "Rather than 30 days or 60 days or even one year, we should give them no days, as in no more chances."[189]

1988 November 17—The *New York Times* begins a five-day series of front-page articles related to drug use and sports. In the opening paragraph of the first article, the authors observe that, "At least half of the 9000 athletes who competed at the Olympics in Seoul used performance-enhancing drugs in training, according to estimates by medical and legal experts as well as traffickers in these drugs. These experts also contend that the drug testing programs of the IOC and other sports associations have had no impact in reducing the use of such drugs." Ben Johnson and the nine other positives in Seoul inspired the series, say the authors.

A number of interesting facts emerge from the series:

1. Dr. Park Jong Sei, director of Olympic drug testing in Seoul, claims that at least 20 other athletes in Seoul tested positive but were not disqualified. According to Juan Antonio Samaranch, the other positives were not at high enough levels.
2. Dr. Robert Voy, chief USOC medical officer, suggests that more than 50 percent of Olympic athletes use performance-enhancing drugs.
3. Underground research/grapevine has enabled athletes to benefit from drugs that the IOC and regular medical communities know little about. The authors estimate that there are approximately a dozen substances in current use that the tests cannot detect.
4. At Seoul, when someone is found positive the test results are sent to a five-member subcommittee of the IOC Medical Committee. Then they go to the full, 23-member Medical Commission that votes on each case. Then the issue goes to the IOC Executive Committee for action.
5. Dr. Robert Voy charges that some sport federations delayed the appeal process in order to continue allowing athletes to compete. He also said, "You can't have a sport test itself and be trustworthy. It's like the fox guarding the henhouse."[190]

1988 November 21—Soviet and U.S. Olympic officials sign a preliminary agreement to establish an exchange program in which athletes from each country could be tested during training by representatives of the other country. U.S. officials must now look at legal issues of civil rights.[191]

1988 November 25—Marat Gramov, chairman of the Soviet State Committee for Physical Education and Sport and president of the Soviet Olympic Committee, announces that approximately 300 Soviet athletes, some of whom are "elite," have been disqualified from national competitions in the past three years. This is announced at a conference in Moscow sponsored by UNESCO. Gramov also suggests holding a world drug conference in the Soviet Union. (Some people at the conference speculate that the Soviet Union's new policy against doping came from the fact that it was falling behind the United States and other countries in doping technology and design. In other words, American athletes now have better drugs, and more access to them.)[192]

1988 November 25—At the Moscow UNESCO conference, sports ministers and other officials from 100 countries meet in Moscow and approve by acclamation an anti-drug charter that establishes guidelines for governments to fight drugs. They also recommend that the IOC set up a panel of drug testers to do random, out-of-competition testing in any country in the world. "This is a big day for the IOC," claims Alain Coupat, a senior IOC official. "It means UNESCO recognizes that the fight against doping must be constructed on a global basis, not by each state and that the IOC is the best organization to direct the fight."

One potential problem with this idea, however, is that the United States and a number of other countries do not belong to UNESCO. Furthermore, some countries have laws forbidding testing on short notice. The Soviet Union, however, strongly supports it and offers multiple entry visas for the drug testers if the committee is formed.[193]

1988 November—IOC publishes "International Olympic Charter Against Doping in Sport."[194]

1988 December 4—Dr. Charles Yesalis of Penn State University publishes a guest editorial in the *New York Times* titled, "Steroid Use is Not Just an Adult Problem." Yesalis discusses his new research study examining the use of steroids by adolescents as young as junior-high-school age. "We estimate that there are up to a half million adolescents (in the United States) who have used anabolic steroids," writes Yesalis.[195]

1988 December 12—David Jenkins, who won a silver medal in the 400-meter relay as a member of Great Britain's team at the 1972 Olympic Games, is sentenced in San Diego to seven years in prison for steroid smuggling. In his trial, which began on November 6, 1987, the prosecutors reveal that Jenkins ran a steroid ring that "at one time dominated the U.S. black market for muscle enhancing drugs."[196]

1988 December 15—The December issue of the *Journal of the American Medical Association* contains the results of a survey of 3,403 high school senior males who completed a questionnaire about current and previous steroid use. The research team, led by William E. Buckley of Penn State University, reports that 6.6 percent of high school males—approximately 1 in 15—use steroids. Of special note is the fact that among the users of anabolic steroids, only 47 percent cite athletic reasons for their use. Twenty-six percent claim that they used the drugs simply to improve appearance.[197]

1989—IOC publishes the proceedings of the 29th Session of the International Olympic Academy meeting held in Lausanne, Switzerland. Included in those proceedings is an article by Anita DeFrantz entitled "Olympic Movement: Youth and Doping" and three other examinations of the IOC's drug testing program.[198]

1989 January 10—Canada's Dubin Commission begins federal hearings into the use of drugs by athletes.[199]

1989—U.S. House of Representatives adopts legislation "to provide for the control of anabolic steroids under the Controlled Substances Act and for other purposes." This act places anabolic steroids under Schedule II of the Controlled Substances Act and it creates an Interagency Coordinating Council on the Abuse of Anabolic Steroids, consisting of the Secretary of Health and Human Services and representatives of the Food and Drug Administration, the Drug Enforcement Administration, the Department of Education, the Department of Defense, and five members of the general public who would work for one year to develop a comprehensive strategy for the control of these substances.[200]

1989 January 10—A bill is introduced at the British House of Commons making it a criminal offense to either take or supply anabolic steroids without a prescription. The legislation also makes anabolic steroids a controlled substance.[201]

1989 March—A Soviet magazine, *Smena*, reports that during the 1988 Olympic Games the Soviet team was pretested aboard the ship *Mikhail Sholokhov*, docked

60 miles offshore from Korea, to be sure they would not test positive at the Games. An athlete quoted in the report claims that she was given drugs by the team doctors and told they were vitamins. "They knew what kind of vitamins these were . . . and that if you refused you'd be thrown off the team. Now," she explains, "I'm practically an invalid . . . constant pains . . . my whole hormonal system is destroyed . . . and my life is still ahead of me. I would have liked to become a mother."[202]

1989 March—IOC releases *Information for Athletes, Coaches and Medical Practitioners on the Permissible Use of Drugs in Amateur Sport.* This publication is an updated position statement and explanation of doping policies.[203]

1989 March 2—Charlie Francis, Ben Johnson's coach, testifies to the Dubin Commission that he administered the steroid furazabol to Johnson before Johnson set a world record in the 100 meters in 1987. He goes on to explain that Johnson has been using steroids since 1981 and that Johnson willingly and knowingly used the drugs to enhance his sprinting ability. Angela Isajenko, a member of Francis' track team who testified about her own drug use to the Dubin Commission, says "All I can say is that I'm happy the truth is finally coming out. . . . Everybody should be straight up and tell the truth. (Francis is) doing a good job of that."[204]

1989 March 4—A lengthy editorial in *The Globe and Mail* ponders the effect of the Dubin Commission's inquiry on sport in Canada.[205]

1989 March 20—Representatives of the USOC and Russian Olympic Committee meet to discuss a new bilateral doping pact. According to USOC president Robert Helmick, the new pact would call for Soviets to test American athletes and Americans to man Soviet labs. "The steroid problem can only be solved by all the countries in the world working together," he says. "There must be a global approach to this problem and by doing this we want everyone to know we're serious about doing something about it."[206] T.M. Wolf examines the legal issues surrounding the new USOC–Soviet Olympic Committee doping agreement in the *Stanford Journal of International Law.*[207]

1989 April 6—The IOC announces that during 1988, more than 1,150 Olympic-sport athletes tested positive for banned substances. A majority of the positives were for anabolic steroids. Forty-seven thousand urine samples were analyzed, according to Dr. Manfred Donike, of the IOC's Medical Commission. There are now 22 IOC-approved labs.[208]

1989 June 5-7—The International Athletic Foundation hosts the World Symposium on Doping in Sport in Monte Carlo. Papers and discussions at the symposium include such titles as: "The Use of Human Chorionic Gonadotropin," "Blood Doping," "A Review of the Seoul Laboratory's Procedures," Code of Ethics for IOC Drug Labs," and the "Psychological Impact of Drug Use by Athletes." The proceedings of the conference are published the next year.[209]

1989 June 16—Ben Johnson takes the stand and, under oath, confesses in the Dubin Commission hearing to having taken anabolic steroids for years.[210]

1989 June 19—Robert Kerr, of Los Angeles, testifies before the Dubin Commission. Kerr tells the investigators that he knew

1. that Eastern-bloc countries had set up centers to investigate masking agents, and

2. that athletes in strength events from Eastern-bloc countries were using small amounts of strychnine as a stimulant 30 to 60 minutes before competition.[211]

1989 June 26—Canadian shot put champion Bishop Dolegiewicz testifies before the Dubin Commission in Toronto. "At the higher levels of competition," says Dolegiewicz, "I would be hard pressed to find the name of an individual who hasn't used steroids." Dolegiewicz testifies that he used steroids throughout the 11 years of his competitive career.[212]

1989 July 30-31—The Amateur Athletic Foundation of Los Angeles hosts the National Consensus Meeting on Anabolic/Androgenic Steroids, a joint effort of the USOC, National Collegiate Athletic Association, National Federation of State High School Associations, and the Amateur Athletic Foundation of Los Angeles. This task force attempts to create a nationwide strategy for research, intervention, education, and rehabilitation in the use of drugs for sport.[213]

1989 August—In a reflective essay published in *Olympic Review,* Canadian IOC member Richard Pound explores the Ben Johnson scandal and its ethical implications. Pound charges that we have entered an era of organized cheating in which athletes, coaches, medical personnel, and sport officials all participate in subverting the doping policies of the IOC. In that same issue of *Olympic Review*, Prince de Merode reports on the progress of the anti-doping movement.[214]

1989 August 30-September 1—In the wake of the Ben Johnson scandal and the beginning of the Dubin inquiry, Prince de Merode attempts to set the record straight on the doping issue in his report to the IOC in Puerto Rico. He reports that in 1988 the IOC laboratories analyzed 47,069 drug screens and found only 2.54 percent positive results. According to de Merode, it was "not 80 percent of athletes who were taking or had taken steroids, but a maximum of 5 percent of athletes who had used this kind of doping." De Merode also addresses the issue of marijuana use in this report, explaining that some sports governing bodies and national federations are asking for its inclusion on the IOC list. In addition, he suggests that the IOC create a mobile drug testing laboratory that could be flown around the world to do random, out-of-competition testing. The IOC approves the basic principle of this flying lab and asks that a budget for the project be submitted in December.[215]

1989 September 4—At a meeting in Barcelona, the IAAF Executive Council votes to remove the world records of all athletes who have admitted under legal oath to using anabolic steroids or other doping agents. This motion is prompted by the Ben Johnson case and the subsequent Dubin Commission hearings in Canada, where Johnson testified to his steroid use.[216]

1989 September 13-16—At the 94th IOC Session in Seoul Korea, Prince de Merode proposes the adoption of a new rule against trafficking in doping substances. He also suggests that an investigation into the use of marijuana be undertaken and that marijuana be considered for inclusion as a banned substance. The IOC Congress passes the new anti-trafficking rule.[217]

1989 September 18—Dr. Arne Ljungqvist, chairman of the IAAF Medical Committee, testifies before the Dubin Commission. According to his testimony, only 25 of the 182 member nations conduct out-of-competition drug tests. He cites

TAC as a particularly bad offender, explaining that TAC conducted their own, internal review before turning test results over to the international federation.[218]

1989 September 19—The Dubin Commission officially ends after eight months of testimony and 120 witnesses.[219]

1989 December 7—Yale medical school researchers Dr. Kenneth B. Kashkin and Herbert B. Klebar announce the discovery of a new form of addiction related to taking anabolic steroids.[220]

1989 December 13—Dr. Claus Clausnitzer, head of East Germany's only drug testing laboratory, tells American reporters that since 1978, East Germany has pretested all athletes selected by officials to compete outside the country. Only three were ever caught at international or Olympic events.[221]

1989 December 13—Eleven nations (the United States, Soviet Union, Australia, Britain, Bulgaria, Czechoslovakia, Italy, Norway, South Korea, Sweden, and West Germany) sign an agreement to test one another's athletes at random. The accord will be supervised by the IOC and will begin on January 1, 1990.[222]

1990–1999

1990—In *From Moscow to Lausanne*, an IOC-endorsed anthology about the Olympic movement in the 1980s, Eric Walter is the author of a chapter entitled, "Doping: Ten Years of Relentless Struggle."[223]

1990—Charlie Francis tells his side of the Ben Johnson story in *Speed Trap: Inside the Biggest Scandal in Olympic History.*[224]

1990—James Wright and Virginia Cowart explore the social implications of drug use in *Anabolic Steroids: Altered States*.[225]

1990—Angela Issajenko, training partner of Ben Johnson, publishes *Running Risks*, her autobiography.[226]

1990 May 5—Edwin Moses, chairman, and three other members of TAC's drug testing committee resign in protest at TAC's unwillingness to take a firm stand on the drug issue.[227]

1990 June 18—Diane Modahl, British half-miler, is found positive for testosterone.[228]

1990 June 28—Jamie Astaphan, Ben Johnson's physician, is formally charged with professional misconduct by the Ontario College of Physicians and Surgeons. Astaphan faces loss of license and possible fines up to $10,000.[229]

1990 August—Butch Reynolds, world record holder in 400 meters, tests positive for anabolic steroid use at a track meet in Monte Carlo and is placed on two-year probation by the IAAF. In subsequent months, Reynolds sues the IAAF and wins a $27 million settlement. However, the IAAF appeals the decision to the 6th U.S. Circuit Court of Appeals. The court overturns the judgment, ruling against Reynolds. Although Reynolds and his attorneys subsequently request it, the U.S. Supreme Court refuses to hear his case.[230]

1990 September 7—The Department of Health and Human Services releases the results of their study on the incidence of steroid use among adolescents. The report estimates that 262,000 students in grades 7 through 12 have used, or currently use, steroids. This averages out to a 3 percent incidence rate among students in grades 7 to 12. More than half the users began using drugs by age 16.[231]

1990 September 11—At the close of the Women's Swimming Championships in Rome, coaches from Australia, Great Britain, Sweden, and Canada appear at a press conference to release a petition signed by officials from 18 countries and the World Swim Coaches Association asking FINA, the world governing body for swimming, to escalate the battle against doping in sport. Canadian coach Dave Johnson tells reporters that although the petition is not meant to single out any particular team, it is, nonetheless, inspired by the achievements of the Chinese team. "The parallels between the East Germans and the Chinese has left everyone with a fairly cynical attitude toward what they are seeing in the pool," Johnson said. U.S. swim coach, Richard Quick, calls the Chinese results "a sham," and adds that if FINA does not deliver on its promise to beef-up its random, out-of-season testing, he will recommend that the U.S. team not participate in next year's World Championships.

On the closing day of the world championships, China wins all three events and sets another world record. Through the course of the entire championships in Rome, Chinese swimmers win gold medals in 12 of 16 events, three bronze and silver medals, and set five world records.[232]

1990 October 5—An article on the front page of *Sport* (Moscow), written by a member of the anti-doping committee of the Soviet Olympic Committee, reveals the names of 38 Olympic athletes who tested positive for drugs. Sixteen were track-and-field competitors. The article does not say if any disciplinary action will be taken against the athletes.[233]

1990 October 28—Three-time Olympian Pat Connolly publishes an editorial in the *New York Times* calling for an end to drug testing. Connolly, a long-time proponent of drug testing, says she has changed her mind because "Drug testing is supposed to help provide for a level playing field, but because of clinical, legal and practical problems, it has actually made the field more tilted in favor of the cheaters." Connolly accuses the USOC of being more interested in its image and fundraising than in protecting either the health of its athletes or the ideal of fair play.[234]

1990 November 28—*Stern* magazine of Germany releases the names of many prominent East German athletes who participated in state-supported drug programs through the Sports Medical Service. The *Stern* report is based on materials from the laboratory in Kreischa, a small town south of Dresden where East Germany's only drug testing facility was located. Kreischa's lab was used for pre-event testing. Among those named in the *Stern* article are six-time gold medalist in swimming Kristin Otto; Ulf Timmermann, the men's shot put champion; Juergen Schult, the men's discus champion; and Christian Schenck, decathlete. Also named are track-and-field stars Heike Dreschler and Torsten Voss (shot put), and swimmers Heike Friedrich and Dagmar Hase.[235]

1991—*Doping-Dokumente* is published by Brigitte Berendonk in Germany. This book chronicles East Germany's comprehensive and official involvement in giving drugs to its Olympic athletes. Berendonk and her husband, Dr. Werner Francke, discovered the secret records of the East German doping doctors, which were hidden in a military facility.[236]

1991—R. Laura and S. White edit a volume of essays entitled *Drug Controversy in Sport: The Socio-ethical and Medical Issues.* Of particular interest is an article by D. Cowan entitled "Biochemical Aspects of Substances Banned by the IOC."[237]

1991—American physician William N. Taylor publishes *Macho Medicine: A History of the Anabolic Steroid Epidemic.*[238]

1991—Former USOC Director of Medical Research Robert Voy publishes *Drugs, Sports and Politics,* an insider's look at the USOC and Olympic drug testing programs.[239]

1991 June—In the *Journal of Sports Medicine and Physical Fitness,* the Olympic Council of Asia reports the results of the drug testing at the 1986 Asian Games. At those Games, 585 samples were collected and tested using the full array of IOC screens. Of these, 3.2 percent were found positive.[240]

1991 July 8—*Sports Illustrated* publishes an exclusive interview with football player Lyle Alzado, who is dying of lymphoma he believes was brought on by his use of steroids and human growth hormone.[241]

1991 October—TAC, the governing body for track and field in the United States, reviews Butch Reynolds' case and rules that he may compete domestically as long as no international athletes are present. The IAAF suspension of Reynolds stands.[242]

1992—The USOC begins testing athletes outside of competition. However, athletes are given 48 hours to report for testing.[243]

1992—Physician William N. Taylor publishes *Anabolic Steroids and the Athlete.*[244]

1992—British journalists Vyv Simson and Andrew Jennings publish *The Lords of the Rings,* a muckraking look at Juan Antonio Samaranch and the IOC Executive Committee.[245]

1992—University of Texas professor John Hoberman publishes *Mortal Engines: The Science of Performance and the Dehumanization of Sport.*[246]

1992—Just before the Albertville Winter Games began, CBS learns that Katrin Krabbe, a former East German sprinter who is the current world champion in the 100 meters, has just tested positive, along with two of her teammates, for substituting "clean" urine for her (and their) own (supposedly "unclean") urine. The story airs and touches off an explosion of media coverage in Europe, particularly in Germany. During the same games, CBS broadcasts a lengthy piece documenting the extent of the state-sponsored drug program in the German Democratic Republic. Another preproduced piece, very critical of the current drug testing procedures, is not aired. According to Alan Weisman, director of CBS's story unit, the decision not to air the piece was made by higher CBS officials who feared the Games would be tarnished by the revelations in the piece and that ratings

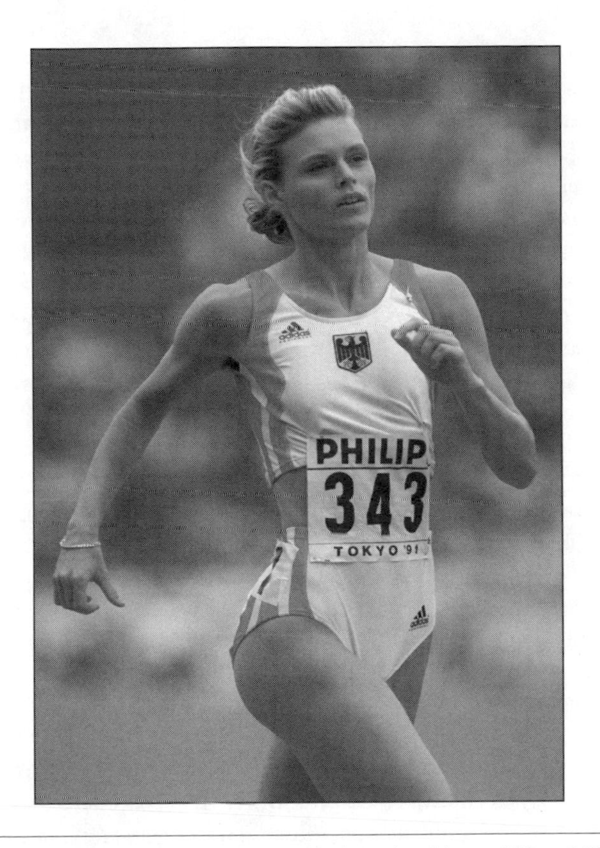

Katrin Krabbe of Germany won the 1991 world championships at 100 and 200 meters. The following year, the IAAF suspended Krabbe after determining that she and two teammates all had submitted the same urine sample for drug testing.
© Gray Mortimore/Allsport

might therefore suffer. *Sports Illustrated*'s report on the Krabbe case appears on March 9, 1992.[247]

1992—Just before the start of the Barcelona Olympic Games, three British athletes are sent home after being found positive for ergogenic aids. Sprinter Jason Livingston was found positive for anabolic steroids after a random test in Britain. Weightlifters Andrew Davies and Andrew Saxton received lifetime bans for having tested positive for clenbuterol in random tests held in June.[248]

1992 June—*Olympic Review* magazine announces that a laboratory in Lausanne, Switzerland, has been added to the list of IOC-approved laboratories.[249]

1993—The IAAF publishes a new guidebook for its athletes and coaches titled *Procedural Guidelines for Doping Control*.[250]

1993—IOC creates the International Council of Arbitration for Sport which replaces the IOC's Court of Arbitration for Sport. Designed to speed up drug appeals, the new council still has no athlete representatives. As Canadian drug testing expert Dr. Mauro Di Pasquale, puts it, "Imagine being tried for a criminal offense by the very people against which this offense was said to have been committed and after being found guilty, your appeals were heard by the same people."[251]

1993 September—Competing in Beijing at a track-and-field championship featuring China's amazing women's team, Wang Junxia turns in the most startling performance in history. In a six-day span, she sets four world records in three separate events—the 1,500 meters, the 3,000 meters, and the 10,000 meters. The world record in the 1,500 meters has stood for 13 years, and was the oldest record in women's track and field. In the 3,000 meters, she lowers the record twice, and runs 16 seconds faster than anyone ever has before. In the 10,000 meters, she trims 42 seconds from the previous record. Nor is she alone. In fact, in the 3,000 meters, five Chinese women break the world record in the preliminary heats. These performances trigger international coverage, much of it negative. Lynn Jennings, for example, the top 10,000-meter runner in the U.S., weeps when she hears the results. Track insiders maintain that the Chinese could not reach such performances without using drugs, whereas the official Chinese position is that they simply trained harder and used such natural substances as caterpillar fungus. There is also speculation that the top Chinese sporting officials have primed their athletes to break these records just a few days before the IOC will vote to determine the location of the 2000 Summer Olympic Games. The argument states that such performances will show potential voters what great athletes the Chinese can produce and thus influence a vote for China over Australia. However, since the IOC is sensitive to negative international press coverage, it is possible that the Chinese plan, if such a plan exists, backfires.[252]

1994 January—IOC publishes an article in its *Olympic Review* titled "Doping: The Historic Agreement," that explores the IOC's policies and presents its position statement.[253]

1994—Before the opening of the Lillehammer Olympic Winter Games, Prince de Merode, head of the IOC Medical Commission, is interviewed on tape by a CBS commentator, and says that he is worried because 60 percent of the athletes are using asthma medications. Another commentator then interviews Dr. Don Catlin, who states he is not sure about the numbers, but that he too is worried about this practice, which he refers to as "low-level doping." One CBS commentator, Terry Todd, then writes a memo to the head of his division urging that such an important story be given major attention and aired immediately. After three days during which no action is taken, Todd does a piece for National Public Radio about the asthma medication. This prompts CBS to cover the story. However, when he is formally interviewed, Dr. Catlin claims that the percentage of those using asthma medication is far less than 60 percent. Notwithstanding Catlin's claim, several members of the CBS "team" had interviewed de Merode's secretary earlier in the day and were told that the figure of 60 percent was indeed accurate.[254]

1994 June—M.H. Williams examines the ethical issues surrounding the use of ergogenic nutritional aids such as creatine in an essay for the *International Journal of Sport Nutrition.*[255]

1994 August—Dr. Don Catlin, head of the UCLA laboratory, tells *The Times* of London that a number of positive results were never reported from the 1984 Olympic Games. The London *Times* piece is prompted by a BBC television documentary that suggests that documents were actually shredded to hide these positives. The source for the BBC's information is Craig Kammerer, Catlin's associate in 1984 in the drug testing lab. According to Kammerer, five of the tests were for anabolic steroids; the others were for testosterone and ephedrine. Kammerer claims that the lab tested the first sample, sent the results to the IOC, and waited for the order to test the second sample. No order was ever received to run the second tests. According to Catlin, the nine positives came during the last two days of the Games when things were hectic. During the last two days, the men's shot put, women's discus, men's 1500, women's 100 meter hurdles, men's marathon, and the boxing finals were held. "We couldn't keep track of each case," Catlin tells the *Times*. "We were so busy. These other things going on didn't sink in until sometime afterwards." In 15 days of operation, the UCLA lab tested 1,502 athletes. Twelve positives were reported, including two medal winners.

According to the BBC report, Juan Antonio Samaranch, president of the IOC; Peter Ueberroth, president of the LAOOC; and Prince Alexandre de Merode, head of the IOC Medical Commission, discussed covering up the positives in a meeting. A fourth person present in the meeting said de Merode did not approve and would not agree to the plan. However, according to Arnold Beckett, a member of the IOC medical commission, before de Merode could follow normal procedures and notify the athletes and their coaches of the positive results, someone broke into his hotel room, stole the document that matched the names to the appropriate lab test numbers, and shredded it. "(de Merode) told us they had taken them and shredded it," says Beckett, (who subsequently was removed from the Commission because of a disagreement at the Barcelona Games). "There was no way to connect the documents with the person." Beckett explains to reporters that he did not speak out earlier because he thought it was best for the Olympic movement. "In retrospect it was a wrong decision. I (finally) broke rank with good intent," Beckett says. "Somebody has got to stop this madness."

Beckett also accuses Primo Nebiolo, head of the IAAF, with attempting to cover up a positive test result on a distance runner in 1984. According to Beckett, several of the other IAAF officials would not go along.[256]

1994 August—Prince Alexander de Merode, head of the IOC Medical Commission, tells reporters that the loss of the records for the nine 1984 drug tests was "an accident." De Merode, speaking in Paris at the IOC's Centennial Olympic Congress, explains that the LAOOC shredded the records in its haste to close operations. De Merode further claims that Dr. Tony Daly, who served as head medical officer for LAOOC, was responsible for the error. However, Daly tells reporters, "we didn't even have shredders. I don't know where he came up with that." Furthermore, according to Daly, the LAOOC did not have access to the sorts of records de Merode claims were destroyed by mistake. "They're his records," says Daly. De Merode "is the only one who gets it."[257]

1994 August 1—In Barcelona, the men's shot put finals are held. For the first time in Olympic history, all three medalists from a sport have formerly been banned from competition for drug use.[258]

1994 September 5—World Swimming Championships open in Rome. Chinese women swimmers raise eyebrows when two of them set world records in the 100-meter freestyle. The winner, LeJingyi, breaks the record by more than half a second. Before LeJingyi, it took athletes 12 years to lower the record by half a second. Chinese swimmers also win the 400-meter individual medley (with the fastest time of the year), and the 800-meter relay. According to the *Los Angeles Times*, "Some experts predict the Chinese will win half of the 16 women's events in the long course championships."[259]

1994 September 9—Dennis Pursley, U.S. Swimming's national team director, accuses the Chinese women swimmers of using performance-enhancing drugs. Pursley meets with a Chinese coach and tells him that he feels drug use explains the phenomenal rise of the Chinese swimmers. Says Pursley, "I have a great deal of respect for the Chinese athletes and their coaches but there is no question the circumstantial evidence is overwhelming that they have an added advantage through drugs."

Swimming officials from Australia, Canada, France, and Sweden ask FINA to establish tighter drug controls.[260]

1994 October 12—Two members of the IOC's drug testing program write opposing editorials for *USA Today*. Don Catlin, head of the Los Angeles laboratory that conducted the drug tests at the 1984 Olympic Games, argues in "Testing Succeeds in Keeping Sports, Athletes Clean" that the IOC's doping program is working. Dr. Arnold Beckett of Great Britain, however, takes the opposing view in, "Incompetent Labs, Unclear Policies Prove Dangerous."[261]

1994 November 16—It is announced that 400-meter freestyle swimming world champion Yang Aihua tested positive for testosterone in a random out-of-competition drug test one week before the Asian Games in Hiroshima. Her testosterone level is nearly three times the allowable limit. She is the fifth Chinese woman swimmer to test positive for a banned substance since 1992. Before the Asian Games end, 10 other Chinese athletes in four sports test positive.[262]

1994 December 19—*Sports Illustrated* calls attention to the high number of Chinese drug positives in a short piece entitled "Great Fall of China."[263]

1995—In an effort to help athletes, coaches, and the public understand the IOC's drug testing policies and its efforts in the war against drugs, the Olympic Committee publishes *Preventing and Fighting Against Doping in Sport.*[264]

1995—During the course of this year, the IAAF will hand down two lifetime bans and 33 four-year suspensions for athletes found positive on drug tests.[265]

1995 February—*Scientific American* focuses on the drug issue with an article by John Hoberman of the University of Texas at Austin and Charles Yesalis of Penn State University."[266]

1995 March—Fifteen-year-old Jessica Foschi is found positive for mesterolone after finishing third in the 1500-meter freestyle at the 1995 National Swimming Championships. U.S. Swimming penalizes her with a two-year probation.[267]

1995 September 4—Dr. Manfred Donike's obituary appears in *Sports Illustrated.* For many years Donike directed the IOC's drug testing program and was responsible for the development of the screening measures to test for exogenous testosterone. Donike died in Africa of heart failure.[268]

1995 October 30—*Sports Illustrated*'s "Scorecard" column explores the IOC's battle to develop a test for human growth hormone.[269]

1996—Andrew Jennings, British journalist and sport reformer, releases *The New Lords of the Rings,* a revised and updated examination of power and corruption in the Olympic movement. The new edition explores in depth the drug testing events surrounding the 1984 and 1988 Games.[270]

1996—T.M. Hoxha examines the legal issues surrounding doping and athletes' rights for *Entertainment and Sports Lawyer.*[271]

1996—IAAF releases a new edition of its *Procedural Guidelines for Doping Control.*[272]

1996—L. Bruunshuus, K. Klempel, D. Cowan, G. Hill, and H. Olesen publish a research article in the *Journal of Chromatography* on drug testing for IOC competitions.[273]

1996—*American Journal of Sports Medicine* publishes a special issue on doping and drug use. Included in that issue are discussions of the prevention of adolescent steroid use through school education programs, an analysis of the ethical implications of doping control, a report on blood doping and erythropoietin use, and an article on creatine use.[274]

1996 February—Jessica Foschi appeals her two-year suspension and demands a hearing with the American Arbitration Association.[275]

1996 April—USOC announces that it will no longer notify athletes ahead of time or give them 48 hours to report for an out-of-competition test.[276]

1996 April—An article in the *Washington Post* explains the drug testing protocol for Atlanta. Every U.S. Olympic athlete will be tested at his/her Olympic trials and at the Pan American Games if he/she competes. However, random, out-of-competition testing, the article explains, will only be done in the sports of weightlifting, cycling, swimming, volleyball, and bobsledding. Other sports do not do out-of-competition tests at this time.

In Atlanta, every medal winner and two members from each medal-winning team sport will be tested. Total cost for testing at the Atlanta Games is estimated at $2 million. That includes 600 people, running 1,800 tests, and the rental of the mass spectrometers and other necessary equipment.[277]

1996 July—British physician Michael Turner tells the BBC that "If you're talking about track and field, you're talking about a situation where the percentage may be 75 or above of Olympic athletes in Atlanta (who) will have taken some kind of performance-enhancing drug." Turner further charges that the drug testing in Atlanta was merely a "cosmetic arrangement." In a press conference, Prince de Merode laughs at Turner's charges, and reports that the IOC conducted 90,000 drug tests in the previous year. De Merode adds, "And another thing I find insufferable . . . is that always now instead of rejoicing when somebody does something extraordinary, pulls off a feat, you'd think people would say, 'Bravo, that's magnificent.'[Instead] . . . everyone points and says, 'Oh, what a cheat, it's not normal, he must have done something really bad to do that.' . . . I think people who say that are sad types, jealous people who wanted to do the same thing."[278]

1996 July—On the fourth day of the Atlanta Games, *Sports Illustrated* columnist Tim Layden laments the fact that mistrust and cynicism over the doping issue are ruining many people's appreciation of the Games. "Drugs, not just by their actual use but also by the possibility of their use, have become a sad, central Olympic theme," writes Layden. "And there remains a sense that the bad guys will always run slightly ahead of the posse, that the drug of choice will simply change and then move from the shot put to the 200-meter freestyle, finding the soft spots in sport and bureaucracy the way a virus finds victims." Perhaps, Layden suggests, "It might be best to simply do away with drug testing, letting the athletes take whatever strength-building, liver-destroying agents they choose."[279]

1996 November—Prince de Merode is interviewed in *Olympic* magazine. De Merode reasserts that the objective of IOC drug testing is to protect the health of athletes.[280]

1997—IOC Executive Board approves the adoption of a single medical code that will be proposed to the international federations. The hope is that sanctions can be applied uniformly across all sports. The IOC will begin implementing the new code at the Games in Sydney, Australia.[281]

1997 October 23—World Swimming Coaches Association chief executive John Leonard charges that FINA, the international governing body for swimming, is not doing what it should to solve the drug problem in swimming. "Eventually, if FINA cannot clean up our sport, the major swimming nations may decide to conduct their own drug testing program and isolate themselves into another form of competition where we can be sure the athletes are clean." Leonard's comments are triggered by the 10 world-record times set at the Chinese National Games in Shanghai when, only one year before at the Olympic Games, China won only one gold medal.[282]

1997 November 28—In the leadup to the 2000 Olympic Games, the Australian Olympic Committee increases the number of drug tests it regularly performs on its athletes. From 2,480 in 1991-1992, the number rises to 3,700 in 1997-1998. As a consequence, an increasing number of Australian athletes are found to be positive. In November, seven different athletes test positive in one month. AOC president John Coates says he has never experienced such a spate of positives at one time but that it is better to "flush out the cheats now rather than suffer the embarrassment of doping scandals in the Olympic Games."[283]

1997 December—A Penn State study, directed by Charles Yesalis, finds that 175,000 high-school women have used steroids in the United States. This represents 2.4 percent of that population.[284]

1998 January 9—With the World Swimming Championships set to begin in Australia, Sydney reporter Jacquelin Magnay examines the high number of drug positives among Chinese women swimmers in a thought-provoking article for the

Sydney Morning Herald. Since 1991, Magnay reports, 23 Chinese swimmers have tested positive.[285]

1998 January 10—Olympic champion swimmer Michelle Smith De Bruin, takes an out-of-competition drug test at her home in Ireland. On April 30 she is informed by FINA that her test is positive.[286]

1998 January—One of the Chinese women swimmers entering Australia for the 1998 World Championships is found to have 13 vials of human growth hormone in her luggage. The swimmer is sent home and banned for four years by FINA. Her coach receives a 15-year ban.[287]

1998 January 23—Prince de Merode announces that the drug testing labs for the 1998 Winter Olympic Games in Nagano will use carbon-isotope machines designed to detect the presence of artificially-administered testosterone. This is the first time these machines will be used at any Olympic games. Drug testers plan to test approximately 800 competitors, including all medal winners.[288]

1998 February 2—IOC president Juan Antonio Samaranch speaks out against U.S. professional sports teams that, according to him, are undermining the anti-doping effort internationally. IOC vice president Anita DeFrantz concurs, noting in an interview, "There are many professional sports organizations in the U.S. that do a tip of the hat and a wink of the eye to drug testing. We wonder how serious the leagues are. I have never heard of a professional athlete banned for steroids. Never."[289]

1998 February 5—The use of ephedrine to increase energy comes under scrutiny following a *Sports Illustrated* report suggesting that 20 percent of NHL players routinely use sudafed, an over-the-counter cold medication that, when taken in sufficient dosages, contains enough ephedrine to act as a stimulant.[290]

1998 February 14—At the Nagano Olympic Games, IOC president Juan Antonio Samaranch defends IOC's new drug test for marijuana use, claiming that marijuana use is an ethical issue and that athletes must be role models. Canadian snowboarder Russ Rebagliati becomes the first Olympian to lose a gold medal for a positive marijuana test. His gold medal in snowboarding is returned, however, when an arbitration panel rules that the IOC failed to follow proper procedures.[291]

1998 March—Sri Lankan sprinter Susanthika Jayasinghe tests positive for nandralone in a random test conducted by the IAAF. The silver medalist in the 1997 IAAF world championships, Jayasinghe denies taking drugs and charges that a conspiracy has been organized against her. Jayasinghe was the first Sri Lankan in 49 years to win a medal at an international competition.[292]

1998 March 18—In Berlin, six former East German sports officials go on trial for administering steroids to teenage female swimmers without their knowledge. The four coaches and two physicians administered the drugs as part of a state-supported program designed to make East Germany into a sports superpower. This trial is the result of several years of investigations that followed the fall of the Berlin Wall and the reunification of Germany.[293]

1998 July 28—American shot putter Randy Barnes and sprinter Dennis Mitchell receive notice from the IAAF that they are suspended from competition because of

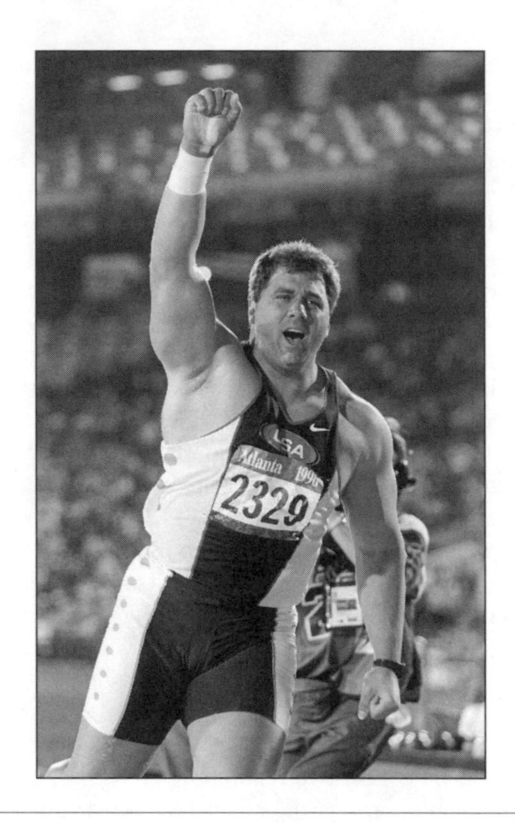

American shot putter Randy Barnes winning the gold medal at the 1996 Atlanta Olympic Games. Barnes missed the 1992 Olympic Games because of a drug suspension. In 1998, the IAAF announced that Barnes had tested positive for androstenedione. Barnes appealed the finding.

positive drug tests administered on April 1, 1998. Barnes is the 1996 Olympic champion and the indoor and outdoor world record holder. Mitchell won the bronze in the 100 meters in the 1992 Games.[294]

1998 Summer—The Festina cycling team is expelled from the Tour de France after it is discovered that their masseur's car contains a supply of EPO, a drug used to enhance cardiovascular efficiency. As the investigations deepens, evidence of widespread doping in the sport of cycling emerges in the press. The ensuing scandal rocks the European sporting community and helps to propel the movement for doping reform in both the cycling community and the IOC. Juan Antonio Samaranch, president of the IOC, adds a new dimension to the scandal when he tells a Spanish newspaper, "The ones to blame are not the athletes but those around them." Samaranch goes on to suggest that perhaps it is time for the IOC to consider removing some of the drugs on its list of banned substances. These statements, seen as a softening of the IOC position on doping, set off demands for Samaranch's resignation. In the ensuing furor, Samaranch retreats and the IOC decides to hold the World Conference on Doping in Sport.[295]

1998 August 18—Prince de Merode, head of the IOC Medical Commission, denounces the views expressed by Juan Antonio Samaranch in the wake of the Tour de France doping scandal.[296]

1998 October 21—USOC Executive Committee asks for "appropriate medal recognition" for the members of the 400-meter medley relay team who placed second in the 1976 Olympic Games. Based on evidence released during the trial of the East German coaches, at least one member of the gold-medal-winning East German team was on steroids at the time of the 1976 Games. Jacques Rogge, IOC Executive Board member, reiterates that the IOC will not retroactively overturn medal decisions because of the new information coming out of East Germany: "We know of course that there was a doping problem in some countries, but at this stage we still have no documented evidence of doping of an athlete on the day of Olympic competitions. You cannot condemn someone because there was a general problem. Not all of them have taken drugs."[297]

1998 October 29—In an attempt to slow the use of the blood booster erythropoietin, the Italian government asks manufacturers to take erithropoetine 4CH—whose active ingredient is erythropoietin—off the shelves. This decision is reached following testimony in an Italian government inquiry into the use of performance-enhancing drugs by athletes. In the inquiry, led by judge Raffaele Guariniello, several athletes testify that they and many others were using a "speedball" made of human growth hormone combined with EPO in the belief that it made growth hormone undetectable in doping tests.[298]

1998 November 28—In Lausanne, representatives of all IOC sports except for soccer, tennis, and cycling agree to adopt a unified drug testing code. The new code calls for a two-year suspension for a first offense and a lifetime ban for a second offense.[299] Such a ban, in the opinion of many people in these three professional sports would be too costly for their athletes and would discourage participation.

1998 December—The International Tennis Federation announces that Petr Korda, winner of the 1998 Australian Open, has tested positive for nandralone at the 1998 Wimbledon Championships. Instead of banning him in accordance with their guidelines, however, the ITF fines him his Wimbledon prize money—$150,000 and his computer ranking points.[300]

1998 December 26—Jere Longman of the *New York Times* explores the growing complexity of the doping scandal in the IOC and its cultural impact in a lengthy special report titled: "Unbelievable Performances: A Special Report—Widening Drug Use Compromises Faith in Sport."[301]

1999 January 10—John Hoberman analyzes the IOC's attempts to quiet criticism of its drug testing program in: "Offering the Illusion of Reform on Drugs," for the *New York Times*.[302]

1999 February 5—Irish swimmer and gold medalist in the 1996 Olympic Games Michelle Smith de Bruin appears before the Council for Arbitration in Sport to appeal FINA's decision to ban her following a positive result during an out-of-competition drug test on 10 January 1998. This will be her second appeal. In July of 1998 she appeared before FINA's doping panel, which denied her appeal and placed her on a four-year probation. The Council rules on June 7, 1999 to uphold FINA's ban.[303]

1999 February 12—IOC vice president Dick Pound denounces baseball star Mark McGwire for his use of androstenedione. "If that had happened at the Olympic Games, there would have been a huge uproar. But in professional sports it doesn't seem to have mattered at all."[304]

1999 February—Mary Decker Slaney appeals her 1996 drug-positive test, which was kept quiet so that she could participate in both the Atlanta Olympic Games and the 1997 World Indoor Championships. Slaney was positive because her testosterone level was too high. USA Track and Field backs Slaney in her quest for reinstatement.[305]

1999 February 3-5—The IOC hosts The World Conference on Doping in Sport in Lausanne, Switzerland. According to the *New York Times*, after three days of debate, "the International Olympic Committee adopted a watered-down declaration on doping that only underscored its eroded authority."[306]

The full text of the "Lausanne Declaration on Doping in Sport" is made available on the IOC's Web site. In summary, it mandates (1) that coaches and other officials will also have to swear the Olympic oath, (2) that educational campaigns will be undertaken to discourage drug use, (3) that the minimum sanction for the use of "major doping substances" or prohibited methods shall be a suspension of two years, (4) that an anti-doping agency shall be in operation by the Sydney Games in 2000 whose mission will be to expand out-of-competition testing, coordinate research, and so on, (5) that the IOC, international federations, and national organizing committees will continue to apply their own doping rules and will maintain authority over the decisions made by the drug testing representatives of their respective organizations, and (6) that arbitration for appeals will continue to be heard by the Court of Arbitration for Sport.[307]

1999 March 13—Prince de Merode, head of the IOC Medical Commission, announces that the IOC will not test for human growth hormone at the Sydney Olympic Games in 2000.[308]

1999 June—*The New York Times* carries a report by Holcomb B. Noble examining the growing use of anabolic steroids and other lipolytic (fat-burning) drugs by teenage girls. According to the article, not all the young women using the drugs do so to enhance athletic performance. Some use the drugs merely to improve their appearance.[309]

1999 October—The U.S. Senate Commerce Committee, chaired by Senator John McCain, begins hearings on how to solve the problem of drug abuse by American athletes. Among those critical of the current policies of the IOC and USOC who testify before the committee are the director of the White House Office of Drug Control Barry McCaffrey and Olympians Frank Shorter, Carl Lewis, and Nancy Hogshead. Shorter testifies, "The IOC has to give up control (of the drug agency) for a myriad of reasons." McCaffrey opposed the IOC's decision at the

February 1999 doping summit to create an internal drug testing unit, and believes that without both independence and governmental support, the likelihood that real reforms can be made regarding the drug issue is low. The IOC is building an institution that is more "public relations ploy than public policy solution," says McCaffrey.[310]

1999 October 24—The USOC, by a vote of 113–0 approves the creation of an independent agency to oversee the testing of American athletes who will participate in the Olympic and Pan American Games.[311]

The View at the Millennium

Olympic sport and the wider world beyond have come to a historic moment—a time in which it is natural to look back and assess the change wrought by the passage of time. Anyone who studies the matter of drug testing for ergogenic substances can see that although there has been a dramatic increase in drug testing during the years covered by this timeline, there has been an even more dramatic increase in the use of ergogenic drugs by athletes who compete in the Olympic sports. This ironic turn of events is a result of several factors: (1) the burgeoning array of ergogenic substances; (2) the concerted efforts of scientists, coaches, and even countries who are less concerned with ethics than with victory; (3) the changeless desire of athletes to improve their performances; and (4) the lack of commitment by sports officials to use all of their resources to fight free of the dread sway of drugs.

Currently, drug-free athletes and scientists who support them often despair when drug-using athletes go undetected because of inadequate testing or the legal vulnerability of the tests themselves. Tests for testosterone are particularly subject to attack, as is the test for nandralone. As of this publication, two potent substances—human growth hormone (HGH) and erythropoeitin (EPO)—remain beyond either the IOC's testing capabilities or their political will. What's more, even the drugs against which testing is sometimes effective can be taken with impunity by athletes willing to subject themselves to such grisly practices as inserting a bag of clean urine into the vagina or intubated anus in order to deceive the watchful eyes of the doping control officers.

This is not to say that the guilty always go unpunished. We have seen more than 30 Chinese swimmers test positive since they began their recent, brutal assault on both the record books and the equanimity of swimming officials around the world. Sometimes, even the most celebrated of athletes is caught. But for every Ben Johnson there are apparently hundreds of men and women who have medals and records they would not have—had they not taken one or more of the hundreds of banned substances—had they not cheated. And it must be admitted that even though the IOC can be justly criticized for its many errors of commission and omission in the area of drug testing, it has done far more than most sporting organizations. Juan Antonio Samaranch, for example, has the right to point to big-time professional sports in the United States and note that their testing programs are far more inadequate.

Often, it seems to outsiders that the rules in Olympic sports are so rigid and unreasonable that simple over-the-counter medications and even coffee must be avoided, the latter because of the ban on caffeine. But thoughtful athletes understand that a significant amphetamine-like boost can be had from such popular products as sudafed or Vivarin tablets. They also know that to test positive for the caffeine in coffee or soft drinks it would be necessary for a person of normal size to consume ten cups of strong coffee in two hours or to drink approximately 20 cans of cola.

One of the most intractable problems in Olympic sport is the growing influence of EPO, a substance that provides advantages to endurance athletes roughly comparable to the advantages conferred to power athletes by anabolic steroids. By increasing the amount of red blood cells in the bodies of endurance athletes, it provides a truly unfair advantage to those who use it. And the scandal surrounding the 1998 Tour de France makes clear how prevalent EPO has become in certain sports.

Many thoughtful observers believe that problems surrounding the use of EPO, human growth hormone, and anabolic steroids can only be attacked by an autonomous and international agency beyond the political reach of any sporting organization, even the IOC—perhaps especially the IOC. Steps have already been taken by the IOC to institute an international anti-doping agency in the 21st century, but their plan would keep them at the head of the organizational chart. In the 30 years of IOC drug testing, only 52 athletes have tested positive out of the tens of thousands of Olympians who competed during this period. This figure—in the face of informed speculation that as many as 50 percent of the men and women who compete in the Olympic Games have taken some sort of banned substance to assist them in training, competition, or both—makes it clear that something drastic must be done.

There are, to be sure, reasons to be hopeful. A new test for testosterone, which can supposedly distinguish naturally occurring testosterone from synthetic testosterone, could close one of sport's largest loopholes. In order to effectively combat the use of EPO, it will be necessary to do blood testing instead of urinalysis, but researchers now believe that they can identify markers in the blood that would allow them to return a "positive" able to withstand the severest legal challenge. Apparently, the human growth hormone loophole could also be closed by a blood test, as several groups of scientists have discovered a procedure that should allow them to identify blood profiles of those who have used exogenous human growth hormone.

Such tests cost money, of course, and they have a political cost as well. Some who follow Olympic sport have already given up on drug testing and argue that the tests should be stopped, since all they really do is to give the appearance of keeping sports clean. Most people who love sporting competition, however, realize that if testing is abolished, athletes will take even more risks with their health than they do now and the playing field will be even less level. Such people ask us to look at the world of elite bodybuilding for an object lesson in what would happen if no meaningful testing were to be done in Olympic sports and if athletes could take anything they wanted to take. It is not a pretty sight.

Further Suggestions

The IOC Web site (**www.olympic.org**) contains a wealth of material on the doping movement, including comprehensive lists of the number of tests done at various Games, information from the Medical Commission, and weekly news bulletins.

Acknowledgments

The authors would like to thank Dr. Wayne Wilson and his excellent staff at the Amateur Athletic Foundation's Paul Ziffren Sport Resource Center for their assistance (and patience) in the completion of this project. We would also like to thank journalist Jim Ferstle for the hundreds of articles he forwarded to us via the internet over the past year. Finally, we would like to thank our University of Texas undergraduate research assistants, Billy Corbin, Matt Harding, and Sarang Desai.

Notes

[1]For information on the early years of the IOC and its medical efforts, see Alan J. Ryan, MD, "A Medical History of the Olympic Games," *Journal of the American Medical Association* 205:715–720.

[2]Wolf Lyberg, *The IOC Sessions: 1956–1988, Volume 2—A Study Made by Wolf Lyberg, Former Secretary General of the NOC of Sweden* (By the author, n.d.), 46. On deposit at Paul Ziffren Sport Resource Center, Amateur Athletic Foundation of Los Angeles.

[3]Terry Todd, "A History of the Use of Anabolic Steroids in Sport," *Sport and Exercise Science: Essays in the History of Sports Medicine* Jack Berryman and Roberta J. Park, eds. (Urbana: University of Illinois Press, 1992), 326–327.

[4]David Wallechinsky, *The Complete Book of the Olympics* (Boston: Little, Brown & Company, 1992 ed.), 258.

[5]Wolf Lyberg, *Fabulous 100 Years of the IOC: Facts—Figures—and Much, Much More.* (By the author, 1996), 375. On deposit at Paul Ziffren Sport Resource Center, Amateur Athletic Foundation of Los Angeles.

[6]"The IOC Medical Commission and the Fight Against Doping," International Olympic Committee Web site, located at: **www.olympic.org/family/ioc/medical/dope_e.html**.

[7]"The Anti-Doping Battle Is Making Good Progress," *Bulletin Du Comite International Olympique, No. 82.* (Lausanne: 15 May 1963). See also: "Doping: Comite International Olympique et presse," *Bulletin Du Comite International Olympique, No. 84* (Lausanne: 15 November 1963).

[8]Wolf Lyberg, *The IOC Sessions: 1956–1988, Volume 2—A Study Made by Wolf Lyberg, Former Secretary General of the NOC of Sweden,* (By the author, N.D.), 99–100. On deposit at Paul Ziffren Sport Resource Center, Amateur Athletic Foundation of Los Angeles.

[9]A.H. Beckett and D.A. Cowan, "Misuse of Drugs in Sport," *British Journal of Sports Medicine* 12 (1979):185.

[10]"Excerpts from the Minutes of the 64th Session of the IOC," *Comite International Olympique, Bulletin 95*, (Lausanne: 15 August 1966), 91–92. See also: "Report Committee on Doping, Sir Arthur Porritt, 3rd March 1966," Annex #15, contained in Reel 45, Box 82 Avery Brundage Collection, Paul Ziffren Sport Resource Center, Amateur Athletic Foundation of Los Angeles.

[11]"Olympic Trackmen Face Drug Tests," *New York Times*, 6 September 1966.

[12]A.H. Beckett and D.A. Cowan, "Misuse of Drugs in Sport," *British Journal of Sports Medicine* 12 (1979):185.

[13]"Olympic Athletes Required to Take Medical Tests," *New York Times,* 9 May 1967.

[14]Bob Goldman, *Death in the Locker Room* (South Bend: Icarus Press, 1984), 27–28.

[15]"Report of the Medical Commission," *Minutes of the 67th Session of the International Olympic Committee, Mexico: October 7th–11th, 1968,* (Lausanne: IOC, 1968), 12–13, A–11. See also: "General Report Presented by Dr. Eduardo Hay, Member of the Medical Commission of the International Olympic Committee, October 1968," in Reel 54, Box 99, Avery Brundage Collection, Paul Ziffren Sport Resource Center, Amateur Athletic Foundation of Los Angeles.

[16]Howard A. Rusk, "Olympic Game Health: Mexico City Events to Be Watched by Scientists for Many Unusual Aspects," *New York Times,* 13 October 1968. For the full breakdown on the kinds of amphetamines tested for in 1968, see: "Report of the Medical Commission Meeting Held on October 1st, at 11:00 A.M." in Reel 54, Box 99, Avery Brundage Collection, Paul Ziffren Sport Resource Center, Amateur Athletic Foundation of Los Angeles. The Brundage Collection contains three other useful documents related to the 1968 doping protocol: "Report Submitted by the Medical Commission to the General Session of the International Olympic Committee," "Communique for the Delegations—Doping," and "Medical Commission of the International Olympic Committee, Reports: Grenoble and Mexico." All three are in Reel 54, Box 99, Avery Brundage Collection, Paul Ziffren Sport Resource Center, Amateur Athletic Foundation of Los Angeles.

[17]Quoted in Bil Gilbert, "Drugs in Sport: Problems in a Turned On World," *Sports Illustrated* (23 June 1969):66.

[18]Terry Todd, "A History of the Use of Anabolic Steroids in Sport," *Sport and Exercise Science: Essays in the History of Sports Medicine.* Jack Berryman and Roberta J. Park, eds. (Urbana: University of Illinois Press, 1992), 327.

[19]Quoted in Bil Gilbert, "Drugs in Sport: Problems in a Turned On World," *Sports Illustrated* (23 June 1969):66.

[20]Quoted in Bil Gilbert, "Drugs in Sport: Problems in a Turned On World," *Sports Illustrated* (23 June 1969):66.

[21]*British Journal of Sports Medicine* 4 (1969).

[22]Quoted in Bil Gilbert, "Drugs in Sport: Problems in a Turned On World," *Sports Illustrated* (23 June 1969):66.

[23]*Minutes of the Medical Commission of the International Olympic Committee, Lausanne, 25th and 26th January, 1969,* (Lausanne, IOC, 1969):4–5.

[24]Bil Gilbert, "Drugs in Sport: Problems in a Turned On World," *Sports Illustrated* (23 June 1969); Bil Gilbert, "Drugs in Sport: Something Extra on the Ball," *Sports Illustrated* (30 June 1969); and Bil Gilbert, "Drugs in Sport: High Time to Make Some Rules," *Sports Illustrated* (7 July 1969); and "Letter from the Publisher," *Sports Illustrated* (23 June 1969):4.

[25]"Letter from Prince de Merode to General Thofelt, President of the Union Internationale de Pentathlon Moderne, 6th March 1969," *Minutes of the 68th Session of the International Olympic Committee, Warsaw, June 6th–10th, 1969* (Lausanne: IOC, 1969): Annex 22. Further details on the adoption of the alcohol test for the modern pentathlon can be found in the Avery Brundage Papers, folder "SP-Medical Commission IOC, 1966-1969." Brundage papers are available in microform at the Paul Ziffren Sport Resource Center, Amateur Athletic Foundation of Los Angeles, Los Angeles, CA.

[26]Terry Todd, "Anabolic Steroids: The Gremlins of Sport," *Journal of Sport History* 14 (Spring 1987):87–107.

[27]"For Athletes Drug Testing Is an Easy Opponent," *Los Angeles Times,* 19 January 1984.

[28]Terry Todd, "Anabolic Steroids: The Gremlins of Sport," *Journal of Sport History* 14 (Spring 1987):87–107.

[29]Michael Janofsky, "Johnson Loses Gold to Lewis after Drug Test," *New York Times,* 22 November 1988.

[30]"Medical Committee Report," *Minutes of the 73rd Session of the International Olympic Committee, Munich, 21–24 August and 5 September, 1972* (Lausanne: IOC, 1972), 31–32.

[31]"People in Sports: New Rx Is No Cure at All," *New York Times,* 6 January 1973.

[32]James E. Wright, *Anabolic Steroids and Sports* (Natick, MA: Sports Science Consultants, 1982), 33; and Terry Todd, "A History of the Use of Anabolic Steroids in Sport," *Sport and Exercise Science: Essays in the History of Sports Medicine,* Jack Berryman and Roberta J. Park, eds. (Urbana: University of Illinois Press, 1992), 328.

[33]Terry Todd, "The Steroid Predicament," *Sports Illustrated* (1 August 1983), 62.

[34]"A Court Case: DeMont Loses, Too," *New York Times* 9 February 1973.

[35]*New York Times*, 25 February 1973.

[36]See "1976 Olympians to Get Steroid Tests" *New York Times*, 7 May 1974; and Allan J. Ryan, "Anabolic Steroids Are Fool's Gold," Symposium presented by the American Society for Pharmacology and Experimental Therapeutics at the 64th Annual Meeting of the Federation of American Societies for Experimental Biology, Anaheim, CA, 15 April 1980. Published in *Federation Proceedings* 40 (October 1981):2685.

[37]"Annex 9: Report from the Medical Commission," *Minutes of the 74th Session of the International Olympic Committee, Varna, 5th, 6th, 7th October 1973* (Lausanne: IOC, 1973):23.

[38]David P. Webster, *The Truth About Drugs* (By the author, 1974).

[39]*New York Times*, 25 February 1973.

[40]See "1976 Olympians to Get Steroid Tests" *New York Times*, 7 May 1974 and "Medical Report," *Minutes of the 75th Session of the International Olympic Committee, Vienna, 21st–24th October 1974* (Lausanne: IOC, 1974):19–20, 44.

[41]"Medical Report," *Minutes of the 75th Session of the International Olympic Committee, Vienna, 21st–24th October 1974* (Lausanne: IOC, 1974):19–20, 44.

[42]Ryan, "Anabolic Steroids Are Fool's Gold," 2685–2686.

[43]"Drug Testers Stiffen Olympic Procedures," *New York Times,* 7 December 1979.

[44]"Effect of Drugs to Aid Athletes Studied by U.S." *New York Times*, 22 August 1976.

[45]*Minutes of the 77th Session of the International Olympic Committee, Innsbruck, 2nd–3rd February 1976* (Lausanne: IOC, 1976), 2, 21.

[46]"Annex 12: Report of the Medical Commission Presented by Prince De Merode," *Minutes of the 76th Session of the International Olympic Committee, Lausanne, 21st–23rd May 1975* (Lausanne: IOC, 1976), 17–18, 49-51.

[47]*New York Times*, 2 August 1976.

[48]"The Blood Scandal," *New York Times*, 1 August 1976.

[49]"Mounting Drug Use Afflicts World Sports," *New York Times*, 20 November 1978.

[50]"Drug Test Positive, Romanian Ousted," *New York Times*, 26 July 1976.

[51]"Steroids: 3 Are Banned," *New York Times*, 31 July 1976. See also "Effects of Drugs to Aid Athletes Studied by U.S," *New York Times*, 22 August 1976 and "Wider Olympic Drug Abuse Is Seen," *New York Times*, 30 January 1977.

[52]Jerry Kirshenbaum, "Steroids: The Growing Menace," *Sports Illustrated* (12 November 1979):33.

[53]"Effect of Drugs to Aid Athletes Studied by U.S.," *New York Times*, 22 August 1976.

[54]"IOC Lifts Some Bans, Not on Steroids," *Physician and Sportsmedicine* 4 (September 1976):20.

[55]"New 'Breakfast of Champions': A Recipe for Victory or Disaster?" *New York Times,* 20 November 1988.

[56]"New 'Breakfast of Champions': A Recipe for Victory or Disaster?" *New York Times,* 20 November 1988.

[57]Neil Amdur, "Wider Olympic Drug Abuse Is Seen," *New York Times,* 30 January 1977.

[58]"West Germans Approve Ban on Steroids for Olympic Athletes," *New York Times*, 12 June 1977.

[59]"Report of the Medical Commission Presented by Prince Alexandre de Merode," *Minutes of the 78th Session of the International Olympic Committee, Prague, 15th–18th June 1977,* (Lausanne: IOC, 1977): Annex 43.

[60]"Five European Athletes Banned for Using Steroids," *New York Times*, 9 November 1977.

[61]"Five European Athletes Banned for Using Steroids," *New York Times*, 9 November 1977.

[62]"Mounting Drug Use Afflicts World Sports," *New York Times*, 20 November 1978.
[63]James E. Wright, *Anabolic Steroids and Sports: A Comprehensive, Up-to-Date Summary and Discussion of the Scientific Findings about the Controversial Drugs Widely Used to Increase Muscle Size and Strength* (Natick, MA: Sport Science Consultants, 1978).
[64]"Mounting Drug Use Afflicts World Sports," *New York Times*, 20 November 1978.
[65]"Mounting Drug Use Afflicts World Sports," *New York Times*, 20 November 1978.
[66]"Mounting Drug Use Afflicts World Sports," *New York Times*, 20 November 1978.
[67]Jerry Kirshenbaum, "Steroids: The Growing Menace," *Sports Illustrated* (12 November 1979):33.
[68]John Vinocur, "East German Tale of Tyranny," *New York Times*, 11 January 1979.
[69]A.H. Becket and D.A. Cowan, "Misuse of Drugs in Sport," *British Journal of Sports Medicine* 12 (January 1979):185–194.
[70]Jerry Kirshenbaum, "Steroids: The Growing Menace," *Sports Illustrated* (12 November 1979).
[71]Steve Cady, "Drug Testers Stiffen Olympic Procedures," *New York Times*, 7 December 1979.
[72]Transcript of interview with Dr. Manfred Donike, 6 February 1982. On file at the Todd-McLean Physical Culture Collection, The University of Texas at Austin.
[73]"Easy Opponent," *Los Angeles Times*, 15.
[74]"Mounting Drug Use Afflicts World Sports," *New York Times*, 20 November 1978.
[75]"Medical," *Minutes of the 82nd IOC Session, Lake Placid, 10th–13th February 1980* (Lausanne: IOC, 1980):24.
[76]L. Barnes, "Olympic Drug Testing: Improvements Without Progress," *Physician and Sportsmedicine* 8 (June 1980):21–24.
[77]"Steroid Bust: Plunknett Loses His Record," *Time* (24 January 1981):66.
[78]"Coe Assails Drugs," *New York Times*, 29 September 1981.
[79]Robert Kerr, *The Practical Use of Anabolic Steroids With Athletes* (San Gabriel, CA: by the author, 1982), 2.
[80]Frederick C. Hatfield, *Anabolic Steroids: What Kind and How Many* (Madison, WI: Fitness Systems, 1982), 3.
[81]Ann Japenga, "Guidebook to Steroid Use Is Called Deceptive and Offensive," *Los Angeles Times*, 31 January 1984, sect. 3, p. 8.
[82]P. Hage, "Caffeine, Testosterone Banned for Olympians," *Physician and Sportsmedicine* 10 (July 1982):15–17.
[83]Robert Pariente, *The Samaranch Years: 1980–1994 Towards Olympic Unity* (1995), 23–24.
[84]"Drug Testing at Issue," *New York Times*, 29 April 1984.
[85]"An Interview With Robert Kerr, MD; The Human Growth Hormone: Is it a Bane or a Blessing, A Prescription for Health or a Portent of Disaster?" *Flex* (June 1983):28–30, 76–77.
[86]Terry Todd, "The Steroid Predicament," *Sports Illustrated* 59 (1 August 1983):62–77.
[87]"Drug Crackdown Prompts U.S. Athletes to Walk Out," *Atlanta Journal*, 23 August 1983. Frank Litsky, "The Other Game: Testing for Drugs," *New York*

Times, 24 July 1984. See also Terry Todd, "Anabolic Steroids: The Gremlins of Sport," *Journal of Sport History* 14 (Spring 1987); and "CBS' Newsmen Dig, Break Story on USA Athletes Leaving Games," *USA Today,* 24 August 1983; and "Cuban Fencer and Dominican Cited for Drug Use," *New York Times*, 27 August 1983.

[88]Frank Litsky, "U.S. Orders Athlete's Drug Tests," *New York Times*, 25 August 1983, B11. See also "Cuban Fencer and Dominican Cited for Drug Use," *New York Times*, 27 August 1983.

[89]Michael Goodwin, "USOC to Seek More Tests for Drugs, *New York Times*, 24 July 1984. See also "U.S. Olympic Group to Weigh Drug Test Plan: 86 American Athletes Failed 1984 Screening," *Chronicle of Higher Education,* 23 (January 1985):3.

[90]Neil Amdur, "Some on U.S. Squad at Caracas Failed Drug Tests Before Games," *New York Times*, 26 August 1983, 1.

[91]Elliott Almond, Julie Cart, and Randy Harvey, "If Athletes Want to Cheat to Get to Olympics . . . There's a Doctor to Help," *Los Angeles Times*, 4 December 1983, sect. 1, 18-20.

[92]Mauro Di Pasquale, *Drug Use and Detection in Amateur Sports* (Warkworth, Ontario: MGD Press, 1984).

[93]Mauro Di Pasquale, *Drug Use and Detection in Amateur Sports: Update Number One* (Warkworth, Ontario: MGD Press, 1986).

[94]S. Chinery, *In Quest of Size* (Toms River, NJ: L&S Research, 1984).

[95]Bob Goldman, Patricia J. Bush, and Ronald Klatz, *Death in the Locker Room* (South Bend: Icarus Press, 1984), 27-28.

[96]Michael Janofsky, "Medical Chief Sees Drug-Free Games," New York Times, 5 February 1984.

[97]Harold Connolly, "Fair Play Through Drug Tests," *Muscle and Fitness* 45 (February 1984):90, 195-196, 199.

[98]"Weightlifter Files Suit," *New York Times*, 21 May 1984.

[99]"Lifter Seeks End to Penalty," *New York Times*, 19 May 1984; and "Weightlifter Files Suit," *New York Times*, 10 May 1984.

[100]"Michaels's Appeal Rejected," *New York Times*, 21 May 1984.

[101]Julie Cart and Randy Harvey, "U.S. Athletes Told How to Take Drug Tests," *Des Moines Sunday Register* 1 July 1984, D1, D3. Anthony Fitton, *Drug Testing . . . So What!! How to Beat the Test* (By the author, n.d.).

[102]Kay Cahill, "Olympic Adviser Linked to Steroid Sale," *Austin American Statesman*, 13 July 1984.

[103]"Michaels Is Named to Olympic Team," *New York Times*, 15 July 1984.

[104]"Michaels Is Named to Olympic Team," *New York Times*, 15 July 1984.

[105]"A California Sports Doctor Defends the Controlled Use of a Fad Drug by Olympic Athletes," *People* (16 July 1984):53-55.

[106] "Cyclist Called Drug Use Error," *New York Times*, 21 July 1984; and "Drug Suspension of Cyclist Is Lifted," *New York Times*, 24 July 1984.

[107]"Drug Suspension of Cyclist Is Lifted," *New York Times*, 24 July 1984.

[108]Frank Litsky, "The Other Game: Testing for Drugs," *New York Times*, 24 July 1984.

[109]"Canadians Ban Two for Drugs," *New York Times*, 30 July 1984.

[110]Allan J. Ryan, "Drug Problem Building Since 1952 Olympics," *Physician and Sportsmedicine* 12 (July 1984):119-121, 124.

[111]"IOC Bans Masseur," *New York Times*, 3 August 1984.

[112]"Drugs Used," *New York Times*, 6 August 1984.

[113]"Swede Loses Silver for Using Steroids," *New York Times*, 6 August 1984.

[114]"Steroid Use Laid to Some Medalists," *New York Times*, 8 September 1984.

[115]Terry Todd, "Sports Rx: The Use of Human Growth Hormone Poses a Grave Dilemma for Sport," *Sports Illustrated* (15 October 1984):6 passim.

[116]"Finn Explains Drug Test," *New York Times*, 27 September 1984.

[117]New York Times, 20 November 1998."American College of Sports Medicine Position Stand on the Use of Anabolic-Androgenic Steroids in Sports," *Sports Medicine Bulletin* 19 (3) July 1984, 13-18.

[118]"Early Deaths of Soviet Athletes Due to Steroids? Magazine Cites 59 Cases in Which Banned Drugs Proved Fatal at a Young Age," *Los Angeles Times,* 6 September 1984.

[119]William N. Taylor, M.D., *Hormonal Manipulation: A New Era of Monstrous Athletes* (Jefferson, NC: McFarland & Co. 1985).

[120]"Canadians Busted For Steroids," *International Olympic Lifter* 8 (August 1984): 29.

[121]"Pisarenko and Kurlovich Nabbed for Steroid Smuggling" *International Olympic Lifter* 9 (September 1984):12–13.

[122]"The Racer's Edge," *Newsweek* (21 January 1985):71. See also: "Olympic Blood Doping," *Sports Illustrated* (21 January 1985):26-27; and Robert Thomas, "USOC Checking Use of Transfusions," *New York Times*, 10 January 1985.

[123]"Cycle Group Bans Use of Blood Doping," *New York Times,* 19 January 1985.

[124]"The Daily Dope Dialogue," *Track & Field News* (February 1985):52.

[125]"Expert Urges Ban on Blood Doping," *New York Times*, 28 March 1985.

[126]G. Legwold, "Blood Doping and the Letter of the Law," *Physician and Sports Medicine* 13 (March 1985):37-38.

[127]Michael Goodwin, "USOC to Seek More Tests for Drugs," *New York Times*, 24 March 1985.

[128]"Powerlifter Sought for Steroid Sales," *Los Angeles Times*, 12 May 1985, Sect. 3, p.14.

[129]Robert Thomas, Jr., "Ueberroth Orders Wide Tests for Drug Use in Pro Baseball," *New York Times*, 7 May 1985, sect. 1, 26.

[130]"Medical Report," Minutes of the 90th IOC Session, Berlin, 4th-5th June 1985 (Lausanne: IOC, 1985), 21-22, 83-85.

[131]"USOC to Begin Tests," *New York Times, 25 June 1985.*

[132]H.L. Nash, "Blood Doping Ban: More Bark than Bite?" *Physician and Sports Medicine* 13 (August 1985):32.

[133]"Tougher Sanctions," *New York Times*, 6 September 1985.

[134]Harold A. Schmeck, Jr. "Gene-Spliced Hormone for Growth Is Cleared," *New York Time,* 19 October 1985.

[135]Terry Todd, "Anabolic Steroids: The Gremlins of Sport," *Journal of Sport History* 14 (Spring 1987):87-107. See also: Terry Todd, "Sports RX: the Use of Human Growth Hormone Poses a Grave Dilemma for Sport," *Sports Illustrated* 60 (15 October 1984):6 passim.

[136]Tom Donohoe and Neil Johnson, *Foul Play: Drug Abuse in Sports* (New York: B. Blackwell, 1986).

[137]H.G. Klein, "Blood Transfusion and Athletics," *New Studies in Athletics* 1 (January 1986):67-71.

[138]Valerie DeBernadette and Terry Todd, "Anabolic Steroids: Black Market and Black Eye," *Medical Advertising News* 5 (15 June 1986):5.

[139]Joseph Durso, "U.S. Plan on Drugs Is Sought," *New York Times*, 27 August 1986.

[140]Joseph Durso, "U.S. Plan on Drugs Is Sought," *New York Times*, 27 August 1986.

[141]"Medical Report," *Minutes of the 91st IOC Session, Lausanne, 12th-17th October, 1986* (Lausanne: IOC, 1986):193-194.

[142]Jonathan Harris, *Drugged Athletes: The Crisis in American Sports* (New York: Four Winds Press, 1987).

[143]Richard H. Strauss, *Drugs and Performance in Sports,* (Philadelphia: William B. Saunders, 1987).

[144]Dan Duchaine, *The Underground Steroid Handbook for Men and Women* (By the author, n.d.), quoted in J.G. Macintyre, "Growth Hormone and Athletes," *Sports Medicine* 4 (1987):140.

[145]J.G. Macintyre, "Growth Hormone and Athletes," *Sports Medicine* 4 (1987):129-142.

[146]"Report of the IOC Medical Commission to the 92nd Session of the IOC" (Lausanne: IOC, 1987).

[147]Michael Janofsky, "Drug Cheaters May Be Winning the Battle With Testers," *New York Times*, 14 September 1988. See also Michael Janofsky and Peter Alfano, "Drug Use by Athletes Runs Free Despite Tests," *New York Times*, 19 August 1987.

[148]Michael Janofsky, "Drug Cheaters May Be Winning the Battle of Wits With Testers," *New York Times*, 15 September 1988.

[149]Michael Janofsky and Peter Alfano, "Drug Use by Athletes Runs Free Despite Tests," *New York Times,* 17 November 1988; Virginia Cowart, "Steroids in Sports: After Four Decades, Time to Return These Genies to Bottle?" *Journal of the American Medical Association* 257 (23-30 January 1987):421-423.

[150]Wina Sturgeon, "The Inside Dope: One of America's Olympic Bosses was Banned for Blood Doping," *Sports Illustrated* (4 October 1999):29.

[151]"Army Studying Blood Doping," *The Tampa Tribune*, 20 March 1987, 6A.

[152]"Tod Einer Sportlerin: Die Wahrheit über den Fall Birgit Dressel," *Der Spiegel* 37 (7 February 1987):228.

[153]J. Eisendrath, "Confessions of a Steroid Smuggler," *Los Angeles Times Magazine* 4 (24 April 1988):8-10. See also: Larry Dorman, "Miami Coach Arrested in Illegal Steroid Web," *Austin American Statesman* 22 May 1987, D1, 11.

[154]Angie Cannon, "Steroid-Using Police Cause Brutality Fears," *Miami Herald*, 19 May 1987, 9A.

[155]John F. Burns, "Johnson Will Tell His Side of Story," *New York Times*, 30 September 1988.

[156]"Deadly Deception: Muscle Mania Stirs Steroids Epidemic . . . and in the End, Users Must Pay the Price," *Pittsburgh Press* 30 August 1987.

[157]"Lewis Continues Plea," *New York Times*, 11 September 1987.

[158]Janet Mohun and Aziz Khan, *Drugs, Steroids and Sports: Understanding Drugs* (New York: F. Watts, 1988).

[159]Michael J. Asken, *Dying to Win: The Athlete's Guide to Safe and Unsafe Drugs in Sport* (Washington: Acropolis Books, 1988).

[160]*Sports Medicine in Track and Field Athletics: Proceedings of the Second IAAF Medical Congress, Canberra Australia, 1987* (Australia: International Amateur Athletic Federation and Australian Institute of Sport, 1988).

[161]"A Pumped Up World," *San Diego Union-Tribune,* 17 August 1997.

[162]Terry Todd and John Hoberman, "China—The Strongest and Smartest," *Austin American Statesman*, 14 June 1992.

[163]"Barred Polish Athlete Protests," *New York Times,* 23 February 1988.

[164]C. Wood, "The Drug Busters. The Expanding Pharmacopoeia of Performance-Enhancing Drugs Represents an Insidious Challenge" *Macleans* 101 (February 1988):122-126.

[165]"Medical Report," *Minutes of the 93rd Session IOC Session, Calgary, 9th-11th February 1988* (Lausanne: IOC, 1988):9-10, 76-77. See also "IOC to Halt Drug-Test Dodging," *New York Times* 28 February 1988, and Michael Janofsky, "Drug Cheaters May Be Winning the Battle of Wits With Testers," *New York Times*, 15 September 1988.

[166]Harrison G. Pope and David L. Katz, "Affective and Psychotic Symptoms Associated With Anabolic Steroid Use," *American Journal of Psychiatry* 145 (April 1988):487-489.

[167]"Drug Abuse: Of Muscles and Mania," *Psychology Today* (September 1987):12; and "And Now the Steroid Defense?" *American Bar Association Journal* (1 October 1988):22-24.

[168]The official report of the Ottawa Conference is contained in a series of appendices attached to the *Minutes of the 94th IOC Session, Seoul, 13th-16th September, 1988*. See in particular "First Permanent World Conference on Anti-Doping in Sport—Ottawa," "Final Declaration," "Principles in the Elimination of Doping in Sport," and "International Olympic Committee Charter Against Doping in Sport." All of these documents are on deposit at the Paul Ziffren Sport Resource Center, Amateur Athletic Foundation of Los Angeles.

For other views on the conference see: "Vote Is Near for Drug Test," *New York Times*, 24 November 1988 and Michael Janofsky, "Drug Plan Gains Approval," *New York Times*, 25 November 1988. See also two articles by S. Newman in Canadian publications: "Anti-Doping Conference. An Interview With IOC Medical Commission Chairman Prince Alexandre de Merode of

Belgium," *Athletics* (October 1988):44-45 and "A Breakfast of Champions: The First Permanent World Conference on Anti-Doping in Sport," *Champion* 12 (Summer 1988):12-21.

[169]Sandra Blakeslee, "Steroid Cheaters are Growing Smarter," *New York Times*, 13 July 1988.

[170]"Weight Lifter Dropped," *New York Times*, 29 July 1988.

[171]"Drug Reprieve," *New York Times,* 14 August 1988.

[172]"Olympic Notebook: Tougher Drug Policy," *New York Times*, 14 September 1988.

[173]"Medical Report," *Minutes of the 94th IOC Session, Seoul, 13th-16th September 1988* (Lausanne: IOC: 1988), 5-6. See also "Plan to Limit Parade Doesn't Last Long," *New York Times*, 14 September 1988.

[174]Michael Janofsky, "Drug Cheaters May Be Winning The Battle of Wits With Testers," *New York Times*, 15 September 1988.

[175]"Myers Appeal Fails," *New York Times*, 18 September 1988.

[176]"U.S. Committee Closes Book," *New York Times*, 18 September 1988.

[177]Laurie Mifflin, "123-Pound Gold Medalist Fails Drug Test," *New York Times*, 2 September 1988; "Ban on Two More Lifters," *New York Times,* 26 September 1988; and "Team Lifted After Second Drug Test Is Failed," *New York Times*, 9 September 1988.

[178]Michael Janofsky, "Johnson Loses Gold to Lewis After Drug Test," *New York Times*, 28 September 1988.

[179]Michael T. Kaufman, "Canada Will Lead Johnson Investigation," *New York Times,* 29 September 1988.

[180]Michael T. Kaufman, "Canada Will Lead Johnson Investigation," *New York Times,* 29 September 1988.

[181]Michael T. Kaufman, "Canada Will Lead Johnson Investigation," *New York Times,* 29 September 1988.

[182]"Weight Lifter Used Drug," *New York Times,* 29 September 1988.

[183]Michael Janofsky, "Citing Drug Use, Olympic Official Proposes a Ban on Weightlifting," *New York Times*, 31 September 1988.

[184]Michael Janofsky and Peter Alfano, "Drug Use By Athletes Runs Free Despite Tests," *New York Times*, 17 November 1988.

[185]"U.S. and Soviet Officials Uniting to Discourage Athletes' Drug Use," *New York Times,* 3 October 1988.

[186]"Canadian Inquiry," *New York Times*, 6 October 1988.

[187]"Myers Suspended," *New York Times*, 18 October 1988; see also: "Angry Myers Insists Drug Tests Incorrect," *Dallas Morning News*, 7 September 1988.

[188]"Coach Is Suspended," *New York Times,* 25 October 1988.

[189]"Ban Proposed for Drug Users," *New York Times,* 17 November 1988.

[190]Michael Janofsky and Peter Alfano, "Drug Use by Athletes Runs Free Despite Tests," *New York Times*, 17 November 1988. Also in the *New York Times,* on 18 November 1988 see "Drugs That May Build Bulk Pull Weight on Black Market"; on 19 November 1988 see "A Guru Who Spreads the Gospel of Steroids"; on 20 November 1988 see "New 'Breakfast of Champions': A

Recipe for Victory or Disaster?"; and on 21 November 1988 see "Victory at Any Cost: Drug Pressure Growing." See also "Olympic Notebook: Tougher Drug Policy," *New York Times,* 14 September 1988.

[191]"Drug Plan Gains Approval," *New York Times,* 25 November 1988. See also, "Vote Is Near for Drug Test," *New York Times*, 24 November 1988; and "Winking at Steroids in Sports," *New York Times,* 22 November 1988.

[192]"Soviet Sports Official Explains Stance on Drugs," *New York Times*, 27 November 1988.

[193]"Drug Plan," *New York Times,* 25 November 1988. See also Anise C. Wallace, "Drug Test Program May Start Quickly," *New York Times*, 29 February 1988.

[194]IOC, "International Olympic Charter Against Doping in Sport," *Olympic Review* 253 (November 1988):628-631.

[195]Charles Yesalis, "Steroid Use Is Not Just an Adult Problem," *New York Times*, 4 December 1988. See also Charles E. Yesalis, "Anabolic Steroid Use: Indication of Habituation Among Adolescents," *Journal of Drug Education* 19 (1989):111-113.

[196]"Steroid Smuggler Gets Prison Term," *Austin American Statesman*, 13 December 1988.

[197]William E. Buckley et al., "Estimated Prevalence of Anabolic Steroid Use Among Male High School Seniors," *Journal of the American Medical Association* (December 1998):3441-3445.

[198]Anita DeFrantz, "Olympic Movement: Youth and Doping," *Report of the Twenty-Ninth Session of the International Olympic Academy* (Lausanne: IOC, 1989):106-111. See also G. Heinze, "The Concept of Doping as a Counterpoint to the Olympic Spirit," 60-66; K. Read, "The IOC Athletes Commission Anti-Doping Campaign," 112-115; and R. Pariente, "The End of Doping: Utopia or Reality?" 116-125.

[199]"Canada to Open Drugs Hearings," *New York Times*, 11 January 1988. See also Howard Witt, "Drug Probe Not for the Faint of Heart," *New York Times,* 26 February 1989.

[200]Draft copy, H.R. for the 101st Congress, 1989. Xerox copy in Todd-McLean Physical Culture Collection drugs file #2.

[201]"British List Bill on Steroid Use," *New York Times*, 11 January 1988.

[202]"Steroid Use Rampant in USSR, Soviet Magazine Says," *Globe and Mail*, 25 March 1989.

[203]IOC, *Information for Athletes, Coaches and Medical Practitioners on the Permissible Use of Drugs in Amateur Sport.* (Lausanne: IOC Medical Commission Paper, March 1989):1-29.

[204]Chris Hall, "Coach Says He Injected Drugs Into Johnson," *The Ottawa Citizen,* 2 March 1989, A1-2; "Amateur Sport Must Clean Up Act Now, Says Olympic Boss," *The Ottawa Citizen,* March 1989, A3. See also: "Johnson Did Use Steroids, Says Coach," *The Ottawa Citizen*, 1 March 1989, B1.

[205]Murray Campbell, "Will Sport Ever Recover?" *The Globe and Mail*, 4 March 1989. D1, 8.

[206]"Russia and U.S. Act to Stamp Out Steroids," *Advertiser*, 3 March 1989 and "U.S., Soviets Near Pact on Joint Steroid Testing," *The Ottawa Citizen*, 2 March 1989, B-2.

[207]T.M. Wolff, "Playing by the Rules? A Legal Analysis of the United States Olympic Committee–Soviet Olympic Committee Doping Control Agreement." *Stanford Journal of International Law* 25 (2:1989):611-646.

[208]"Increase in Positive Tests," *New York Times*, 6 April 1989.

[209]P. Belliotti, G. Benzi, and A. Ljungqvist, eds., *Official Proceedings of the International Athletic Foundation World Symposium on Doping in Sport, June 5-7, 1989* (Italy: International Athletic Foundation, 1990).

[210]"Ben Johnson Confesses," *New York Times,* 17 June 1989.

[211]Michael Janofsky, "Doctor Says He Supplied Steroids to Medalists," *New York Times*, 20 June 1989.

[212]Michael Janofsky, "Canadian Shot Putter Tells of Steroid Role," *New York Times*, 27 June 1989.

[213]"Report of the National Consensus Meeting on Anabolic/Androgenic Steroids," Amateur Athletic Foundation, Los Angeles, July 30-31, 1989.

[214]Richard Pound, "Reflections on Cheating in Sport," *Olympic Review* 262 (August 1989):390-391 and Prince de Merode, "The Fight Against Doping: Ongoing Evolution," *Olympic Review* 262 (August 1989):383-384.

[215]"Medical Report," *Minutes of the 95th IOC Session, Puerto Rico, 30th August-1st September 1989* (Lausanne: IOC, 1989):10-12, 85-86.

[216]"Group Votes to Erase Johnson's Records," *Austin American Statesman* 5 September, 1989, D3.

[217]*Minutes of the 94th IOC Session, Seoul, 13th-16th September 1988 (Distributed to Members of the IOC, 1988), 5-6.* See also "Rule Against the Trafficking of Prohibited Drugs, Approved by the IOC Executive Board 11.9.88," attached as Annex 9 to the *Minutes*.

[218]"Probes Produce Bleak Outlook for Olympic Control Over Drugs," *Globe & Mail*, 19 September 1989.

[219]"Canadian Inquiry Ends," *New York Times*, 20 Sept 1989.

[220]Warren E. Leary, "Users of Steroids Risk Addiction, Two Researchers at Yale Report," *New York Times*, 8 December 1989.

[221]Michael Janofsky, "Image-Conscious East Germany Ran Drug Tests before Trips," *New York Times*, 15 December 1989.

[222]"Eleven Nations in Drug Test Accord," *New York Times,* 14 December 1989.

[223]Eric Walters, "Doping: Ten Years of Relentless Struggle," in *From Moscow to Lausanne* (Lausanne, Switzerland: International Olympic Committee, 1990).

[224]Charlie Francis and Jeff Coplon, *Speed Trap: Inside the Biggest Scandal in Olympic History* (Toronto: Lester & Orpen Dennys Ltd., 1990).

[225]James Wright and Virginia Cowart, *Anabolic Steroids: Altered States* (Carmel, CA: Benchmark Press, 1990).

[226]Angela Issajenko with Martin O'Malley and Karen O'Reilly, *Running Risks* (Toronto: MacMillan of Canada, 1990).

[227]"Moses and Three Others Quit T.A.C. Drug Panel," *New York Times*, 5 May 1990.

[228]Randy Harvey, "Obscure Sprinter's Rise, Fall Symbolize Doping Nightmare," *Los Angeles Times*, 3 September 1994.

[229]"Astaphan Accused," *New York Times*, 28 June 1990.

[230]Dan Giesin, "U.S. Sprinter Reynolds Held at Standstill by IAAF," *San Francisco Chronicle*, 3 April 1992. The best legal discussion of the Reynolds case is found in "Those Who Don't Run, Sue," *California Lawyer* (July 1996):18.

[231]"Steroid Use by Teen-Agers Cited," *New York Times*, 8 September 1990.

[232]Randy Harvey, "Coaches Call for Escalation of Drug Battle," *Los Angeles Times*, 12 September 1994.

[233]"38 Soviet Athletes Fail Drug Tests," *New York Times,* 6 October 1990.

[234]Pat Connolly, "It's Time to Ban Punitive Drug Testing," *New York Times*, 28 October 1990.

[235]Michael Janofsky, "Drug Use by Prominent Athletes Reported," *New York Times,* 29 November 1990.

[236]Brigitte Berendonk, *Doping-Dokumente: Von der Forschung zum Betrug* (Berlin, Heidelberg, New York: Springer-Verlag, 1991).

[237]R. Laura and S. White, eds., *Drug Controversy in Sport: The Socio-ethical and Medical Issues* (Sydney: Allen and Unwin, 1999).

[238]William N. Taylor, *Macho Medicine: A History of the Anabolic Steroid Epidemic* (Jefferson, NC: McFarland, 1991).

[239]Robert Voy, *Drugs, Sports, and Politics* (Champaign, Illinois: Leisure Press, 1991).

[240]J. Park, "Doping Test Report of 10th Asian Games in Seoul," *Journal of Sports Medicine and Physical Fitness* 31 (June 1991):303-317.

[241]Lyle Alzado and S. Smith, "'I'm Sick and I'm Scared,'" *Sports Illustrated* (8 July 1991):20-24, 27. See also Anne P. Davis, "Lyle Alzado has Come Clean," *USA Today,* 5 July 1991.

[242]Giesin, "U.S. Sprinter Reynolds Held at Standstill," *New York Times,* 3 April 1992.

[243]"USOC Guide to Prohibited Substances and Methods, May 1997," *Inside the USOC* Web site. Located at **http://www.olympic-usa.org/inside/in_1_1_4_6_5.html**.

[244]William N. Taylor, M.D., *Anabolic Steroids & the Athlete* (Jefferson, NC: McFarland & Co, 1992).

[245]Vyv Simson and Andrew Jennings, *The Lords of the Rings: Power, Money and Drugs in the Modern Olympics* (London: Simon & Schuster, 1992).

[246]John Hoberman, *Mortal Engines: The Science of Performance and the Dehumanization of Sport* (New York: Maxwell Macmillan International, 1992).

[247] Interview with Alan Weisman, 29 February 1992; See also W.O. Johnson and A. Verschoth, "Testy Times in Germany: Katrin Krabbe and Two Other Track Stars Were Banned for Drug-Testing Improprieties They Hotly Deny," *Sports Illustrated* 76 (9 March 1992):51-52 and Dick Patrick, "Krabbe Cleared to Run By German Federation," *USA Today,* 31 March 1993, 11C.

[248]"Three Brits Kicked Out for Drug Use," *San Diego Union-Tribune,* 30 July 1992.

[249]"Lausanne Gets Its Accreditation," Olympic Review 296 (June 1992):297.

[250]International Amateur Athletic Federation, *Procedural Guidelines for Doping Control* (London: IAAF, 1993).

[251]"Those Who Don't Run, Sue," *California Lawyer* (July 1996):18.

[252]Terry Todd, "Drug News," *Flex* (March 1994):129-130.

[253]"Doping the Historic Agreement," *Olympic Review* 315 (January/February 1994):15-16.

[254]Interview with Terry Todd, 10 April 1998.

[255]M.H. Williams, "The Use of Nutritional Ergogenic Aids in Sports: Is it An Ethical Issue?" *International Journal of Sport Nutrition* 4 (June 1994):120-131.

[256]Elliott Almond, "Olympic Cover-Up Alleged," *Los Angeles Times*, 23 August 1994, sect. C.

[257]Elliott Almond, "Officials Conflict on 9 Drug Tests," *Los Angeles Times*, 2 September 94.

[258]Julie Cart, "Drugs Dim Glow of Victory for U.S. Shot Putters," *New York Times,* 1 August 1992.

[259]Randy Harvey, "China Makes Big Splash With 100 Freestyle Record, Controversy," *Los Angeles Times*, 6 September 1994.

[260]Randy Harvey, "U.S. Swim Chief Confronts Chinese With Drug Claims," *Los Angeles Times,* 10 September 1994; see also Randy Harvey, "Coaches Call for Escalation of Drug Battle," *Los Angeles Times,* 12 September 1994.

[261]Don Catlin, "Testing Succeeds in Keeping Sports, Athletes Clean" *USA Today*, 12 October 1994, 8C and Arnold Beckett, "Incompetent Labs, Unclear Policies Prove Dangerous," *USA Today,* 12 February 1994, 8C.

[262]Elliott Almond, "Chinese Woman Tests Positive, May Face Ban," *Los Angeles Times*, 17 November 1994 and Phillip Whitten, "China Drug Bust," *Swimming World and Junior Swimmer*, (January 1995): 70.

[263]"Great Fall of China," *Sports Illustrated* 81 (19 December 1994):19.

[264]International Olympic Committee, *Preventing and Fighting Against Doping in Sport* (Lausanne, Switzerland: IOC, March 31, 1995).

[265]Tim Layden, "Damning of Champions," *CNN-Sports Illustrated,* 22 July 1996. Lo-cated at: **http://cnnsi.com/events/1996/Olympics/daily/july22/column.html**.

[266]John M. Hoberman and Charles E. Yesalis, "The History of Synthetic Testosterone," *Scientific American* (February 1995):60-65.

[267]Christine Brennan, "FINA Plans Review of Foschi's Probation," *Washington Post*, 1 March 1996, sect. B. See also Karen Allen, "Foschi Suspension Weighs Heavily on Ruling Board," *USA Today,* 15 February 1996, 10C.

[268]"No Dope: Dr. Manfred Donike," *Sports Illustrated* 83 (4 September 1995): 22-24. See also "In Memory: Manfred Donike," *SportEurope* 6 (September 1995):48.

[269]"The Olympian Battle Over Human Growth Hormone," *Sports Illustrated* 83 (30 October 1995):17.

[270]Andrew Jennings, *The New Lords of the Rings: Olympic Corruption and How to Buy Gold Medals* (New York: Pocket Books, 1996).

[271]T.M. Hoxha, "Atlanta '96 and Athlete's Rights: An Update on Drug Testing and the International Olympic Committee," *Entertainment and Sports Lawyer* 14 (Spring 1996):7-10.

[272]International Amateur Athletic Foundation, *Procedural Guidelines for Doping Control* (France: IAAF, 1996).

[273]L. Bruunshuus, K. Klempel, D. Cowan, G. Hill, and H. Olesen, "Transmission of the Results of Tests for International Olympic Committee-Defined Drugs of Abusc," *Journal of Chromatography* 687 (1) 6 December 1996, 157-182.

[274]See D. Elliot and L. Goldberg, "Intervention and Prevention of Steroid Use in Adolescents"; S. Oliver, "Drugs in Sport: Justifying Paternalism on the Grounds of Harm"; B. Ekblom, "Blood Doping and Erythropoietin: The Effects of Variation in Hemoglobin Concentration and Other Related Factors on Physical Performance"; "Effects of Creatine Supplementation of Performance," *American Journal of Sports Medicine* 24 (6 Supplement, 1996): 2.

[275]"Foschi Files for Arbitration," *Washington Post,* 17 February 1996. See also Karen Allen, "Foschi Probation Turned Into Suspension," *USA Today,* 14 February 1996.

[276]"USOC Passes Stiff Antidrug Program," *USA Today,* 15 April 1996, 3C. See also "USOC Guide to Prohibited Substances and Methods. May 1997" *Inside the USOC* Web site. Located at: **http://www.olympic-usa.org/inside/in_1_1_4_6_5.html**.

[277]Thomas Heath, "Drug Testing Performance Enhanced: High-Tech Equipment, Better Methods, But Will Abusers Slip Through?" *Washington Post,* 23 April 1996.

[278]Reuters Information Service, "IOC Laughs off British Doping Allegations," *Olympics Features Page, The Sports Page.* Located at **http://www.nando.net/newsroom/sports/oth/1996/oth/oly/feat/archive/071596/oly33745.html**. See also "Top Australians Doubt Drug Claim," AAP Info Center Web site. Located at: **http://www.aap.com.au/service/393a.html**.

[279]Tim Layden, "Damning of Champions," CNN-*Sports Illustrated,* 22 July 1996. Located at **http://cnnsi.com/events/1996/Olympics/daily/july22/column.html**.

[280]"Our Objective Is to Protect the Health of Athletes," *Olympic Magazine* 11 (November 1996):40-42.

[281]"Latest from the IOC." Located at: **http://www.wfsgi/latest_from_ioc12_sep_97.html**.

[282]Associated Press, "Swimming: World Coaches Association's Leonard Threatens to Break From FINA." Located at **http://www.sportserver.com/newsroom/ap/oth/1997/oth/mor/feat/archive/102397/mor46976.html**.

[283]Louise Evans, "More Positive Tests to Come, Warn Experts," Sydney Morning Herald on the Net, 28 November 1997. Located at **http://www.smh.com.au/daily/content/971128/sport/sport10.html**.

[284]"Winning the Right Way," *Chicago Sun Times*, 18 December 1997.

[285]Jacqueline Magnay, "Drugs and the Chinese," *Sydney Morning Herald,* 9 January 1998. Located at **http://www.smh.com.au/daily/content/980109/sport/sport103.html**. For other information on Chinese drug positives, see Karen Allen, "China's Road to Success Hits Its Share of Hurdles," *USA Today*, 4 June 1998, 5E; "IOC President Says Chinese Sports Programs 'Very Clean,'" *USA Today*, 6 October 1994, 2C; and "U. S. Coach: Chinese Swimmers Not Clean," *USA Today*, 19 July 1996, 4E.

[286]Jere Longman, "De Bruin, Irish Swimmer Is Facing New Questions," *New York Times,* 30 April 1998.

[287]Associated Press, "Nagano Goes High-tech to Catch Drug Cheats," CNN-*Sports Illustrated*, Posted 23 January 1998. Located at **http://cnnsi.com/Olympics/events/1998/nagano/news/1998/01/23/doping_controls/**.

[288]Associated Press, "Nagano Goes High-tech to Catch Drug Cheats," CNN-*Sports Illustrated,* Posted 23 January 1998. Located at **http://cnnsi.com/Olympics/events/1998/nagano/news/1998/01/23/doping_controls/**.

[289]Associated Press, "IOC: U.S. Pros Ignoring Doping Issue," CNN-*Sports Illustrated* Web site, posted on 2 February 1998. Located at **http://cnnsi.com/Olympics/events/1998/nagano/news/1998/02/02/Olympics_doping**.

[290]"IOC Warning Label: Stay Off Sudafed," Nando Sportserver. Located at **http://www.nando.net/newsroom/ap/oth/oly/feat/archive/020598/oly49061.html**.

[291]Jill Lieber, "Snowboarders Not Too Shy About Defending Rebagliati," *USA Today*, 12 February 1998, 3E. See also: Associated Press, "Two More Athletes Test Positive for Marijuana," CNN-*Sports Illustrated* Web site, posted on 19 February 1998. Located at **http://cnnsi.com/Olympics/events/1998/nagano/news/1998/02/19/marijuana_tests**. See also Associated Press, "Fundamental Values Are at Stake," CNN-*Sports Illustrated* Web site, posted on 14 February 1998. Located at **http://cnnsi.com/Olympicsc/events/1998/nagano/news/1998/02/14/ioc_news**.

[292]Reuters Limited, "Jayasinghe Denies Drug Charge," CNN-*Sports Illustrated* Web site, posted on 3 April 1998. Located at **http://cnnsi.com/athletics/news/1998/04/03/jayasinghe_denial/**.

[293]Associated Press, "Steroid Trial: Former East German Sports Officials Face Charges for Doping." CNN-*Sports Illustrated* Web site, posted on 17 March 1998. Located at **http://cnnsi.com/more/world/news/1998/03/17/egerman_doping/**. See also Reuters Limited, "Steroids Under Attack, Lawyers Want Doping Case against East Germans Dropped," CNN-*Sports Illustrated* Web site, posted on 18 March 1998. Located at **http://cnnsi.com/more/world/news/1998/03/18/egerman_drugs/**.

[294]Thomas Heath, "Drug Tests Rock U.S. Track World," *Washington Post*, 28 July 1998.

[295]Christopher Clarey and Samuel Abt, "The Tainted Tour: A Special Report—Drug Scandals Dampen Cycling's Top Event," *New York Times*, 3 July 1999.

[296]Philip Hersh, "Olympic Medical Chief Blasts Samaranch for Views on Drugs," *The Tribune*, 18 August 1998.

[297]Associated Press, "IOC Official Rejects U.S. Medal Claim," Nando Media Web site, posted on 21 October 1998. DIALOG(R)File 858:AP NEWS JUL(c) 1999 ASSOCIATED PRESS. All rts. reserv. 04708100 0135 **IOC official rejects U.S. medal claim** BY: TONY HARPER DATELINE: SYDNEY, Australia PRIORITY: Rush WORD COUNT: 0408Associated Press DATE: October 21, 1998 04:56 EDT

[298]James Christie, "Government Bans Off-the-Shelf Medicine Containing Ingredient in Tour de France Controversy," *Globe and Mail*, 29 October 1998.

[299]Associated Press, "Federations Look for Common Ground on Doping," Nando Media Web site, posted on 27 November 1998.

[300]Don Cronin, "Court Rules Against Korda," *USA Today*, 26 March 1999, 27C. See also "Korda Launches Legal Challenge," 15 January 1999, Drug Download file, The Todd-McLean Physical Culture Collection, The University of Texas at Austin.

[301]Jere Longman, "Unbelievable Performances: A Special Report—Widening Drug Use Compromises Faith in Sport," *New York Times,* 26 December 1998.

[302]John Hoberman, "Offering the Illusion of Reform on Drugs," *New York Times,* 10 January 1999.

[303]Don Cronin, "Drug Ban Upheld on Irish Swimmer," *USA Today*, 8 June 1999, 13C. See also Tom O'Riordan, "D. Day for de Bruin's Appeal," 6 January 1999. Drug Download file, The Todd-McLean Physical Culture Collection, The University of Texas at Austin.

[304]Associated Press, "Olympics Official Blasts McGwire Again Over Andro," 12 February 1999. Nando Media located at **http://www.sportserver.com**. For other reactions of the IOC to McGwire, see Mike Dodd, "McGwire's Use of 'Andro' Concerns IOC," *USA Today,* 15 September 1998, 2C.

[305]Gary Graves, "Slaney Challenges Reliability of Test," *USA Today*, 29 January 1999, 3C. See also "Slaney Suing IAAF in Dispute Over a Drug Test," *New York Times*, 14 April 1999 and Jill Lieber, "Slaney Numb Over Latest Suspension News," *USA Today*, 12 June 1997, 16C.

[306]Paul L. Montgomery, "IOC Falters in Doping Bid as Summit Ends," *New York Times* 5 February 1999. See also Dick Patrick, "Drug Czar Calls for Rebuilt IOC," *USA Today,* 2 February 1999, 18C; "Drug Test Credibility Debated," *USA Today,* 3 February 1999, 8C; Dick Patrick, "IOC Drug Chief's Proposal Blasted," *USA Today,* 1 February 1999, 17C; "Compromise Reigns," *USA Today,* 5 February 1999, 14C; and Paul L. Montgomery, "IOC Credibility Questioned as Drug Meeting Starts," *New York Times*, 3 February 1999.

[307]"Lausanne Declaration on Doping in Sport," 4 February 1999. Located at **http://nodoping.org/Declaration_e.html**.

[308]"Sydney 2000: Growth Hormone Test Is Ruled Out," *New York Times,* 14 March 1999.

[309] Holcolmb B. Noble, "Steroid Use by Teenage Girls Is Rising," *New York Times,* 1 June 1999.

[310]Richard Sandomir, "Olympics: IOC's Drug Plan Criticized at Hearing," *New York Times, 21 October 1999.* See also Amy Shipley, "McCaffrey, IOC Testify on Anti-Doping Efforts," Washington Post, 21 October 1999, D2.

[311]Buddy Martin, "USOC Authorizes New, Independent Agency to Supervise Drug Tests," *New York Times,* 24 October 1999. For background see Rachel Alexander, "USOC Moves on Anti-Doping Program," *Washington Post*, 23 October 1999, D2.

5

CHAPTER

An Ethical Analysis of Drug Testing

Angela J. Schneider, PhD, and Robert B. Butcher, PhD
University of Western Ontario

In Canada, since Ben Johnson's positive test for steroid use in the Seoul Olympics, we have seen a royal commission, a ministerial task force, a parliamentary committee, a federally sponsored report on values and ethics in amateur sport, and the creation of a new anti-doping agency (Dubin Commission, 1990a,b; Blackhurst, Schneider, and Strachan, 1991); and the Canadian Centre for Drug-Free Sport, created by the federal government in 1992, it is now the Canadian Centre for Ethics in Sport (CCES). At the international level, the International Olympic Committee (IOC) recently hosted a World Conference on Doping in Lausanne, Switzerland, in February 1999, in order to launch a new international anti-doping agency called the World Anti-Doping Agency (WADA). Despite all this activity there still remain some serious unanswered ethical questions. Surprisingly, the first of these questions is just why it is that we should ban drug use from athletic competition in the first place. We have discussed this matter at length elsewhere (Schneider, 1993; Schneider and Butcher, 1994). This chapter concentrates on something rather different, although intimately connected to this matter. The focus in this chapter is on the ethical ramifications of enforcing any ban on drugs, substances, or practices. The ethical consequences of dope testing are related to (1) the content of the banned list—just what it is we are testing the athletes for, (2) the methods used for testing, and (3) the penalties that are levied in the event of a positive test.

Most of the arguments in favor of dope testing are related to issues of "harm." We concentrate on these arguments because the primary purpose of this chapter is to pose a second question about the potential for harm caused by bans and their required enforcement. We argue that the invasion of privacy caused by effective anti-doping measures cannot be justified solely by the good those measures seek to attain. This leads to an impasse. For drug-free sport we need effective enforcement. But the steps required for effective enforcement can be too invasive of athletes' rights, particularly the personal right to privacy. We offer a proposal for a way out of this deadlock, a way that shares ownership of the rules of sport, and the methods for enforcing those rules, with those most affected by them: the athletes.

The Invasion of Privacy Caused by Bans

If one bans drugs or practices from sport, one must necessarily take steps to enforce those bans. It has become apparent to those involved with doping control that, despite some "in-competition" positive tests, the only effective way to test for banned substances is to introduce random, unannounced out-of-competition testing (RUT). This is because some substances, for instance anabolic steroids, can be discontinued before competition and still retain their effects, and also because of the prevalence of masking agents and the method of urine substitution (e.g. catheters and condoms).[1] The demand that athletes be prepared to submit to urine testing at any time, with no notice, is a serious breach of their civil and human rights in North America. As we will argue, that sort of intrusive intervention in people's lives could only be warranted by the need to protect others from serious harm. It is questionable whether the depth of harm required to warrant such extreme interference with personal liberty can be established at the present time. Let us look first at the sorts of substances and practices that are banned and the steps required to enforce those bans, and then go on to see if those measures can be justified from the moral point of view.

Training Enhancement Versus Performance Enhancement

It is helpful to distinguish between the types of drugs and practices for which testing is required. Broadly speaking, a banned substance or practice may be intended to enhance performance on the day of competition or to enhance training. The vast majority of performance-enhancing substances such as stimulants, depressants, and narcotics, can, with some degree of reliability, be tested at the competition site, but certainly not all of the banned substances can be tested for at the time of performance with any accuracy. For example, the entire group of peptide hormones and analogues cannot be detected with the current testing procedure, and the IOC has added substances to the list for which they know there is no possibility of testing right now.[2] In addition, and crucially for our purposes, some performance enhancers work, not by directly improving performance on the day of competition, but rather by enhancing prior training.

Until now, in-competition testing has been the primary form of testing. However, in-competition tests are of limited value in detecting training enhancers. Athletes may use a training-enhancing substance, for example, anabolic steroids. The use of a sophisticated drug regime, with the discontinuation of the training enhancer before competition, renders the detection of these compounds extremely difficult at the time of competition. This is so, despite the contemporary use of endocrine profiles that allow changes in the body to be traced. (The logical problem is that endocrine profiles are only useful as a testing criterion for those with a long history of previous tests.) In-competition testing is thus seen to be largely ineffective against training-enhancing drugs, and current trends appear to indicate an increasing use of training enhancers.

To detect training enhancers, out-of-competition testing is essential. Also, to prevent athletes from using masking techniques to hide their drug use, the testing must be unannounced. Ultimately, training enhancers improve performance, but as Ben Johnson's coach, Charlie Francis, testified at the Dubin Inquiry when defending himself and Johnson against the use of so-called "shortcuts," anabolic steroids are not a lazy person's method, for what they do is allow you to work harder, not less (Dubin, 1990a). These considerations are the basis for introducing RUT.

The randomness of RUT is necessary because the expense of testing everyone is too great. However, the randomness may be modified; not all sports and not all national team members have the same chance of being tested. Problem sports have been identified, for example, weightlifting and track and field, and so the probability of an athlete in these sports being tested is greater than the probability for an athlete in other sports. In addition, the question of targeting specific athletes is still open. It is not clear if individual athletes are selected on the basis of hearsay. If so, then the testing is not random but on the basis of suspicion. Note the difficulties. If testing is targeted toward individuals on the basis of rumor, the scene is ripe for vindictive campaigns of harassment. Start a rumor about your primary rival for selection and you could make his or her life quite a bit more difficult. On the other hand, if the testing agency does not follow up on rumors and test accordingly, it runs the risk of being accused of turning a blind eye to so-called "known" abuses and abusers.

Enforcement of Bans and the Privacy of Athletes

Enforcement of bans on doping requires that athletes be prepared to submit to a dope test at any time, anywhere, without warning. Not only will the athlete be tested for a wide range of substances, which include recreational drugs such as marijuana and cocaine that have no conceivable training-enhancing properties (as opposed to the performance-enhancing properties of cocaine), but which do carry criminal penalties for ownership or possession. The consequences of a positive test are enormous.

Let us look at a couple of examples where the testing process and the results management has gone seriously awry, with painful personal consequences for those concerned.

Ross Rebagliati

A recent case involved Canadian snowboarder Ross Rebagliati, who was stripped of his Olympic gold medal (in Nagano in 1998) for testing positive for marijuana.

The Canadian Olympic Association (COA) launched an appeal to the independent court of arbitration (a panel established by the IOC to try to avoid legal challenges to its rulings). The COA argued the appeal on two grounds, the first that Rebagliati's positive test came as a result of second-hand smoke, and the second that the IOC ought not to be testing for marijuana in the first place.

The second-hand smoke argument was greeted, when announced at a press conference, with predictable groans and snickers. This defense ranks right up there with the "I smoked but did not inhale" approach favored by some famous U.S. politicians. The second argument is far more interesting—should the IOC be testing athletes for marijuana use?

This case raises some serious questions for the IOC and its drug policy. No one seriously argues that marijuana improves training or performance. If anything, its use is likely to impair performance, so why does the IOC test for it? Marijuana was not on the IOC's list of banned substances, but rather on a list of restricted substances. These restricted substances are not banned outright, but their use may be tested for at the request of the international federation of the sport concerned. But still the question arises, Why? Why would anyone care if a snowboarder has smoked a joint? Why is marijuana on any sort of IOC list and why was it tested for in Nagano?

Testing and punishment for marijuana use in sport has a controversial history. (The history of general prohibitions against marijuana use is equally interesting.) In Nagano, the vote of the IOC Medical Commission was only 13-12 to penalize Rebagliati, and the vote of the IOC Executive was only 3-2 to uphold that decision. The history of the inclusion of marijuana on the IOC restricted list was controversial from the beginning. One story has it that the IOC Medical Commission originally voted 32-1 against including marijuana on the restricted list but that decision was overruled by the IOC Executive Committee.

Quite simply, the IOC has no good grounds for including marijuana on a restricted list, or for testing for its use. The mandate of the IOC for drug testing is to ensure that athletes compete fairly. The rules against drug use are to ban performance-enhancing substances—marijuana is not a performance-enhancing substance, so the IOC has no business testing for it.

Some people might argue that the use of marijuana is illegal (and perhaps also immoral) and so the IOC is justified in testing for its use. But what possible grounds are there for suggesting that the IOC has a role in enforcing the law? The IOC is a sports organization, not a law-enforcement agency. Similar arguments apply if we suggest that the IOC has a role to play in enforcing morals. In all sorts of areas, community moral standards are contested and open to debate. There are many people throughout the world who believe that homosexuality is morally wrong—yet it would be both absurd and immoral to suggest that the IOC has a role in testing for, and prohibiting from competition, anyone who has engaged in same-sex sexual activity. As a vast and powerful social institution the IOC has an obligation to uphold and respect our basic human rights. These rights involve the fundamental right of each of us to choose how we will live our lives (providing we do not harm others), and they involve respect for the worth and dignity of each human being. We have a basic right to privacy, as well.

The system went wrong because it was intruding into something that is beyond its jurisdiction and its moral authority. It is unfair to athletes to test for more than is required to ensure fair competition. Drug testing in sport is an intrusion into an athlete's privacy. That intrusion requires an athlete's consent, something that is, and should be, freely given when the test is conducted in order to ensure fair competition. However, the demand for consent to test for something that is irrelevant to sport is unfair and coercive. The demand for consent to test for marijuana is unfair because marijuana is irrelevant to sport and it is coercive because unless the athlete consents to testing he or she is prohibited from competition.

The COA should have made these arguments in Ross Rebagliati's appeal. Even if we agree that Rebagliati has an obligation to obey even bad rules, the punishment is in no way commensurate with the "crime." But the COA's (or any other National Olympic Committee's) position in Nagano would have been much more convincing if there were a history of consistently supporting athletes' rights in these and other areas. There is no such history. Athletes tend to be viewed as interchangeable commodities, subject to the control of those who run sport. Our athletes deserve support and commitment to their personal rights, but they need it not just at the Games and not just when a gold medal is at stake.

Even a two-year ban for drug use can spell the end of a competitive athletic career. Not only does this mean the loss of sporting opportunity but, for some athletes in high-profile sports, this can also mean the loss of enormous commercial possibilities.

It should also be remembered that this was an in-competition test. It could be argued that prudent athletes, knowing that in competition they may be tested, would scrupulously avoid marijuana for some time preceding the event. But the intrusion into personal liberty is even greater for out-of-competition tests. In Canada, the state is not permitted to subject its citizens to random tests for the use of illegal drugs. There is no compelling reason why a sports organization would have a power denied to the state.

Silken Laumann

The second example of a system that seems to have gone seriously awry is that of Silken Laumann and her positive drug test at the Pan Am Games in 1995 for the use of an over-the-counter cold medication.[3] The tragedy of Silken Laumann's doping infraction with an over-the-counter cold remedy raises a number of questions about cheating, morality, and sport, what constitutes fairness in sport, and just what it is doping rules are intended to achieve. Let us have a look at some of these questions.

Did Silken Laumann cheat? What exactly is cheating? Cheating is the intentional violation of rules to gain an unfair advantage while trying not to get caught. Did Silken intentionally violate the rules? No, by all accounts she tried to find out if the substance she was using was against the rules, and she has a history of scrupulously avoiding drug use in her rehabilitation from a severe leg injury for the 1992 Olympic Games.

Did Laumann try to hide the fact that she was taking this cold medication? No, again by all accounts she listed the medication she was taking on the appropriate forms.

Did Laumann gain an unfair advantage over her opponents? It seems clear that she did not intend to gain an unfair advantage and it is obvious that this crew did not need one at this level of competition (the Pan American Games are not especially competitive for women's rowing) because they predictably won by 11 seconds, which is not just a win, but an annihilation. It is a separate question as to whether Laumann, in fact, gained an unfair advantage, whether she intended to or not. It is highly likely that she did not gain an unfair advantage. Benadryl decongestant, as well as containing the banned substance pseudoephedrine, contains substances that inhibit athletic performance. But, of course, no one tests for those substances.

So, it seems that Laumann did not cheat and did not gain an unfair advantage. If the doping test had been done in Canada, Laumann would have received a positive test but not a doping infraction because the CCES rightly takes the athlete's intention into account. Silken would have been given a warning for inadvertent drug use. So why was she publicly humiliated and she and her crew stripped of their medals?

Who is to blame? There was enormous energy spent on this question in Canada, when in fact it is pointless. Ultimately, athletes have to be responsible for what goes into their bodies. Adult athletes should not be treated like children. Yet, we all count on medical advice in all sorts of areas. Laumann sought medical expertise and did not simply read the substances listed on the box and in the manual given to all athletes by the CCES. The physicians thought she was referring to benadryl and not benadryl decongestant and did not ask to see the substance. So both sides made an error, but instead of spending their resources on finger pointing in this case, those involved should have been asking why would the innocent use of an over-the-counter cold remedy resulted in stripped medals, press conferences, public recrimination and an assault on a Canadian heroine? The current system and current list of banned substances confuses the goals and glory of sport with a misguided attempt to protect athletes from themselves and an unfounded notion of sporting purity.

So far, we have argued that there can be serious harm done to athletes by testing them. Now we must ask if that harm is justified. Athletes, like all people, have some right to privacy. Under what circumstances can the state, or other agencies, interfere with the autonomy of its members? It would seem that an intervention, such as a drug test, must be justified by its advocate. An intervention can be justified two ways.[4] First, intervention can be justified by an overwhelming need to pursue other moral values: the moral value of privacy is superseded by some other moral value, such as harm to others. Second, intervention can be justified by permission. Therefore, if consent is gained for an intervention, then that individual has waived his or her right to privacy. In Canada, all carded athletes (elite athletes who receive government

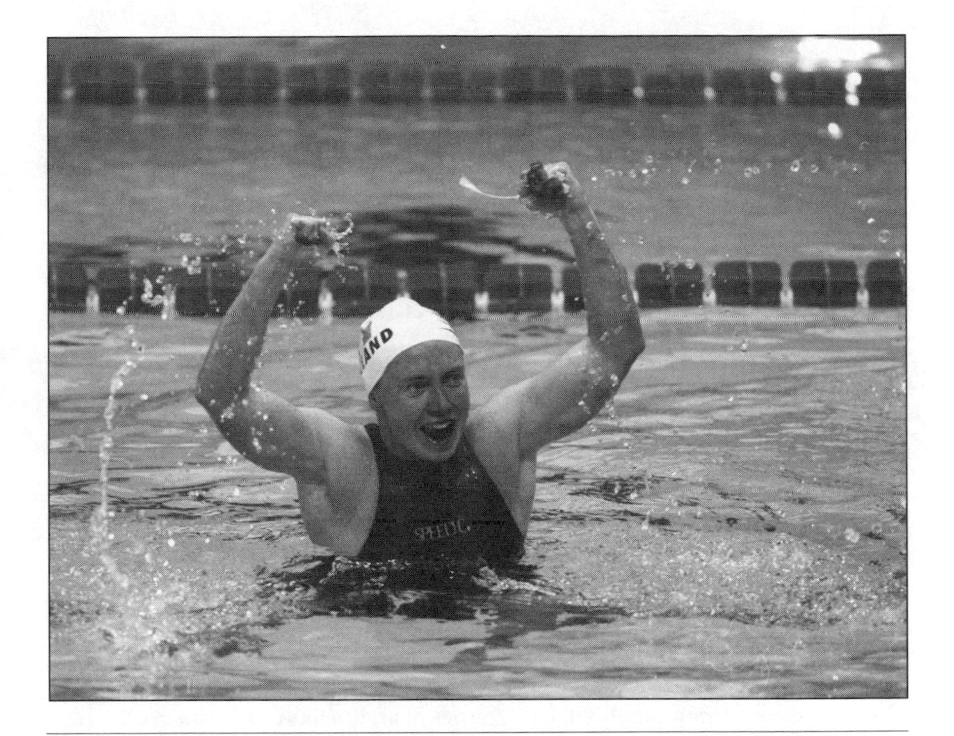

Ireland's Michelle Smith de Bruin won three gold medals at the 1996 Atlanta Olympic Games amid charges of drug use. In 1999, the international swimming federation banned de Bruin for four years, charging that she had tampered with a urine sample provided to drug testers.
© Michael Cooper/Allsport

financial support) are required to sign a contract agreeing to the testing (and many other things) in order to receive their funding. (Similar agreements are required by many national sport organizations and federations—the organizations in charge of selecting athletes to compete internationally.)

The suggestion that there is an overwhelming public interest that could supersede the assumption of privacy is implausible. Such an interest in public safety was postulated in Canada in 1991, when then Transport Minister Doug Lewis proposed the introduction of random drug testing for workers in the transport industry. The proposal was amended, since public interest sufficient to justify the random testing of transport workers and pilots was not perceived to exist. However, the principle of overwhelming public interest in safety is accepted in the case of random roadside breath testing for alcohol use (RIDE programs). If the public interest in safety is insufficient to justify random testing of transport workers, then the public interest in doping-free sport is likely to be insufficient to justify random testing of athletes. In the case of transport workers, the feared harm had to do with causing accidents, and the evidence was not there. Let us look at the arguments that are designed to show that doping should be banned because of the harm it causes to see if there is a sufficient justification to warrant the intrusions into privacy caused by enforcing bans through the required drug testing.

Arguments From Harm

During the Royal Commission of inquiry into drug-use in sport (the Dubin Commission), launched by the federal government of Canada as a result of the Ben Johnson scandal, many important players, such as Richard Pound, IOC vice president, testified on the subject.

> THE COMMISSIONER: And if you read the detailed list as I read it, in every case there is some reason for it apart from the ethics, a health reason.
>
> THE WITNESS: Yes, we think so [Richard Pound, IOC vice president].
>
> THE COMMISSIONER: And we know what all the side effects are, and as I understand certainly Sports [*sic*] Canada's policy of prohibiting the use of these drugs is twofold: One, because this is cheating. And secondly, because of health . . . one may put a higher priority on the other, probably health first (Dubin, 1990a: 13644).

One of the most commonly cited categories of arguments used to justify the bans on doping are those from harm. In this section we will look at four types of arguments from harm: (1) harm to users, (2) harm to other athletes, (3) harm to society, and (4) harm to the sport community. The purpose of this section is to analyze these arguments to see if they will work to justify RUT.

Harm to Users

The argument from harm to the user, in its simplest form, looks like this:

> Premise 1: Substance or practice X harms its user.
> Premise 2: Its user needs to be protected.
> Premise 3: The user can be protected by banning the substance.
> Conclusion: Therefore the substance should be banned.

It should be pointed out that the harm argument needs to be applied on a substance-by-substance basis. As we have seen, we cannot simply assume that all substances and practices on the current banned list cause harm to their users. Let us, however, consider, for example, the general argument in regard to adult rational athletes and the particular substance, anabolic steroids. We can examine it in three quite different ways.

Strictly speaking, the assertion that any steroid use harms the user is not scientifically, soundly proven because the medical evidence is mixed. Much of the evidence concerning harm is derived from anecdotal testimony of athletes using very high doses in uncontrolled conditions. On the other hand, the hard medical evidence from controlled low-dose studies tends to show minimal harm (Dubin, 1990a). Our society's abhorrence of the practice has prevented the gathering of hard, scientifically validated evidence because such research has yet to pass ethics committees when volunteers, who are already using steroids, come forward just to be monitored.[5] For premise one of the argument to work we would require far better data than is currently available. There are two elements to the harm charge: bad effects and the causal linkage of these to steroid doping. Currently it has not been scientifically proven just what bad effects come from steroid doping. This question about the truth of the first premise is, however, insufficient for us to dismiss the argument. So let us grant, for the sake of argument, that steroids do indeed harm their users, because it is not implausible, as we have heard now from testimony from the criminal trials in Germany on the former East German high-performance machine.

The second premise fails for different reasons. The desire to protect some other "competent" adult from the consequences of his or her own actions is paternalistic.[6] Banning doping, in the present context, would be a form of paternalism if it were done in order to protect the athlete. Paternalism has acceptable and unacceptable forms. For example, some argue that banning doping for minors is acceptable and banning doping for adults is unacceptable. However, there are cases in society where we ban practices for adults (e.g., driving without seat belts, or use of marijuana or cocaine, but not steroids). The question that must be addressed is, is banning steroids and other substances and practices an example of acceptable paternalism?[7]

In this section, because the focus is on adults, we will be referring to Feinberg's "hard" paternalism, the view that paternalism is sometimes justified even if the action is fully voluntary (Feinberg, 1977: 106-124).[8] Both R.L. Simon and W.M. Brown suggest that paternalistic interventions in the lives of adult competent athletes are unwarranted (Brown, 1980; Brown, 1984a; Brown, 1990; Simon, 1984a). In "Paternalism, Drugs, and the Nature of Sports," Brown describes his position as follows:

> At this point, we may resort to something like a principle of "hard" paternalism if we are to persist in our efforts to control the choices and options of [adult] athletes. We are in effect seeking to impose on those who resist it an alternative set of values. But what would justify such an imposition? There seems no reason to suppose that taking risk in sports, even great risk, is inevitably irrational, self-destructive, or immature, as we have seen. Nor is it plausible to suggest that we forbid all of the sports that involve such risk, such as mountain climbing, skydiving, or even boxing. As Mill (1859) argued, such intervention in people's lives would itself be a greater wrong than the possible injury of activities voluntarily chosen. We can indeed forbid the use of drugs in athletics in general, just as we do in the case of children. But ironically, in adopting such a paternalistic stance of insisting that we know better than the athletes themselves how to achieve some more general good, which they myopically ignore, we must deny in them the very attributes we claim to

value: self-reliance, personal achievement, and autonomy (Brown, 1984a: 20–21).

In "Good Competition and Drug-Enhanced Performance," Simon also reminds us of J.S. Mill's position. However, if we accept the "harm principle," which is defended by such writers as Mill, paternalistic interference with the freedom of others is ruled out. According to the harm principle, we are entitled to interfere with the behavior of competent, consenting adults only to prevent harm to others. After all, if athletes prefer the gains that the use of drugs provide along with possible side effects to the alternative of less risk but worse performance, external interference with their freedom of choice seems unwarranted. (Simon, 1984a: 8)

Generally we foster and value independence and the right to make the important choices that affect our own lives. We value autonomy.[9] Much of the thrust of modern North American medical ethics has been directed precisely against medical paternalism. To ban steroids solely to protect their competent adult users is to treat those athletes as children unable to make the choices that most affect them. As Brown (1980, 1984a,b, 1990) points out in all of his writings on this topic, this position is generally inconsistent with the limit-pushing nature of high-performance sport. The question to be asked is, why this inviolable boundary?

This second premise is unsuccessful for other reasons too. It is inconsistent at the least, and maybe even hypocritical, for sports governing bodies to attempt to justify a ban by appealing to the athlete's health and well being. There are many training practices and indeed many sports that carry a far greater likelihood of harm to the athlete than does the controlled use of steroids.[10] If the reason for banning doping in sport really were a concern for the health and well-being of athletes, there would be many sports and many more practices that should be banned. So at the very least, it seems inconsistent to argue in favor of the bans on doping and not the myriad other practices that are also harmful to the athletes.

One might try to argue that risks that are incurred by the nature of the sport, say, brain damage from having one's head pummeled in boxing, are different from risks that are incurred from practices that have nothing to do with competition in the sport per se, such as liver damage from steroid use. This suggestion works from the idea that we can distinguish between risks necessary in some sport and risks that are not. This is a promising suggestion, but one that is not yet complete. What is required is a method for distinguishing between a sport's necessary risks and those that are unnecessary. But this distinction is not going to be based on health.

Finally, the third premise fails because there is no evidence to suggest that banning steroids really would protect athletes. As long as a subculture exists that indicates that using steroids brings benefits and that it is an occupational hazard of high-level competitive sport, athletes will continue to use them in clandestine, unsanitary, and uncontrolled ways. Rectifying this is not just a matter of better enforcement of the ban, rather, it requires a change in values, and this will only happen after a logically consistent position for the ban has been put forward and the subculture in some sports changes.[11, 12] Presumably the ban would be intended as part of a larger process aimed at producing just such a change in values. Given the ban, for example, doping is cheating, so the negative value placed on cheating would be extended to doping, which might change athletes' attitudes toward doping but for different reasons. Further, even if it were argued that we might protect some, if not most, athletes from harm and that this makes the ban worthy of enactment, there are other harms caused by drug testing to enforce the bans—the violation of privacy—that must be weighed against this consideration.

Taken singly, the counterarguments motivated by our antipathy to paternalism and the inconsistency of a ban predicated upon the desire to protect athletes, are sufficient to show that the first argument from harm does not work. The justification of banning drugs such as steroids based on protecting "competent" and consenting adult users from harm stands in need of considerable strengthening.

Harm to Other Athletes

The second form of the argument from harm is based not on the harm that the steroids cause to their users, but on the harm their use causes to other athletes. The "others" in this argument are usually deemed to be other, "clean," athletes ("clean" simply means not doped). Sometimes this argument is called the "coercion" argument and it is more difficult to dismiss quickly. The same liberal tradition that prohibits paternalistic intervention permits interventions designed to prevent harm to others. The crucial questions will concern how great the harm is to other athletes and how severe the limitation on personal action. The argument runs like this:

Premise 1: An athlete's use of substance X causes harm to "clean" athletes.
Premise 2: Those people need protection.
Premise 3: Banning substance X will protect those people.
Conclusion: Therefore substance X should be banned.

In order to assess this argument we need to consider whether or not the potential coercion of clean athletes outweighs the infringement of the liberties of all athletes caused when a substance or practice is banned. Clean athletes are harmed, so the argument goes, because the dopers "up the ante." If some competitors are using steroids then all competitors who wish to compete at that level will need to take steroids or other substances to keep up.

T.M. Murray has argued that the competitive sport environment is inherently coercive in "The Coercive Power of Drugs in Sport." Murray says that because some athletes choose to take drugs to give them a competitive edge, others will be pressed to do likewise, or resign themselves to either accepting a competitive disadvantage or leaving the endeavor entirely (1983: 24). This limited choice is considered a genuine threat to athletes' life plans or their freedom, and further, it is a serious threat to human flourishing according to Murray. Thus, drug use is wrong because it is coercive, because of its potential for harm, and because it advances no social value (Murray, 1983: 30). Because we are dealing with health, harm, and drug testing in this chapter, the focus will be on Murray's first two points.

The problem with Murray's position, and others like it, is that elite-level competitive athletics is already a very high-stakes game. In order to compete effectively one has to dedicate oneself totally and submit to a minutely controlled training regimen that will dictate almost all aspects of one's life. Why is the upping of the ante caused by the use of steroids qualitatively different from the upping of the ante caused by the increasing professionalization of athletes and coaches and the mechanization of athletes that elite-level competition now requires? It might be argued that this criticism rests on the assumption that one must either ban all bad things, or none, and can be met with the reply that if we ban this one bad thing, that will at least be one bad thing the less. But, what remains to shown, is what it is about doping that is, in fact, the bad thing.

Although there is no question that elite athletes face the pressures that Murray is concerned about, and steroid use is definitely one of them, why single any of them out? One possible answer to this question may be that one particular practice is especially coercive, that the coercion is somehow more extreme. This reply is not very plausible. Any effective training practice "ups the ante," and many training practices are extremely onerous. Further, both Simon (1984a) and Brown (1984a) have argued that the choice of whether the risk of drug use is worth the gain should be left to the individual athlete to make, just as in the case of other risky training techniques.

The feeling that somehow steroid use is worse than longer and ever more specialized training just raises the question of why it is worse. Some may argue that the question really is: Why can't an athlete accept two "raises of the ante," but not accept a third, or an unlimited number? The answer to this question relies on a demand for consistency. There must be some reason why this, rather than that, practice is the one that is banned, and that reason cannot be merely that it was the third or the *n*th raise of the ante. This is a qualitative question, not a quantitative one, which necessarily requires an explanation for the rejection of the third raise of the ante, when there has been no rejection of the first two. It may be argued that the answer could be simply that two is acceptable but three is too many. But then we must ask which two, and the answer will inevitably appeal to a qualitative distinction.

Harm to Society

A second potential group that could be harmed by doping by athletes is the general public, in particular, children. People look up to athletes and view them as role models. If elite athletes (such as Ben Johnson and Mark McGwire) take drugs such as steroids, they are no longer suitable as role models and the general public has lost a significant benefit. There are several things to say in response here. The first will examine just why it is that steroid use disqualifies one from acting as a role model. The response might be that those who use steroids are cheats, and of course cheats cannot be role models. And, of course, this is true, because steroids are currently banned, but this just begs the question as why steroids have been banned in the first place. (The discussion about banning them was not raised until the late 1960s, even though it was well know that they were used in the 1950s. Further, another similar example can be found with blood doping, which was not banned until after 1984, and it is well known that many gold medallists have admitted doing it.)

A further response to the suggestion that athletes should be role models, and in particular "moral" role models, is to ask just why that should be so. We currently expect widely varying things of our public figures. No one seriously expects musicians or actors and actresses to be moral role models; why should athletes be singled out for special treatment? There is apparently quite widespread use of beta-blockers by concert musicians, yet there has not been the hue and cry and media circus that followed the revelations of drug use by athletes (Wolfe, 1989). Why do we expect more from athletes than from other public figures?

Paul Weiss (1969) argued that sport is one of the very first arenas young people experience and in which they hope to gain excellence: the excellence of their heroes.[13] From a societal perspective, if this hero is morally despicable, this will be a negative influence because young people will not separate the athletic abilities of their heroes from the quality of their personal lives, especially when fame and glamour surround the hero. Weiss also points out that the achievement of excellence in athletics comes before, and will influence greatly, the achievement of excellence in other arenas such as business, academia, and politics. Perhaps for these reasons we are more concerned about the moral image of athletes than that of other public figures.

First, what is not clear is why drug-assisted performance or excellence is negatively perceived (assuming we can put cheating aside for the moment until we establish a justification for the proscription on doping).[14] If it were public knowledge that, for example, Karen Cain, a famous Canadian ballerina, used painkillers to get through her excellent performance of "Swan Lake," would we hear the same outcry? Are fashion models less beautiful (if they are in fact beautiful) if they have used diuretics or "uppers" to lose their weight? Weiss's point is well taken, but what is it about drug use in sport that we find morally repugnant? For example, no one else is prevented from using cold remedies, even if they drive public transportation, or from using caffeine as a stimulant to work harder. So it is not even the case that we want athletes to meet the standards every one else meets, but rather, that we want them to meet more rigorous standards in regard to substance use.

The best avenue we have open to us to explore and strengthen this argument is that regarding athletes as role models for children. The recent example of Mark McGwire's drug use is a good case to strengthen this argument. There is apparently a good deal of anecdotal evidence to suggest that there was a marked rise in drug use by children in the United States; apparently these children aspired to be like McGwire. If a causal linkage could be determined, we could well be on the way to satisfying Mill's principle of sufficient harm. However, the work required to establish a causal linkage in this case, is yet to be done. Should this work be completed, we would definitely have grounds to reopen this argument.

It is sufficient to say at this point, as Simon has clearly stated, that until a clear and cogent reason is put forward to justify treating athletes differently from other public figures and until a causal link between their actions and harm to others has been demonstrated, we do not have a justification for RUT based on this argument alone.

Harm to the Sport Community

One other group that is potentially harmed is the sports-watching public. These people have been harmed because they have been cheated. They expected to see dope-free athletes battling it out in fair competition and they were denied this entertainment. This harm can be removed in other ways than through banning steroid use. One could remove the expectation that athletes are dope-free. If you do not expect them to be dope-free, you cannot be harmed if they are not. The feeling of being cheated is dependent on the idea that what was expected was a particular type of competition. But this response may be too quick. If what spectators want is doping-free competition, then their desire is not met by warning them that what they want is not to be found at the Olympics. At best, it is simply proposed (if not required) that they settle for less than what they really want. If they do not expect athletes to be dope-free, then indeed they do not suffer the harm of deception if they are not. But they might suffer other harms, for example, loss of the chance to watch doping-free competition. The question we need to answer is, why do they value doping-free competition? We do think that there is a very good answer to this question and have tried to capture in other work, as it requires a full and thorough discussion (Schneider and Butcher, 1994).

We have now examined the main variants of the harm argument. None has been found convincing. Of course, someone might argue that there are other harms caused by athletic doping (e.g., tempting the athlete to use recreational drugs), but it is doubtful that any of these harms would be sufficient to outweigh the harm *caused* by banning and testing for drugs and or other potential performance or training enhancing substances.

There is thus an insufficient justification in the harm caused by doping, itself, to warrant the intrusion caused by enforcing those bans. That leaves open the second option; that we might allow dope testing because the athletes consent to it. Unfortunately there are some challenging complications with gaining legitimate consent.

Problems With Consent

The following section considers several difficulties with the concept of legitimate, informed consent, as well as problems in obtaining it.

Consent and Autonomy

For consent to be valid, it has to be freely given (i.e., without coercion), informed, and made by a person competent to consent. Consent, like privacy, does not stand alone. It is assumed here that the requirement of consent, for example, for medical intervention and treatment, is grounded in the desire to protect and promote patient autonomy. The discussion of autonomy centers on the rights of individuals to make choices and to have control of their own lives. These rights have corresponding duties. If you have a right to be left alone, we have a duty not to interfere. The limits of these rights and duties could equally as easily have been approached from the standpoint of duties rather than the rights. Kant's (1985) discussion of autonomy is couched in these terms. For Kant, respect for autonomy entails that one cannot treat others as means but as ends only. What does this mean? One obvious meaning is that one cannot "touch" or interfere with a person without that person's permission. If you touch someone without their permission you violate their integrity, which in turn, violates their autonomy. Veatch, in *A Theory of Medical Ethics*, puts it like this:

> From the standpoint of one committed to the principle of autonomy, consent is required independent of the calculations of consequences if a person is to be touched, if privacy is to be invaded, or if the person is to be used in research, therapy, or preventative medicine, if a person is to be treated as an end and not as a means only, then permission is needed when that person is brought into the professional medical nexus. (Veatch, 1981: 201)

Veatch is here emphasizing that if one takes any action that involves another person, in order to prevent the possibility of treating people as means rather than as ends in themselves, one must first seek the other person's permission. The principle of autonomy, however, is stronger than this. The requirement of permission before interference could be met by simple assent to a minimal physical description of the procedure to be followed. This, however, would not be sufficient to satisfy the positive aspects of autonomy. Acquiescence is not autonomous choice. For example, it is possible to argue that the current method of gaining consent from Canadian athletes to test them is invalid because they are told that if they do not sign, they will not get any money and they will be ineligible for selection to Canadian teams, so they acquiesce. Further, a stronger claim regarding this method of gaining consent would be that athletes living below the poverty line are actually coerced into signing because they cannot continue to compete without financial aid, unlike the more wealthy athletes. This does not mean, however, that a person cannot autonomously choose to forgo either information or indeed the decision making itself, for example, to let the coach decide. It might be argued that it is perfectly acceptable for a person to request that someone else make a decision for them. What is not acceptable is for the coach or team physician to assume athlete compliance and merely present a course of action for acquiescence.

However, to satisfy the stronger aspects of autonomy a person must make decisions that affect his or her welfare. Athletes, therefore, are the ones who have to decide if they will follow the procedure. To satisfy the demands of autonomy, athletes cannot simply acquiesce to the procedure chosen by the coach or team physician; they must actively choose the procedure in the first place. Respect for autonomy thus requires that the consent doctrine have two distinct parts. The first, and weaker, requirement is that one cannot act upon, or interfere with, other people without their permission. If one does, one breaches the area of inviolability, which is an integral part of personal integrity and autonomy. The second, and stronger, requirement is that people should make all decisions that pertain to their welfare, indeed that they should decide just what it is that comprises their welfare. As a final word on the way autonomy may ground consent, if the model assumed in the coach/physician/athlete relationship is contractual, the model itself presupposes that the contractors are autonomous. One cannot enter into a binding contract unless one is an autonomously acting agent.

Consent and Minors

Another important issue involves consent and minors because many of the federally funded athletes are minors. Any person consenting to an intervention must be competent to do so. It is generally assumed that adults are competent, unless shown to be otherwise, and that minors are not. In the latter case, usually a parent or a guardian may consent to an intervention on behalf of a minor. This has worked well enough in the case of consent to medical treatment designed to benefit a minor. In Canada, however, recent court cases have ruled that a parent or guardian is not in a position to give consent for interferences related to research that do not have the prospect of direct benefit for the minor. This is usually referred to as "nontherapeutic research." For example, it is currently impossible in Canada to get a valid permission to draw blood from healthy children to establish a "normal" baseline from which to measure abnormal deviations in subsequent tests. Urine testing in RUT has clear similarities to nontherapeutic research on children. It may therefore be that it is impossible to get a valid consent on behalf of a minor to RUT in Canada at this time. The consequence of this is that a minor, tested in the absence of a valid consent, could be in a position to sue the testing agent for assault, not unlike a case involving touching without consent.

The Scope of Consent

The scope of consent may also be difficult to determine. The inherently coercive power imbalance between an individual and a state agency that requests consent for a drug test has already been alluded to. This imbalance is exacerbated by the possible consequences of the test result. Testing positive for steroid use can ruin an athletic career and, in some cases, destroy a livelihood. This may be viewed as an appropriate result given that the purpose of RUT is primarily to deter steroid use. However, the banned list currently contains a variety of drugs that are also used for recreational purposes, in particular cocaine and marijuana. These substances do not appear to have any training-enhancing properties, and their possible performance-enhancing properties are irrelevant outside competition. In giving consent to RUT, an athlete is consenting to being tested at any time for drugs that have no relation to his or her training, but which do carry the risk of criminal prosecution. The potential consequences of a consent to RUT may have the result that it is impossible for an athlete to give a consent that is genuinely informed.

Consent, Coercion, and the Role of Government

First, the Canadian government has taken specific steps to limit its own intrusion into the privacy of Canadian citizens. The *Privacy Act* exists, at least in part, to recognize the extreme imbalance in power between governments and individuals. This imbalance renders some requests by governments for permission from individuals inherently coercive. The Privacy Commissioner argues that in seeking permission for RUT, the government would be breaking its own rules established in the *Privacy Act* and in the *Charter of Rights and Freedoms* (*Charter*).

> One can hope that Justice Dubin will recognize that athletes should not be forced to abandon their *Charter* rights at the locker room door—no matter how many may be willing to do precisely that in order to compete in their sport. *Charter* rights also apply to federally funded athletes: random mandatory drug testing of athletes would be found to violate sections 7 or 8, or both, of the *Charter*. On almost all counts, random mandatory testing of athletes would fail to measure up. Thus, not only would such a program fail to comply with the *Charter*, it would, if conducted by Sport Canada, be a violation of the *Privacy Act*. (1990: p. 43)

This interpretation of the *Charter* and the *Privacy Act* has not, naturally enough, met with universal acceptance. Justice Dubin himself took the view that the Privacy Commissioner's views were wide of the mark. One answer might be that if the *Charter* prevents the government from making sure that the athletes are doping-free, then it should stop funding athletes altogether. This is in fact the position that Dubin takes. We do not need to judge the legal aspect of this argument, however; if we take the view that unreasonable search and seizure provisions of the *Charter* and the *Privacy Act* are designed to protect autonomy, then the position of the Privacy Commissioner is surely right. Government insistence on testing would be coercive and unjustified.

All of these difficulties are predicated on the assumption that the method of testing requires a urine sample. There is an additional invasion of privacy (one quite often cited by athletes as troubling) because the sample must be produced under the observation of the testing agent. Currently, there is a trend toward adding blood tests. Although this will save athletes' modesty, it will introduce an invasive testing procedure, one that enters the body, to replace one that did not.

One objection to the requirement of consent is that sport is somehow different, in that the usual requirements of consent fail to apply. These arguments are unconvincing, but they warrant our attention.

Sport Is Different

The Canadian government, Justice Dubin, and Sport Canada, in discussions of the topic have suggested that "sport is different." They have argued that, because of this difference, the limitations imposed by the requirements of consent do not apply. The suggestion is that participation in "high-performance" sport is a privilege, not a right. In chapter 24 of the *Dubin Report* on athletes' rights, in which Ken Read (a former Olympian) and Dubin claim that participation in sport is a privilege not a right, it is argued that the imposition of otherwise unjustifiable conditions is acceptable as a precondition of participation in sport (1990b: 490-491). Their argument is that athletes are not deprived of their rights if they are deemed ineligible because they will not submit to a drug test, because they do not have a right to participate in the first place. The serious consequences of this argument is that it would allow the imposition of any rules no matter how absurd, for it says that the authorities may impose whatever rules they like, but would not have to *justify* such rules.

Further, this argument is unclear. It may mean that no person has the *right* to be selected for a national team or for carding support. This is certainly true, but it is also true that there is some obligation to select the best available people for national teams and, barring income tests (which are currently not performed), for carding too. It could then be argued that the "best available person" means the best person available who abides by the rules of the sport, one of which is the requirement that athletes consent to RUT. However, the rules of sport are not arbitrary and they themselves are open to moral scrutiny. Just as a rule of eligibility that barred people on the basis of race would be objected to on moral grounds, other rules of eligibility for sport are open to similar moral assessment. If, therefore, RUT is unacceptable on the moral ground that it invades privacy, it would be unacceptable for there to be a rule of eligibility that required RUT. Sport may well be different, but nothing is so special or different that it can escape all moral scrutiny from those outside of sport.

Summary

The harm arguments, on the surface, appeared quite powerful. After all, the one generally accepted limitation on individual liberty is that one's actions might harm others. But as we saw, the harm argument comes in a variety of forms, some of which are more potent than others. There are also important limitations on the arguments from harm, limitations that stem from the requirements of consistency and balance.

The argument that seeks to justify RUT on the basis of the harm doping causes to the adult user is paternalistic and inconsistent. Although some cases of paternalism may be justified, we argue that this case is not. With athletes who are competent adults there are no grounds to intervene to prevent them from harming themselves through doping. The argument is inconsistent because there are many other risks of harm that are not banned. (Even if we accept that some of those risks are inherent in the sports themselves, and therefore somehow justified, others, such as the risk of injury through excessive training, are not.)

Harm to other athletes is the most cogent form of the harm argument. The best form of this argument is that doping harms other athletes in that it coerces them into accepting risks of harm that are not essential to the sport being practiced. Banning, and the measures required to enforce it, is justified to protect other athletes. This argument provides a strong argument for banning certain drugs or practices (for example, the use of strychnine by marathon runners). However, the argument has its limitations. The first is that it needs to be applied practice by practice, drug by drug, and sport by sport (indeed, it may even be necessary to evaluate not just substances but amounts ingested or methods of administration). The second is that not only would it only work for some items on the banned list, but consistent application would require that we ban other nonessential but harmful practices (for instance, we might wish to limit training). Third, the harm caused by the practices concerned has to be weighed against the harm caused by enforcing bans through drug testing. Although the harm caused by enforcing a ban on a performance enhancer, a test on the day of the competition, is relatively minor, the requirements of enforcing bans on training enhancers are quite onerous. In this case it might turn out that the harm caused by enforcing a ban outweighs the harm caused by the banned practice itself. The conclusion here is that although harm to other athletes may well feature in the justification for banning certain elements of doping, it cannot stand alone as the whole story.

A further major problem with random, unannounced out-of-competition mandatory testing is that it may not be possible to establish a selection procedure for testing that would have, as eligible candidates, all and only prospective national team athletes. For example, it would be unfair if an athlete were able to avoid testing, perhaps through training outside of the country, or by refusing to accept government support or carding. Examples of this sort of unfairness could lead to challenges to the validity of the entire doping control protocol.

Against all of these drawbacks, however, is the most cogent consideration in favor of RUT, which is that one cannot have doping-free sport without it. That is, one cannot have doping-free sport without RUT given the value system that now prevails among athletes and their coaches, but that value system might change, or be made to change.

There is thus an impasse; the value of privacy indicates that RUT is unacceptable, yet, given the current bans on doping, fair high-performance sport requires it.

Possible Solutions

The following section contains several changes that could be made to current policy and procedures that might provide solutions to the current problems in testing.

Athlete-Driven Testing

All of the discussion so far has been based on the idea that the governing bodies of sport and governments decide on rules and then impose them on those who would play. An alternative is to turn part of the formulation of rules, in particular rules of eligibility, over to the athletes, the ones to whom the rules apply. There is some evidence that the majority of athletes would prefer doping-free sport if it could be guaranteed that the competition is fair. What is missing is the guarantee. Often athletes feel compelled to take drugs to even-up the competitive playing field.

If athletes agree that they want doping-free sport, and if they also agree that they are prepared to take the necessary steps to achieve the thing they want, then they could be in the position to request an agency to conduct testing on their behalf. Thus, instead of governments and the governing bodies of sport imposing rules, the athletes would set their own rules and request that an outside agency enforce them. Thus, athletes would be limiting their own liberty while their autonomy is clearly unfettered. They take steps to curtail their liberty in the short term in order to preserve or enhance their liberty in the long run. One possible way of constructing this reasoning and decision-making process is to use the prisoner's dilemma model.[15] To avoid the less than optimal outcome that results from self-interested decision making in a prisoner's dilemma, athletes could collectively request testing to gain an outcome they all in fact want, but which none can individually achieve. In this way, the agency conducting the testing is not acting on behalf of governments or sports bodies, but on behalf of athletes. The government or governing bodies of sport cannot then be seen as interfering in the lives of its citizen athletes. (In terms of moral philosophy the approach we are proposing is contractarian. This means that the power of the justification relies essentially on genuine athlete agreement. Whether this agreement could be found is an empirical question.) However, to achieve this sort of agreement, steps would have to be taken to minimize the negative impact of bans and testing.

Minimizing the Athlete's Loss of Freedom

For an athlete-driven system of testing to gain the maximum acceptance by athletes, it should permit only the minimum intrusion required to obtain the desired effect. The desired effect of RUT is to eliminate the use of training-enhancing drugs. Logically, then, one does not need to test for performance-enhancing drugs out of competition.

There are four advantages to athlete-driven testing: (1) Athletes and other interest groups could create a system to choose and enforce doping-free sport. (2) Athletes retain their freedom; in other words, they request RUT to preserve something they want. (3) The intrusion into athletes' lives is minimized by only testing for training-enhancing substances out of competition. (4) Government cannot be accused of unfairly interfering in the private lives of its citizens. However, the prerequisites for this model are hard to meet: (1) A proper survey of athletes' opinions on this topic would have to be undertaken. (2) Strong support among athletes would have to exist in order for a genuinely athlete-driven model to work. (3) Governments and national sport organizations would have to share their power in the realm of testing. Although they would still be responsible for in-competition testing, they would not have control of RUT. (4) A great deal of international cooperation on this topic would have to exist. It is not clear that athletes from countries that adopted this model would wish to compete with athletes from countries that did not. (5) The proposal does not deal with the problem of consent from minors.

The new international doping agency, WADA, has a fundamental choice before it. There is unprecedented international agreement that doping control measures should be effective. There does seem to be some evidence that athletes want doping-free sport. The choice facing the new agency is whether to proceed with business as usual, with the content of the banned list devised by sports administrators and imposed on athletes, or to actively seek a genuine athlete agreement that gives power over the content of the banned list—and the means of enforcement—to those to whom the rules apply. If athletes view the rules as imposed from the outside and fundamentally against their own personal self-interest, we will be doomed to the ultimately fruitless and self-defeating game of tester against cheat. The outcome of that game will be the eventual abandonment of doping control—in just the same way that the IOC abandoned amateurism.

There are immense practical difficulties in introducing an athlete-driven system that would provide the protection athletes want while truly honoring their autonomy and their privacy. However, we believe that the values of sport and of personal autonomy and privacy are such that we should try to take those steps, and we also believe that the majority of athletes truly want a doping-free system.

Acknowledgment

The authors would like to thank the Canadian Centre for Ethics in Sport for partial funding for the research of this article.

Bibliography

Blackhurst, M., Schneider, A., and Strachan, D. 1991. *Values and Ethics in Amateur Sport*. London: Fitness and Amateur Sport, Canada.

Breivik, G. 1987. The doping dilemma: Some game theoretical and philosophical considerations. *Sportwissenschaft* 17(1): 83-94.

Breivik, G. 1992. Doping games: A game theoretical exploration of doping. *International Review for Sociology of Sport* 27: 235-252.

Brown, W. 1980. Ethics, Drugs, and Sport." *Journal of the Philosophy of Sport* 7: 15-23.

Brown, W. 1984a. Paternalism, drugs, and the nature of sports. *Journal of the Philosophy of Sport* 11:14-22.

Brown, W. 1984b. Comments on Simon and Fraleigh. *Journal of the Philosophy of Sport* 11: 33-35.

Brown, W. 1990. Practices and prudence. *Journal of the Philosophy of Sport* 17: 71-84.

Dubin, C. 1990a. *Commission of Inquiry into the Use of Drugs and Banned Practices Intended to Increase Athletic Performance*. Transcripts. Toronto.

Dubin, C. 1990b. *Commission of Inquiry into the Use of Drugs and Banned Practices Intended to Increase Athletic Performance*. Ottawa: Canadian Government Publishing Centre.

Feinberg, J. 1977. Legal paternalism. *Canadian Journal of Philosophy* 1: 106-124.

Gaylin, W. 1984. Feeling good and doing better. In T.H. Murray, W. Gaylin, and R. Macklin, eds., *Feeling Good and Doing Better: Ethics and Nontherapeutic Drug Use*. Totowa, New Jersey: Humana Press, pp. 1-10.

Gledhill, N. 1982. Blood doping and related issues: A brief review. *Medicine and Science in Sports and Exercise* 14(3): 183-189.

International Olympic Charter Against Doping in Sport. 1990a. Lausanne, Switzerland.

International Olympic Committee. 1987. *The Olympic Movement*. Lausanne, Switzerland.

Kant, I. 1985. *Critique of Pure Reason*. N. Kemp Smith, trans. London: Macmillan Publishers.

Luce, R., and Raiffa, H. 1967. *Games and Decisions*, New York: John Wiley and Sons.

Mill, J. 1978. *On Liberty*. Indianapolis: Hackett Publishers.

Murray, T. 1983. The coercive power of drugs in sport. *The Hastings Center Report* 13: 24-30.

Murray, T. 1986a. Drug testing and moral responsibility. *Physician and Sportsmedicine* 14(1): 47-48.

Murray, T. 1986b. Human growth hormone in sports: No. *Physician and Sportsmedicine* 14(5): 29.

Murray, T. 1987. The ethics of drugs in sport. In R.H. Strauss, ed., *Drugs and Performance in Sports*. Philadelphia: W.B. Saunders, pp. 11-21.

Privacy Commissioner of Canada. 1990. *Drug Testing and Privacy*. Ottawa: Supply and Services Canada.

Schneider, A.J. 1993. Doping in sport and the perversion argument. In G. Gaebauer, ed., *The Relevance of the Philosophy of Sport*. Berlin: Academia Verlag, pp. 117-128.

Schneider, A.J., and Butcher, R.B. 1991. The mésalliance of the Olympic ideal and doping. In F. Landry, M. Landry, and M. Yerles, eds. *Sport . . . the Third Millennium*. Sainte-Foy: Les Presses de l'Université Laval, pp. 495-504.

Schneider, A.J., and Butcher, R.B. 1994. Why Olympic athletes should avoid the use and seek the elimination of performance-enhancing substances and practices in the Olympic Games. *Journal of the Philosophy of Sport* 20 and 21: 64-81.

Schneider, A.J., and Butcher, R.B. 1998. Fair play as respect for the game. *Journal of the Philosophy of Sport 25*: 1-22.
Simon, R.L. 1984a. Good competition and drug-enhanced performance. *Journal of the Philosophy of Sport*. 21: 6-13.
Simon, R.L. 1984b. Response to Brown and Fraleigh. *Journal of the Philosophy of Sport* 21: 30-32.
Simon, R.L. 1991. *Fair Play: Sports, Values and Society*. Boulder, CO: Westview Press.
Sport Canada. 1985. *Drug Use and Doping Control in Sport*. Ottawa: Fitness and Amateur Sport.
Veatch, R. 1981. *A Theory of Medical Ethics*. New York: Basic Books.
Weiss, P. 1969. *Sport: A Philosophic Inquiry*. Carbondale, IL: Southern Illinois University Press.
Wolfe, Mary L. 1989. Correlates of adaptive and maladaptive musical performance anxiety. *Medical Problems of Performing Artists*, March, 49-56.

Notes

[1]This is still true despite more positive tests. The game of testing and masking is constantly evolving. If one knows when one is to be tested one has a far greater opportunity to seek to thwart the test.

[2]Notably, the IOC has dropped the criterion of "performance enhancement" from any justification for the banned list because scientists have pointed out to them that the evidence is mixed in regard to the performance-enhancing abilities of the substances and practices on the banned list.

[3]Under the doping class of stimulants in the IOC *International Olympic Charter Against Doping in Sport* (1990), products like these are listed on page 2.4: "Thus no product for use in colds, flu or hay fever purchased by a competitor or given to him/her should be used without first checking with a doctor or pharmacist that the product does not contain a drug of the banned stimulants class."

[4]Later in this article, we will examine the suggestion that doping could be banned on the paternalistic ground that it is good for the athletes concerned. At this stage we are concentrating on the testing procedures themselves.

[5]Personal communication from N. Gledhill who testified as an expert witness on doping from the sport sciences at the Dubin Inquiry.

[6]The basic notion is that individuals are deemed to be competent to make their own decisions unless they are minors or are demonstrated to be "incompetent" from a medical/legal perspective.

[7]For the purposes of this chapter, we will concentrate on the justification of bans imposed on competent adults. We will leave open the discussion of whether it may be possible to prohibit minors from doping. Most writers assume that this is possible. This raises an interesting difficulty. If we ban doping for minors, but

do not ban it for adults, and if adults and minors compete against each other in the Olympic Games (which they do in some sports), then we would have the odd situation of different rules applying to different competitors. This would not be fair. One might therefore conclude that doping should be banned for adults so that the competition between them and children might be fair. An alternative would be to ban minors from competing in the Olympic Games (there are currently minimum age requirements but they are well below the standard age of majority, e.g., 13 in some cases). Given the enormous amount of time and commitment required to reach Olympic levels, permitting children to compete may well be placing an intolerable burden upon them—a burden they are not fully able to consent to or to choose.

[8]It should be made clear at this point that this argument from paternalism operates only in the case of so called "competent" adults; different considerations come into play when the people one seeks to protect are children or are deemed not to be competent to make their own decisions. We are not going to engage the philosophical problems surrounding the issue of competence in this study as it deserves a full study itself.

[9]Once again, as with the issue of competence, we will not be discussing all of the philosophical problems with definitions of the concept of autonomy because the discussion of this topic is too large for the scope of this chapter.

[10]One need only note the deaths in cycling, boxing, and alpine skiing.

[11]The concept of "positive deviance" is proposed to account for this type of behavior by some sociologists of sport.

[12]We have argued extensively in "Fair Play as Respect for the Game" (Schneider and Butcher, 1998), that in sport there is an essential connection between playing and outcome. Doping does not enhance playing, and only enhances outcome when one competes against someone who does not dope. See also Schneider and Butcher, 1994.

[13]Weiss only refers to heroes but presumably he would also include heroines. We will treat his work as if it does include both males and females.

[14]Brown believes that the reason drugs in sport continue to be an issue is a result of North American's obsession with drugs in our society in general (1990: 71).

[15]See Schneider and Butcher, 1994.

6
CHAPTER

Comparative Analysis of Doping Scandals: Canada, Russia, and China

Bruce Kidd
University of Toronto
Robert Edelman
University of California, San Diego
Susan Brownell
University of Missouri, St. Louis

This collective essay is not about doping itself. Rather, it seeks to examine official discourses about doping in three very different national contexts. We are not in a position to judge guilt or innocence in any particular case, nor are we able to reveal deeper, especially state-sponsored, conspiracies. Our intention is simply to demonstrate how the attitudes of sport officials about the use of performance-enhancing drugs reveal larger truths about the Canadian, Russian, and Chinese understanding of their place in the global community. As rapid globalization changes each nation's often conflicted sense of itself, reactions to doping incidents turn out to be significant markers of each country's position in the world diplomatic order.

As is inevitable in comparisons of this type, we want to identify what elements are generic in official reactions to doping scandals and which are specific to each country. Embarrassment appears universal. No one says, "We dope and are proud." Similarly, the appearance of scandals in three such different political systems and cultures demonstrates the close, perhaps inevitable, link between elite sport and performance-enhancing drugs. Yet, when confronted with charges made by international authorities, officials in each nation have felt their moral values challenged, but each country has responded differently to scandal. Here Canadian shame, Russian uncertainty, and Chinese outrage reveal much about national identity and self-image. As the global political and cultural environment has changed rapidly, officials and citizens of all nations have had to reexamine their relationships with the outside world. In this sense, the doping scandal becomes a useful and revealing litmus test. At the same time, this comparison can show those concerned with the problem of performance-enhancing drugs the difficulties of making sense of the problem in sharply differing settings.

Canada

Canadians pride themselves on one of the strictest regimes of doping control in sport. Since 1984, when mandatory domestic testing was introduced for athletes in amateur and Olympic sport, the number of annual tests has risen tenfold to the point where approximately 2,000 urine samples are examined each year by the Canadian Centre for Ethics in Sport (CCES), the independent agency created by the federal government for the purpose, at a cost of $2C million, or 5 percent of the federal sports budget.[1] About 75 percent of these tests are "unannounced," away from competition. Any nationally ranked or Canadian Interuniversity Athletic Union athlete may be required to provide a sample for the CCES's roving doping control officers either on the spot ("no notice") or within 36 hours ("short notice"). An athlete who is suspected of drug use may be "target tested" on an unannounced basis. Stars like Olympic sprint champion Donovan Bailey may undergo as many as 15 unannounced tests a year (in addition to the domestic and international in-competition tests they are required to take).[2] The sanctions imposed for a positive result tend to be far more severe than those meted out elsewhere in the sport world. For example, there is an automatic minimum four-year suspension for first infractions, when the penalty for similar infractions in most international federations is two years. Any coach convicted of a doping offense is banned for life. The Canadian government has also forged provincial and international agreements to extend the scope of doping control as broadly as possible.[3]

These measures enjoy widespread support. In national public opinion surveys in 1989 and 1991, the majority of respondents indicated that "it is more important to compete fairly than win at all costs." Eighty-seven percent of those interviewed said that it is "extremely important" that Canadian athletes compete without cheating or bending the rules, even though 40 percent believed that international sport is not a "level playing field" because of the use of performance-enhancing drugs. The majority of respondents said that the primary purpose of sport should be character building and fostering personal development. Subsequent surveys have found much the same.[4] During the 1990s, the effort to stamp out doping in sport stimulated an agonizing reappraisal of the Canadian sport system and enabled major challenges to the Canadian sport power structure and long accepted practices of training and competition. It shifted the dominant discourse among sport leaders from "the ideology of excellence,"[5] the unabashed pursuit of the podium, to the commitment to "values-led" and "athlete-centered" sport.

This section of the paper will briefly describe and analyze the impact of doping on Canadian sport. It will be argued that the deep concern with sport doping in Canada can be explained by the convergent trajectories of amateurism, nationalism, and the state, on the bifurcated landscape of Canadian sport. None of the CCES's doping controls apply to the highly salaried athletes who labor in the commercial (and for the most part continental) sport cartels, such as the Canadian Football League, Major League Baseball, the National Basketball Association, and the National Hockey League. The burden of moral leadership in sport, and arguably the society as a whole, is borne entirely by the state-led sector of Olympic sport.

Johnson, Dubin, and the Search for Integrity

Canada's anti-doping regime sprang directly from the perceived national disgrace associated with revelations that athletes were enhancing their natural abilities with drugs. In the fall of 1983, positive tests by Canadian and other athletes at the Pan American Games in Cuba, and the arrest of four members of the Canadian weightlifting team in possession of a large quantity of contraband steroids at the Montreal airport, raised fears that drugs were rife in Canadian sport. Almost immediately, the federal Ministry of Fitness and Amateur Sport ordered sport governing bodies receiving federal financial assistance to establish their own testing regimes and provided funds to the Sport Medicine Council of Canada to conduct the testing. By the summer of 1988, it also won agreement for what became the International Charter Against Drugs in Sport, signed by 28 countries on the eve of the Seoul Olympics.

Yet many in the sport community feared that these measures were ineffective, and that some Canadian sport and government officials were turning a blind eye to steroid use among prominent Canadian athletes. These fears seemed to be borne out when four Olympic weightlifters were found to have steroids in their system before leaving for Seoul. When Ben Johnson won the 100-meter final in Seoul with a record-shattering run, several prominent athletes and coaches refused to stand for the Canadian anthem during the victory ceremony. "I refuse to stand up for a cheater, even if he does beat the tests again—it sends a distorted signal about what sport should be about," distance runner Paul Williams said at the time.

Johnson's disqualification for steroids just 36 hours after the victory ceremony turned the "speaking bitterness groups" within the amateur sport community into an intense national debate. Among the public, his victory unleashed a weekend of heady celebration. The triumph of a humble, working-class immigrant of color, encouraged in his abilities by a popular public program, in the most elemental and accessible of sporting events, reassured Canadians about their ability to succeed in the age of fiercely competitive globalization. The previous year, Johnson's world-record championship dash in Rome and Team Canada's thrilling victory in the Canada Cup hockey tournament were believed to have had the same effect. Sensing this in Seoul, at a reception just a few hours after Johnson's run, Lyle Makosky, the deputy minister for amateur sport, gleefully told me that "now the prime minister can call the (free trade) election."[6]

In Canada, news of the disqualification on a hungover Sunday morning turned pride and elation into anger and disgrace, reawakened fears about the future of the country, and brought the whole sport system into question. To be sure, because it took almost a year before Johnson himself admitted to steroid use, denial, doubt, and conspiracy theories (e.g., Carl Lewis changed the bottles; the IOC Medical Commission sought a scapegoat to salvage its reputation for complicity) were among the responses. Despite what has been alleged, few blamed Johnson, or rejected him as an immigrant.[7] To defuse the concern and uncertainty, the federal government immediately appointed a commission of inquiry, chaired by the then associate chief justice of Ontario, Charles Dubin.

The Dubin Commission galvanized the country. Daily hearings were held in Toronto and Montreal, with front-page coverage and a national television audience. Athletes and coaches gave emotional accounts of the economic difficulties they experienced and pressures they faced to win. While some asked for sympathy, confessing to the embarrassing intimacies of obtaining, injecting, and masking steroids, others called for harsh penalties for users. Perhaps, given the symbolic dimension of the crisis and Dubin's conservative leanings, the inquiry was headed one way from the beginning.[8] But it did face a concerted attempt to normalize the use of performance-enhancing drugs and techniques. Johnson's coach, Charlie Francis, was virtually alone in arguing for an end to the doping protocol with his own version of competitive fairness—everyone else is doing it, so why shouldn't we?[9] But others such as Angela Schneider (in interventions similar to those she made at this conference) wondered about the contradictions implicit in the increased application of science to some aspects of training and the prohibition on applying it to others; the privileging of doping controls as the measure of the "level playing field" while widening class, gender, and regional inequalities were ignored; the health risks involved in "driving steroids underground"; and the economic and social costs of policing. The Olympic movement and governments such as Canada's were seen to be sharpening these contradictions by heightening the rewards of victory.[10] These complexities led one senior official of the Canadian Olympic Association, a physician, to wager privately that before the year 2025 the IOC will "return the gold medal Ben Johnson won in Seoul, just as it returned the gold medals Jim Thorpe won in Stockholm."

For Dubin, however, the issue was cut and dried: The use of banned performance-enhancing drugs to improve performance beyond one's own natural ability is cheating. Cheating is the antithesis of sport. The widespread use of such drugs has threatened the essential integrity of sport and is destructive of its very objectives. It also erodes the ethical and moral values of athletes who use them, endangering their mental and physical welfare while demoralizing the entire sport community.[11]

Dubin cited "the failure of many sport-governing bodies (including the IOC and Sport Canada) to treat the drug problem more seriously and to take more effective

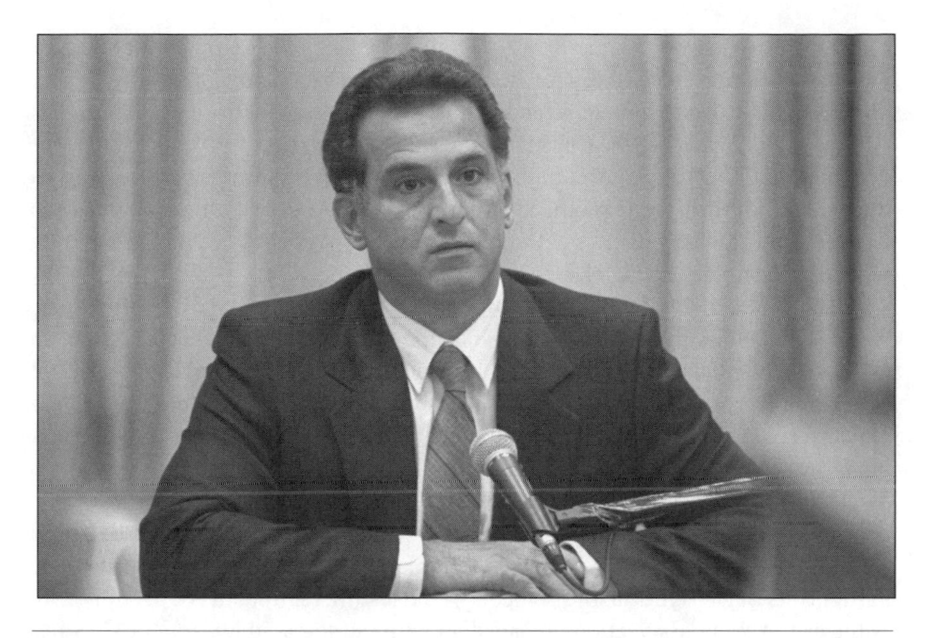

Dr. Jamie Astaphan, who supplied Ben Johnson and other Canadian athletes with banned performance-enhancing drugs, testifying during the Dubin Inquiry.
© Allsport UK/Allsport

means to detect and deter the use of drugs by athletes." Among his 70 recommendations, he called for a value-based approach to public funding, the creation of an agency independent of government and the sport governing bodies to assume responsibility for doping control, an emphasis upon unannounced out-of-competition testing, and the criminalization of anabolic steroids, with greater penalties for illegal possession, importation, and trafficking. Clearly, the athletes and coaches who had characterized doping as a "moral crisis" requiring a stern response had won his ear. In the months following the report's publication, other inquiries, seminars, and conferences were undertaken to consider, mediate, and implement its recommendations—in the House of Commons, in the Ministry of Fitness and Amateur Sport, in the Canadian Olympic Association, and among schools, colleges, and universities. As a result of these discussions, a strong consensus that opposition to performance-enhancing drugs should be a matter of national priority emerged among coaches, civil servants, sport administrators, and the public.[12]

Toward the "Athlete-Centered System"

The most enduring legacy of Johnson and Dubin has been the creation of the testing regime administered by the Canadian Centre for Ethics in Sports (CCES). First known as the Canadian Anti-Doping Organization, and then as the Centre for Drug-Free Sport, the Centre was established in 1991 to assume the responsibilities previously carried out by the Sports Medicine and Science Council of Canada, which felt compromised because it also appointed physicians and other health professionals to national teams, and actively supported sport science research.[13] Although it is funded by the Canadian government, it is responsible to an independent board of directors. The authority for its activities is contractual: it stems from the constitutions of the participating sport governing bodies, which adopted the Centre's anti-doping policies and rules as their own as a condition of continuing federal government financial support.[14]

The Centre quickly implemented the "no notice" and "targeted" testing recommended by Dubin. Initially preoccupied by the methodology of test analysis, in an effort to ensure the accuracy of results, it gradually mounted an ambitious series of educational programs and services, including an 800-number "hotline" where athletes, coaches, and physicians can inquire about the composition of pharmaceuticals. An important concern is the apparent widespread use of performance-enhancing drugs among young athletes. A 1993 survey of students from sixth grade and above estimated that 2.8 percent of the school cohort, or 83,000, had used steroids during the previous year.[15] Most recently, it has sought to strengthen participants' legal rights in the protocols of the testing regime. In cooperation with Athletes CAN, an association of Canadian national team athletes, the CCES has undertaken to improve procedural fairness, helping to establish an Alternate Dispute Resolution Program for Amateur Sport and other safeguards.[16]

The realization of the other changes sought by Dubin has proven more elusive. The Chief Justice recommended that federal sport policy "reflect a commitment to broad participation in sport, not solely a focus on elite sport," and actively assist women, disadvantaged groups, and persons with disabilities, while ameliorating regional disparities. He also recommended that "individuals and organizations in receipt of government funding meet the ethical standards as well as the performance standards required for funding."[17] In the aftermath of the commission's report, several attempts were made to achieve these goals. Perhaps the most heroic effort to do so was the Canadian Sport Council, a pan-Canadian federation created to provide a collective voice on all matters of policy and collaborate with government in national planning.

The Canadian Sport Council grew out of three consecutive post-Dubin forums held on the outskirts of Ottawa. Whereas most previous "national" policy discussions were confined to senior federal and sport governing body officials from Ottawa, Montreal, and Toronto, the Sport Forums involved athletes, coaches, aboriginal sport leaders, athletes with disabilities from across the country, and representatives of the provinces, territories, and municipalities. After three days of intense debate, Sport Forum II agreed that a new national body was needed, and Sport Forum III was organized as the constituent assembly to create it. The "guiding principles" of the Canadian Sport Council affirmed broad accessibility, "athlete-centeredness," linguistic duality (French and English), gender equity, and the "essential role" of athletes and coaches in positions of leadership. By "athlete-centeredness," Council leaders meant that the primary focus and measure of the

Canadian sport system at all levels was to be the ethical and healthy growth and development of participants.[18]

The Council was to be led by a 17-member board, responsible to an annual assembly. Member organizations were entitled to send up to four persons to each assembly, but delegations of two or more were required to include one athlete and one from each gender, with a goal of equal participation. Delegations of three or more were required to include one coach.[19] In the heady atmosphere of the forums, it was expected that the Council would be able not only to broaden federal sport policy well beyond the pre-Seoul preoccupation with high performance, but help disseminate and implement a more "athlete-centered" approach across Canada's broad distances and networks of institutions and associations.

The Canadian Sports Council soon foundered and collapsed, however, a victim of the savage cuts the federal government administered to Sport Canada (and the greater public sector as a whole), and by extension, the national sport organizations, and the reassertion of the interests of high performance. In 1994, Sport Canada completely eliminated funding for some 50 national organizations, most of which were outside the Olympic family, and significantly reduced the funding for 36 others, according to a ranking scheme heavily weighted toward international performances. (The Sport Recognition Policy, as this scheme is called, simply adds to the burden athletes carry into major competitions: they must not only compete for families, friends, teammates, and coaches, but the very material conditions of their sport!) Similar cutbacks have occurred in most provinces. As a consequence, member organizations no longer could or no longer wanted to support the new Council and its goal of increased participation. The resulting vacuum has given Sport Canada and the Canadian Olympic Association, which helped initiate Sport Forum I and then withdrew its sponsorship because the Forum process was becoming too radical, a new lease on life. Today, Sport Canada, the Canadian Olympic Association, and the Coaching Association of Canada, jointly control the most significant current initiative, the creation of national training centers in major cities, a measure focused upon the athletic elite and high performance. These trends are reinforced by the voluntary sector's increasingly desperate search for corporate sponsorship.

Nonetheless, so deep was the post-Dubin consensus regarding the need for a "values approach" that these aspirations continue to be reflected in the dominant discourse, regardless of the day-to-day reality. In meetings, posters, leadership development sessions, speeches, awards ceremonies, and commercial advertisements, Canada's commitment to educational, drug-free sport is stressed over and over again. Moreover, a number of organizations remain committed to actually realizing the "athlete-centered approach"' espoused by the Canadian Sports Council. One is Athletes CAN, created out of athletes' frustration with the limited role they could play as members of the COA's Athletes' Advisory Council. In its brief existence, Athletes CAN has won a 25 percent increase in federal funding for national team members, the right to bank tuition waivers, and other benefits and has initiated several new protections, including the insertion of an independent athlete advocate on Canadian teams at the Commonwealth and Paralympic Games.[20]

Other organizations include the Canadian Association for the Advancement of Women and Sport and Physical Activity (CAAWS), which took advantage of the Sport Forum's spirit of inclusiveness to persuade many national organizations to adopt gender equity guidelines, and the National Association of Professional Coaches, which has developed a code of conduct for coaches and a training manual to help coaches realize "athlete-centered" training and competition.[21] Perhaps the most influential is the CCES, created in 1995 from the merger of the Centre for Drug-Free Sport and the Fair Play Commission of Canada (formed in the 1980s to combat violence in men's ice hockey). Although the organizations that rose in the post-Dubin period lack the power and resources of Sport Canada and the COA, they have certainly succeeded in winning support for an alternative voice. When the Canadian public was jolted in 1996 by another disturbing sport scandal—the sexual abuse of athletes—it was the CCES and CAAWS to which the affected organizations turned for help and which coordinated the response. CCES and CAAWS are now widely recognized as among the most progressive centers of Canadian sport.

Two qualifications must be inserted here. First, the discourse of "athlete-centered" sport goes largely unheard in the mass media, which provide most Canadians, including young athletes, parents, teachers, and coaches with most of their information about sport. In most cities the lion's share of print and electronic coverage and commentary is devoted to the masculinist, continentalist, commercial cartels, and revolves around scores, standings, and salaries. On those rare occasions when reporters cover Olympic or university athletes, with a few important exceptions they do so with the corporate frame of reference.[22] Moreover, the changes I have described did not originate solely from the moment of reform created by Johnson's disqualification and the Dubin Inquiry. Other factors contributed to the conditions out of which they grew, including the panic about new street drugs such as crack, and cheating in many other spheres of North American society in the depressed aftermath of the takeover-induced inflationary cycle; the hegemony in Canada of the neoconservative variant of the attack on the state, with its concern for strict morality (alongside unrestricted commerce); and the major triumphs of the Canadian women's movement in pay equity, employment equity, and the achievement of sexual harassment codes throughout both public and private sectors.

Yet probably the most important factor in ensuring that "steroid business as usual" did not occur in Canada was the persistence of the intertwined ideologies of Canadian nationalism and amateurism. The amateur and Olympic sports constitute Canada's oldest and most visible nationalist movement. In a country still bitterly divided by the legacy of the wars of European colonization, now overwhelmed by the invasion of American corporations and popular culture, there are few opportunities for exuberant nation-building and the expression and celebration of pan-Canadian achievement. But ever since the mid-19th century, the amateur movement has provided such occasions, consciously grafting the familiar sporting precepts of self-discipline, teamwork, and respect for authority onto the aspirations of Canadian independence. In a society that has always privileged "the gospel of order" and civility—remember the enabling clause of the Canadian constitution is "peace, order and good government," not the "life, liberty and the pursuit of happiness" of the American Declaration of Independence—it has been a potent mixture. Amateur sport is thus a sphere of public culture representative of the social good. It was the symbolic links between amateurism, nationalism, and pan-Canadian unity that led a succession of governments in the 1960s and 1970s to invest heavily in amateur sport.[23] Today, in the unsettling world of the Free Trade Agreement, the North American Free Trade Agreement, and perhaps the Multilateral Agreement on Investment, the symbolic burden on Canadian athletes in international competition is greater than ever before. Canadian society remains deeply attached to the values of fairness and order: the drive to succeed must be balanced by a respect for others and authority in the way espoused by the traditional amateur ideal. The confluence of these aspirations and beliefs has impelled governments and sport leaders to ensure that Canadian athletes compete "clean."

Russia

Throughout the history of both the Russian Empire and the Soviet Union (USSR), state officials viewed the West with ambivalence. Russia, and later the USSR, were diplomatic outsiders, and the many peoples who lived in these lands were constantly reminded that they were perceived as backward. This fanned xenophobia and fostered feelings of cultural inferiority toward an imagined West. For educated Russians, their country's position posed an ongoing dilemma. Was this backwardness to be overcome by emulating Europe or by finding a specifically national path to the future?

This most cursed of historical questions did not disappear with the revolutions of 1917. It did, however, assume a special political inflection, given the proletarian character of the new Soviet state. Diplomatically isolated between the wars, the USSR was not part of the Eurocentric councils of global politics, nor were the Soviets any more active in the various organizations controlling world sport. After World War II, however, the USSR did come to participate in international competitions, including the Olympics, achieving what appeared to be a dominant position. However, this success was tainted in the eyes of many outsiders who charged the Soviets with unfair methods, including phony amateurism and, of course, the use of drugs.

It is by now a truism that Soviet sporting victories were seen both domestically and internationally as proof of the USSR's embrace of modernity. Yet, the rumors of drug use only served to reinforce the Soviet Union's outsider status, and a significant number of positive tests seemed to confirm the illegal practices. As a result, it took several decades of contentious international participation for Soviet sport officials to become players in global ruling bodies. Acceptance, however, was more a product of their athletes' success than recognition of the officials' political suitability. Accordingly, Soviet sport bureaucrats continued to feel like outsiders despite the formal respect they had come to receive.

After the collapse of the USSR, well-placed post-Soviet sport officials (most of whom had been well-placed Soviet sport officials) saw a new opportunity for international acceptance. They announced their eagerness to become part of what Russians were then calling the "normal" and "civilized" world—a world that, at least officially, frowned on the use of illegal, performance-enhancing substances. In the years after the breakup, Russian sport leaders did little to defend athletes who tested positive. However, after 1996, those same officials, charged with maintaining performance under eroding conditions and sensitive to the political pressures of Russian proto-democracy, came to experience conflicting nationalist emotions. Today, it is now common for coaches, federation presidents, and Russian Olympic Committee members at least to give the appearance of protecting the interests of athletes who are caught transgressing international norms.

We now know that doping played a significant role in Soviet high-performance sport. Still, there have not been the kinds of all-encompassing exposés that emerged after the unification of Germany. Soviet-era archival materials pertaining to these matters remain closed, in large part because of the continuity of officialdom. Recent Russian journalistic accounts, however, do give the impression that Soviet doping, although extensive, was neither so rigorously organized nor systematically imposed as it was in the German Democratic Republic. Officials, team doctors, and pharmacologists made drugs available to coaches who were under enormous pressure from the Communist Party to produce winners. Facilities and assistance, especially preemptive testing, were provided to ensure that athletes could escape both detection and death (not necessarily in that order). If an athlete's pharmacological preparation was bungled, that athlete would be withdrawn from an upcoming international competition with the public excuse of injury or illness. Positive tests and other scandals were minimized. Still, a regular stream of athletes did manage to get caught.[24]

The use of performance-enhancing drugs in the USSR may have been less organized than it was in the German Democratic Republic, but it is also clear that for many highly placed people in the Soviet sport world, doping and elite sport were inseparable. Recently, Dr. Sergei Portugalov, who was responsible for the pharmacological preparation of several Soviet national teams over a 15-year period, told the leading Russian sport monthly,

> I am categorically against the use of stimulants in youth sport, but high performance sport is a very special case. First of all it has nothing in common with matters of health. It is, if you will, an experiment which people consciously undertake. The question of how an athlete can lift 300 kilos or set a record in the 100 meters interests everyone—scholars, equipment makers, television and, of course, pharmacology.[25]

Portugalov continued,

> Not every coach can set up a scheme that will prevent overdoses and avoid risk. Basically, the question of a drug test's result has no meaning whatso-

> ever . . . if a test is negative it only means that the pharmacological preparation was done correctly. If it is positive, then the coach is an idiot.[26]

This level of cynicism was echoed by Vladimir Ilyin, an elite-level weightlifting coach from Ukraine who trained several Soviet Olympians:

> If your goal is to prevent all weightlifters from using illegal methods, then the matter should be turned over to professionals who are well paid. Now, as a rule, the control stations are worked by "volunteers." If you offer them a sum that is five times the salary of a teacher or a lawyer in Italy or Germany, they will do what is asked of them. I'm not talking about those who work in doping control in Russia or the former USSR. It's enough to offer them a nice meal. I, of course, am judging from my own experience, but in all the time I worked with the national team there never was an instance when I did not know the results of a test . . . several days before they were on the desk of the head of the doping commission.[27]

Although it is entirely possible both Portugalov and Ilyin exaggerated the extent of Soviet-era drug use in order to create journalistic sensation, their statements are typical of the broader societal corruption and cynicism during the last decades of the Soviet Union.[28] Late in 1993, the great weightlifter, Vassili Alekseev, who coached the national team from 1989 to 1992, told one Russian newspaper, "We received the funds for obtaining them [drugs] openly from Goskomsport [the State Sport Committee]."[29]

When the Soviet Union came apart, thousands of bureaucrats, coaches, and athletes throughout the successor states suddenly found themselves with neither the controls nor the resources of the old system. It became harder to acquire performance-enhancing drugs, and, with the state far weaker, controls virtually disappeared. The result was a rash of doping incidents in the first post-Soviet years. Russian officials, eager to curry favor with their counterparts in other nations, were only too eager to turn over transgressors to the punishments of international sport's ruling bodies, and virtually no attempt was made to defend those who were caught.

Given the widespread rumors, it can hardly be surprising that Russian athletes received special scrutiny in the first years after the Soviet Union's break-up.[30] The world-class sprinter, Irina Privalova, complained to the Russian press that she was repeatedly required to be tested when others were not:

> Right after Stuttgart [1993 World Championship] at a meet in Berlin they drew blood from me and Margarita Ponomareva and no one else. We went on to Brussels. I finish second. They test me but not Gwen Torrence who won. This summer there were four doping controls at Grand Prix meets. I was required to be tested at three of them. It's hard to believe this was just the luck of the draw.[31]

Yet, numerous Russian athletes and others from the former Soviet Union were caught between 1992 and 1995, and neither the Russian Olympic Committee nor the appropriate federation officials took up the cudgels on their athletes' behalf.[32]

Russian functionaries demonstrated particular passivity during the two most visible scandals of the early post-Soviet period. One involved the hurdler, Liudmilla Narozhilenko. The other centered around three weightlifters. Narozhilenko tested positive early in 1993 after an indoor meet in France.[33] The year before, she was one of four Russian athletes forced to leave Sweden when their coach's luggage was found, on passing through customs, to contain numerous steroids. At that time, the athletes tested negative and were cleared.[34]

In May, 1993, Narozhilenko protested the four-year ban she had been given the previous month by the International Amateur Athletic Federation (IAAF). She presented a letter from her former husband and coach, Nikolai, whom she had left for her new manager and lover, Johann Engquist, a citizen of Sweden, where Narozhilenko had now taken up residence. Nikolai testified he had given Liudmilla the drugs without her knowledge as revenge for her leaving him. The Russian Track Federation acknowledged receiving Nikolai Narozhilenko's statement but refused to take action, claiming the letter he had sent was not a legal document. Vladimir Usachev, general manager of the federation, claimed there were no grounds for reinstating Liudmilla Narozhilenko because any positive test, regardless of the circumstances, was grounds for disqualification. Hiding behind the fig leaf of international norms, Usachev told reporters, "We must act according to the rules, which are very strict and do not give us the right to reinstate athletes who have tested positive for drugs."[35] One could easily surmise that the Russian federation's unwillingness to defend Narozhilenko was influenced by her relationship with a foreigner who had come to manage several other former Soviet track athletes. Nevertheless, the Russians' position was consistent with their actions in other cases during the first post-Soviet years.

That fall Narozhilenko took her case against the Russian federation to a Moscow court, which heard her ex-husband's testimony and ruled in her favor.[36] Although a Russian court had no standing with the IAAF, her ban was eventually reduced, and she was able to compete in the 1996 Olympics for Sweden under the name of Engquist, whom she had married in the interim. Russian permission was required for her to take part, but after some ritual foot-dragging, she was allowed to run at Atlanta where she won the gold medal for her new country.

When three Russian weightlifters, Maxim Apitov, Andrei Matveev, and Ramzan Musaev, were caught by international doping controls in the fall of 1993 and given life bans, the ensuing scandal produced an orgy of mutual accusation but no defense of the athletes. The weightlifting federation had to pay $50,000 to retain the team's right to participate in the world championships, but the president, Viktor Poliakov, told the Russian press, "We are upset with what has occurred but we support the action of the international federation. There will be no appeal."[37] Instead, Poliakov placed the blame on the head of the federation's medical committee, Vitaly Semyonov, for failing to catch the guilty before they fell into the clutches of international authorities.

Semyonov admitted he knew that virtually the entire team was taking steroids. Yet, he claimed, this situation made it meaningless for him to name specific individuals, since anyone could have been caught. Semyonov noted he had gotten the federation to promise funds for doping control in light of the rise in steroid use on the team after 1991, but Semyonov blamed Poliakov for never actually coming up with the money.[38] Soon thereafter, Vassili Alekseev joined the fray. Alekseev, the greatest of all Soviet lifters, had been a coach on the national team during the 1980s and was head coach from 1989 to 1992. He was removed after the Barcelona Olympiad for, in his words, "struggling against doping." He claimed virtually every team member used performance-enhancing substances. Funds, said Alekseev, were made available by Goskomsport. He also charged that his predecessor, Aleksei Medvedev, had personally organized the pharmacological preparation of each team member.[39] When Alekseev became coach, he was aware of the full extent of drug use, but he claimed he could do little to stop it. Alekseev knew the Barcelona superheavyweight champion, Alexander Kurlovich, had tested positive in Russia on the eve of the Games, but he risked letting him go to Barcelona in the hope that Kurlovich would test negative, which he did. As for himself, Alekseev admitted only to dabbling briefly in drug use early in his career.

It is safe to say that between 1992 and 1996 there was no Russian policy on doping. Controls were weakened first by political instability and then by a lack of funds to support enforcement measures. Russian officials sought to put the best face on their increasing impotence by claiming they were eager to cooperate with the IOC's campaign against drugs. This was, after all, what "normal" and "civilized" sport bureaucrats did. Soon before the Atlanta Games, however, these attitudes began to change. In part, this shift may have been influenced by that spring's presidential elections. Nationalist and Communist claims of excessive subservience to the West had touched a chord with the electorate, and government sport officials were not immune to these pressures.

When the middle-heavyweight lifter, Alexei Petrov, tested positive at the November, 1995 World Championship, he was threatened with a lifetime ban.[40] He was not, however, left by Russian officials to twist in the wind. They revived Narozhilenko's "jilted lover" scenario, claiming Petrov's abandoned fiancee, herself an aerobics competitor and a medical student, had given Petrov the drugs after he had called off their engagement.[41] Alexander Kozlovsky, long a senior Soviet sport bureaucrat and still a major player on the Russian Olympic Committee, told Reuters,

> We know that he did not take the drug. We know that somebody did something. He was the victim. . . . Our athletes leaving the country for foreign competition go through our laboratory and they are clean. Then they come and compete, and they are with drugs.[42]

That May, Kozlovsky, on a visit to Atlanta, claimed the Olympic drug testing facilities were inadequate, revealing in the process an exasperation with international authorities. This new Russian truculence would prove effective in getting Petrov reinstated for the Olympics where he won a gold medal.[43]

However, Russian authorities were operating in a new, post-Soviet age in which the old consistency and unanimity had disappeared to be replaced by ambivalence. Two days before the Atlanta Games began, another lifter, Iurii Myshkovets, was booted off the Russian team after failing a test administered at the Russian training camp. His coach, Armen Nalbandian, was publicly unforgiving:

> After being burned several times before, we do not trust anyone, even ourselves. We are very tough now and decided to test everyone.[44]

Some Russian officials were still willing to throw athletes on the mercy of the international federations, but when four Russians were caught at Atlanta using the recently banned drug, bromantan, the Russian Olympic Committee mounted a spirited and ultimately successful defense.

Bromantan had been added to the list of illegal substances on the very eve of the Games, and Russian press accounts have speculated this step might not have been taken at all had the drug not been viewed by the IOC as a product of the "Soviet bloc." Regardless of anyone's motives, there can be no doubt about bromantan's origins. It was developed in 1982 at the State Institute of Military Medicine by Iurii Morozov who received a state prize for his work. According to *Sportekspress* monthly magazine, the State Institute of Pharmacology entered into an agreement with the Olympic Committee to supply athletes with the drug, and it was widely used at Albertville and Lillehammer. Although it has been called a stimulant, Russian pharmacologists regarded the drug primarily as a restorative after heavy exercise, especially in harsh climatic conditions. It also strengthens the body's immune system which would obviously be useful to soldiers fighting in a climate like Russia's. Outside specialists, who were largely unaware of bromantan's existence until early in 1996, have placed a great deal more emphasis on the drug's use as a masking agent for steroids.

Four Russian athletes, including two bronze-medal winners, tested positive for bromantan. They were disqualified and had their awards stripped. Immediately, the Russian Olympic Committee went into overdrive. Vitaly Smirnov, the committee's long-time president, seemed to be dusting off classic Soviet rhetoric when he told the press, "I believe that someone does not like the success of the Russian National Team in Atlanta and in my opinion it is a matter of putting psychological pressure on our sportsmen."[45] Other officials mobilized with an energy not seen in the post-Soviet era, causing one Russian journalist to muse that had these events not taken place on the worldwide stage of the Olympics, no such effort would have been made. Gathered together in Atlanta with sport bureaucrats from the world over, these post-Soviet apparatchiki felt their honor impugned and their hard-won respectability threatened.[46]

The matter was taken to the newly created Court of Arbitration for Sport. Kozlovsky presented the Russian side with the help of lawyers retained for the case. Outside experts were brought in to evaluate the effects of bromantan, but because the West had just recently become aware of the drug, there was only the most limited scientific literature available in languages other than Russian. No attempt appears to have been made in the course of the proceedings to translate any material on bromantan from the Russian. Mention was made of the limited effectiveness of the drug as a stimulant. More emphasis was placed on its positive impact on the immune system, but there was no discussion in the proceedings of bromantan's possible use as a masking agent. Ultimately, because the drug had been banned just before the Games and because the literature available to the Court was ambiguous, all four athletes were cleared, and the two medal-winners were allowed to keep their prizes.[47]

In return for the exoneration of their athletes, Russian officials agreed to furnish additional scientific information about bromantan and to clamp down on any further use of the drug. It appeared the post-Soviet sport bureaucracy had won an important victory. The years of accepting the decisions of international authorities seemed to have ended. Russian officials were simultaneously defending their athletes and promising to enforce international norms. It seemed there actually might be a Russian drug policy emerging. As a result, the next scandal to hit was even more bizarre and demoralizing.

The cross-country skier, Liubov Iegorova, who had dominated the competition at Albertville and Lillehammer, tested positive for bromantan at the 1997 world

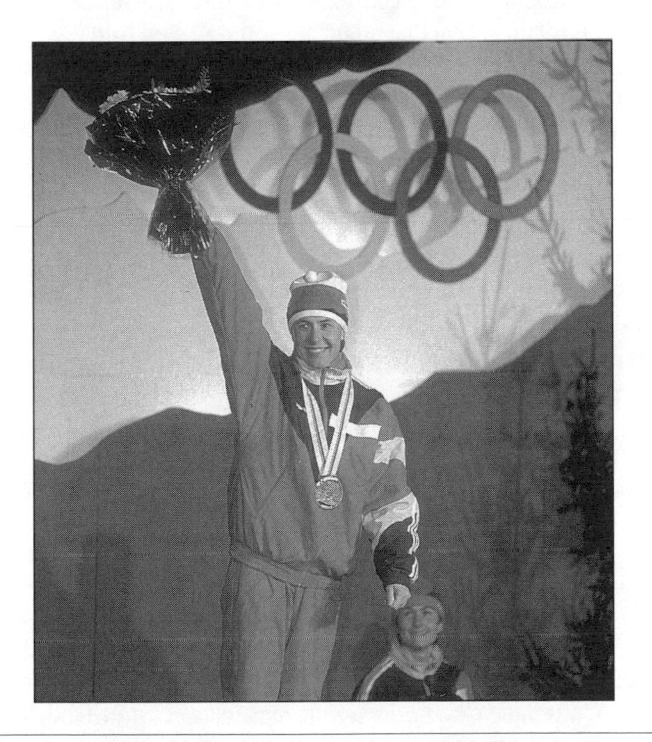

Cross country skier Liubov Iegorova, of Russia, won nine medals at the 1992 and 1994 Olympic Winter Games. She was suspended following a positive test for bromantan at the 1997 world championships, but returned to competition in 1999.

championship in Norway. She immediately admitted taking two bromantan tablets on the eve of a race that she subsequently won. Iegorova, whose victories had received enormous attention in Russia, had taken 1995 off. When she returned to competition, she experienced severe pain in her legs. Initially, the problem was thought to be minor, but a surgical procedure revealed serious neurological difficulties and a second more complicated operation was required in the summer of 1996, during the Atlanta Games. When Iegorova was reproached for not knowing bromantan was on the banned list, she defended herself, fairly lamely, by claiming she was in the hospital when the announcement was made.[48] It was all the more improbable that no doctor, coach, or official had ever informed her of the change.

At first, the Russian skiing federation and her teammates shunned Iegorova, who had recently been surpassed at the top of the Russian team by her less-than-friendly rival, Ielena Valbe.[49] Press reaction back home was similarly negative, but by the spring, Iegorova's situation had improved. The national sport daily, *Sportekspress,* ran an interview in which she defended herself, and the Russian skiing federation took up her case when punishment was meted out by the international federation that June.[50] Russian officials denounced Iegorova's four-year ban as too severe and announced plans for an appeal that might allow the 32-year-old Iegorova to resume her career in time for the 1999 world championship. Left unmentioned throughout the entire episode was bromantan's possible effectiveness as a masking agent, which, if true, cast an enormous shadow over Iegorova's previous successes.

Russian officials' mixture of embarrassment and subsequent defiance in this case perfectly encapsulated their historically ambivalent feelings about the outside world's opinion, sentiments made all the more profound by the complexities of post-Soviet life. Sport bureaucrats in the country formerly known as the Soviet Union, indeed all government officials, no longer speak with a single voice. A weakened state is no longer able to control either drug use or official reactions to it. As a result, there still is no real drug policy—no real control. In the near future Russian athletes will likely continue to use drugs and get caught, while Russian officials will probably continue to react with inconsistency and uncertainty.

China

On April 4, 1981, the Propaganda Department of the Chinese State Sports Commission issued Document Number One, which included the "Athletes Regulations."[51] This document contained 10 articles outlining the basic rules that governed the lives and behaviors of elite athletes. The first and most important article, #1, read, "Support the Communist Party, love our socialist ancestral land, love physical culture work, bravely scale the peaks, win glory for the nation." Article #7 required athletes to "Place top importance on work, postpone courtship, and marry late." Other articles enjoined athletes to "care for the collective," "oppose liberalism," and "oppose anarchism."

The 1981 Athletes Regulations also included the first rule against drug use. Article #6 stated, "Do not smoke cigarettes, do not drink alcohol, dress neatly and tastefully, conscientiously resist the corrosive influence of bourgeois ideology."

These regulations illustrate several important points about the history of drug policies in the State Sports Commission. In 1981, China was just recovering from the end of the Cultural Revolution (1966-1976). Elite sport development was at a standstill. At a time when systematic drug use was well-established in the Eastern Bloc, and informal drug use was well-established in the capitalist nations, cigarettes and alcohol were the major drug problems on Chinese sport teams. Today, nicotine is still probably the most commonly consumed drug in sport, since smoking is almost universal among Chinese men. These regulations also make clear that in 1981 the sport authorities were still far more concerned with infractions of political thinking than they were with drug violations. The period of rebuilding in the 1980s was the foundation upon which the sport system of the 1990s was built. Chinese government organizations are not known for their forward-looking abilities. The State Sports Commission, like the other ministries, is not organized around a codified set of rules. Policies are created in response to problems that already exist. Government is primarily exercised through the promulgation of documents such as the Athletes Regulations, which very often are drawn up to deal with problems that have existed for quite a while and have reached a crisis point.

In sum, Chinese government tends to be reactive, not active. To a large extent, this is what has characterized the history of anti-drug policies. Formal regulations were not put into place until after the problem came to international attention with the 11 positive drug tests among Chinese athletes at the 1994 Asian Games in Hiroshima, Japan. The general attitude toward drug use is strongly shaped by the director of the State Sports Commission. The director who rebuilt the sport system after the Cultural Revolution was Li Menghua, who moved from vice director to the chief position in 1981. Li Menghua's primary concern was the reform of the economic structure of sport, and the sport system was one of the first state systems to implement a bonus system to reward good performances. The reformed financial infrastructure was said to be responsible for the rapid improvement in elite sport. Yet it would seem that Li Menghua was far too preoccupied with economic matters to devote much attention to the issue of drug use.

It may be significant in understanding Chinese attitudes toward performance-enhancing drugs to note that the Chinese translation for performance-enhancing drugs, *xingfenji,* in a literal translation implies something like "a preparation for making one happy and energetic." The words actually have fairly positive connotations.

The use of steroids and other drugs was certainly known by 1988; the use of stimulants was discussed in a controversial exposé of the sport system, Zhao Yu's "Superpower Dream."[52] Zhao Yu's story reveals a lesson about the lack of transparency in the State Sports Commission—as in Chinese politics generally. Zhao had joined a provincial cycling team in 1975 at the age of 20, and he was the team captain. His distance was the 100-kilometer event. He first heard about performance-enhancing drugs while lying in his bed in the dorms one night, when one of his teammates, a son of a doctor, started talking about them. Another teammate revealed that when some athletes took medicines, they performed like machines. Aghast to realize that they were competing under unfair conditions, that all their hard training was for nothing, they resolved to find and take drugs themselves. They requested friends outside the team to buy medicines for them. In the evening, Zhao hid under the blankets and read what little material he could find on the matter. The stories he read made his hair stand on end: the deaths of Dutch [*sic*—he was Danish] and British cyclists in 1960 and 1967, and an American female bodybuilder who abused her husband. Confused, he did not dare ask his coach for advice. Behind his coach's back, he approached a childhood friend who had become a doctor, and the friend supplied him and three teammates with a stimulant.[53] The teammates took it for an important road race, but the result was a disastrous performance.

Zhao Yu went on to describe what happened since that time. However, it is important to remember that at the time he wrote the article, he was no longer employed in the sport world and, so, was an outsider. He wrote that the pursuit of medals compelled local team coaches and athletes to seek out doctors, pharmacists, and friends, and to consume concoctions like "golden pills," "great strength pills," placenta, and fetuses from early miscarriages. He commented that a friend in the sport world told him, "On behalf of that medal, huh!, besides dirt, there's nothing that they won't eat." Zhao identifies a drug testing team sent to the competition venues of the November 1987, National Games as the State Sports Commission's first action on the issue. He relates that many athletes were upset at the fact that, since names were drawn at random, some athletes were not tested. For the first time, anonymous letters accusing competitors of drug use were mailed to the organizations in charge. He did not relate the results of these first drug tests, except to note that they gave full evidence of the clever technology of the apparatus.

Zhao concluded that drug use does violence to the Olympic spirit and should be eliminated. In particular, he remembered the way that thoughts about drugs tormented his mind because he felt trapped in a no-win situation: if his competitors were taking drugs, he couldn't win without them; if he took drugs, he endangered his health. His account is interesting for several reasons. First, in this case, athletes acquired and took drugs without the knowledge of their coach. Second, his mention of the outrage of the athletes at the 1986 National Games, and their anonymous letters to the organizers, indicates a desire by the athletes themselves to rid their sport of drugs. Finally, he only mentions stimulants and traditional Chinese drugs—but not steroids, hormones, and so on, or at least not by their Western names. The traditional medicines he mentioned may have similar effects.

However, what is perhaps more significant is what happened to Zhao Yu. A few leaders in the State Sports Commission attempted to block circulation of the article, criticized it in internal publications, and threatened to sue Zhao. Zhao remarked at that time that the State Sports Commission was unable to retaliate against him because he was not employed in the sport system and did not live in Beijing. A year and a half later, however, the enemies he had made were able to get their revenge in the wake of the 1989 student demonstrations, in which Zhao played a role as an organizer. He was imprisoned for three months in the ensuing crackdown. After that, he abandoned investigative reporting and has maintained a low profile in the years since. These were the risks of investigative reporting on sport in 1988. It is not clear to what extent this situation improved in the 1990s.

During her dissertation research in the late 1980s, Susan Brownell heard steroids discussed on three different occasions by female track athletes at the National Team Center in Beijing, the Zhejiang Provincial Team, and the Shandong Provincial Team. As was then typical in U.S. track and field, these stories were always second-hand stories told about other athletes by athletes who represented themselves as "clean." In two of these cases, athletes claimed to know of cases where coaches gave athletes steroids without informing them what they were. One of them, a javelin thrower from Shandong province, said that the doctors on the team would give them injections and tell them it was to prevent hepatitis. She joked that when their voices got deeper and whiskers grew on their faces, they would say, "What kind of hepatitis medicine is that?" Although these are only anecdotes, it may be significant that in these three stories, two involved athletes who were not informed about what they were taking, and the third involved athletes who knew what they were taking and did not want to, but gave in to pressure from coaches and doctors. Relationships between coaches and athletes in the Chinese system are based on the model of the authoritarian parent figure. The parent (usually the father) knows what is best for the children and acts accordingly with small regard for the feelings of the child. This kind of relationship makes it more possible for coaches to require athletes to take substances that they may not understand.

Ironically, at the world sprint championships just before the Calgary Olympics, at about the same time that Zhao Yu's article was published, speedskater Ye Qiaobo produced China's first positive drug test (for anabolic steroids) and suspension. In contrast to Zhao Yu's openness, China's major sport newspaper, *Sports Daily* (*Tiyu bao*), merely reported midway through the speedskating competitions that she and her teammate had been injured before the start of the competitions and returned home. At the Albertville Winter Olympics in 1992, in the press conference after winning her silver medal, she told reporters that in 1987 the entire team was told to take medicines, but they were not informed what kind of medicine it was. She was extremely bitter about having to miss the Calgary Games.[54]

In the late 1980s, there was clearly drug use among Chinese athletes, but there has never been any evidence that China had a centrally administered drug system like that of East Germany. For one thing, the Chinese sport system as a whole was highly decentralized, with a great deal of rivalry between the provinces, and between the provinces and the national team. Provincial coaches highly resented the national team coaches who got top preference for international assignments, and who could try to take away their best athletes. Teams kept the secrets of their success to themselves, and drugs were likely one of these secrets.

Chinese sports medicine was at a standstill during the Cultural Revolution and has been playing catch-up with the rest of the world since the late 1970s. In the early 1980s, sports medicine training was offered and specialists were first assigned to provincial teams. The State Sports Commission's Sports Medicine Research Institute was established in 1987, and its Drug Testing Center in 1989.[55] This lab became the first IOC-accredited drug testing lab in China before the 1990 Asian Games. Although research on the use of Chinese herbal medicines had been carried out since the 1980s, it was not until around 1990 that scientists began to attempt to establish whether Chinese medicines contained banned substances.[56] Sports medicine researchers were slow to turn their attention to this topic because of the stereotype that Chinese herbal medicines were "natural" and qualitatively different from those used in Western medicines. Many people assumed they would be legal until athletes tested positive at international meets for substances consumed in teas or herbal medicines. Because of the late development of sports medicine in China, it may well be the case that the difference between Chinese athletes and those in the West is that the Chinese are so unsophisticated as to get caught when they use drugs.

When China won only five medals in the 1988 Olympic Games in Seoul, Li Menghua was replaced by Wu Shaozu as director of the State Sports Commission. Informed observers (coaches and officials) in Beijing said that from the start, Wu Shaozu had always taken an open stand against drug use. In 1989, he promulgated the "Three Strict" policy (strictly prohibit, strictly test, strictly punish).[57] It was this stance that protected him from losing the directorship in the wake of the 1994 Asian Games scandal. But when asked how drug use could have gone on in the face of his opposition, they said that his opposition had been superficial. In fact, he had not implemented any strict policies against it, and the State Sports Commission had turned a blind eye to it. When asked if this meant the State Sports Commission knew about drug use and refused to do anything about it, sportspeople said that things were not this simple. The sport authorities didn't want to know. They were under a great deal of pressure to produce more Olympic medals, and so they refused to face the issue directly. This is highly reminiscent of the will-to-ignorance in the Canadian Sports Ministry and Sport Canada, as described by John MacAloon in his article on the Dubin commission.[58] What happened, then, when the Chinese State Sports Commission was finally forced to act?

In 1989, the first track-and-field athlete to fail a drug test seems to have been female 800-meter runner Sun Sumei. From 1989 through 1993, a total of 10 Chinese track-and-field athletes failed drug tests, and 6 more failed tests in 1994. In 1992, the 10-member Chinese Anti-Doping Committee, a division of the Chinese Olympic Committee, was created. Yuan Weimin, vice director of the State Sports Commission and vice chairman of the Chinese Olympic Committee, was appointed the director. This is significant because Yuan, the coach who led the women's volleyball team to their first world victories in the 1980s, is a national hero known for his integrity. As someone who rose up in Chinese politics based on his successes as a coach and his national popularity, not on his political abilities, he has always remained above the moral compromises made by insiders.

An interesting side note is that political dissident Wei Jingsheng, in a recent interview, stated that he believed he was given growth hormones before his brief release from prison in 1993. He stated that this was done to make him look robust, as if he had been well-treated during his 14 years in prison.[59]

Scandal at the 1994 Asian Games

During the Asian Games, *Sports Daily* reported that the president of FINA, the international swimming federation, Mustapha Larfaoui, had criticized the *American Swimmer's World* magazine for refusing to consider Chinese swimmers in its world rankings. The article attributed to Larfaoui statements that some Western nations, led by the United States, had accused the Chinese of drug use, and that they were renewing their attack in Hiroshima. Larfaoui reportedly defended China, and said that coaches were accusing Chinese women swimmers "just to cover up their own defects."[60]

Eleven Chinese athletes tested positive from the 1994 Asian Games in Hiroshima. The Western press is riddled with conflicting reports and even clear errors, and the Chinese press did not report the details. Therefore, the following account is by no means definitive. According to different accounts, in the week before the 1994 Asian Games a positive result was reported from a random drug test done on discus thrower Qiu Qiaoping. The Chinese authorities did not allow her to attend the Asian Games. *Sports Daily* tersely reported that she and two other female track and field athletes (a javelin thrower and a heptathlete) did not go to Hiroshima because their "physical condition was poor."[61] At the Games themselves, seven swimmers (four men and three women), two canoeists (male), a cyclist (female), and a hurdler (female) had positive drug tests. Chinese swimmers had won all 15 titles in Hiroshima.

In addition, at the world championships in women's weightlifting two months later, two gold medalists tested positive. All but one of the athletes were found to have taken DHT (dihydrotestosterone), for which a test had only recently been developed. A number of other athletes were found to have elevated DHT levels, but not enough to be declared positive.[62] Two of the female swimmers were gold medalists in the 1994 Rome world championships, Yang Aihua and Lu Bin. The swimmers received two-year bans on competition, which extended through the 1996 Olympics. The weightlifters were banned for life. The bans for the other athletes were not stated, but all would have been determined by the respective international sport federations, not the Chinese.

Qiu Qiaoping was sent home to await punishment; Wei Jizhong said that the Chinese Olympic Committee might impose a life ban far in excess of the four-year ban required by the IAAF,[63] but this was never confirmed. Her coach, Bai Lin, was suspended and called to Beijing for questioning.[64]

All of the athletes protested their innocence. Lu Bin reportedly said that she had used no substance and she had no idea why she tested positive.[65] Fu Yong, one of the men, also declared after his return in 1997, "I want to prove I was innocent."[66]

FINA banned the swimmers from competition for two years. Coach Zhou Ming also maintained his innocence, arguing that he was not Yang Aihua's full-time coach, and that, as the Asian Games coach, he had only coached her in the period immediately preceding the Asian Games. He said that his suspension should have shown that the Chinese officials were serious.[67]

At the time the Asian Games tests were made public, Chinese officials and the press reacted with denials and then counterattacks. At first the validity of the tests was questioned, then the Japanese were accused of being racist against the Chinese and engineering the tests to improve their medal standing, and finally official involvement was denied and responsibility laid on the shoulders of individuals.[68] The Chinese Olympic Committee said it was "shocked and upset."[69] Wei Jizhong, head of the Chinese Olympic Committee, stated that they also had their doubts, and would like to find out what happened, adding that no one could show that the Chinese government, Olympic Committee, or national federations organized these things.[70] The Foreign Ministry said it was "an act by individuals," which was taken to mean athletes.[71] Guo Qinglong, secretary general of the Chinese Swimming Association, also claimed that these were the acts of individuals. He denied that the swimmers were part of a systematic doping program and that officials of his federation sanctioned illicit drugs. He denied that drug abuse was more of a problem in China than elsewhere. He said these were the acts of athletes, and perhaps coaches, who were tempted by monetary incentives to use substances available on the black market.[72] He explained that the use of banned drugs has entered China like flies coming through windows, but they would never tolerate it or yield to it.[73]

It appears that the coaches involved were instructed to say to foreign reporters that it was the act of individual athletes, team doctors, or coaches, having nothing to do with state policy.[74] FINA and the Olympic Council of Asia sent a special seven-member delegation to Beijing to interview Lu Bin and others and to assess the situation. The delegation concluded that there was no proof that China had a systematic doping program. They decided that the problem was "purely individual cases which cannot be generalized for other athletes who have performed and shown their talents and abilities in all fairness."[75]

Again, media coverage in China was sparse. *China Sports Daily* simply issued another series of terse reports. On December 5, 1994, on page one, under the simple headline, "Statement by the Chinese Olympic Committee," it was reported that the Olympic Committee had received the news that eleven Chinese athletes had positive tests at the twelfth Asian Games and had given it utmost attention.[76] The official statement issued by the Olympic Committee was then reprinted in whole. "On this account," it said, "the Chinese Olympic Committee is deeply surprised and regretful." It was reported that the Anti-Doping Committee had formed an investigative group. A brief history of the anti-doping effort was recounted. The tone of the statement then became defensive. It noted that, according to past findings, athletes mistakenly take medicines because they lack knowledge. Although the eleven positives were a small fraction of the athletes at Hiroshima, the Chinese Olympic Committee called on sport associations to further develop their anti-doping rules and strengthen education and management. Like their sport friends around the world, the Olympic Committee wanted to cooperate tirelessly in controlling drug use to preserve the purity of Olympic sport.

In an editorial on December 21, *China Sports Daily* continued this defensive vein. It noted that the use of performance-enhancing drugs originated in the Western world. "When our country began to fully return to the world sport stage in the 1980s, we faced this international sport world already polluted by banned drugs." Along with the fresh air, this fly entered China's window.[77]

There were some hints of a crackdown on press reporting of the drug scandal. According to *Asia Week* (published in Hong Kong), *The New People's Sports Daily* in Shanghai was criticized by the propaganda bureau at the Shanghai municipal government for publishing a report about the athletes who tested positive in Hiroshima, and a deputy chief editor who had been in the job six months was demoted.[78] There was coverage in the most widely-read newspapers in Beijing: the *People's Daily,* the *Beijing Youth Daily,* and the *China Sports Daily.* Therefore it appears that it was well covered, if perhaps not objectively analyzed. It is not clear whether the names of the guilty athletes were ever published; in any case, they were not published in the initial reports in *China Sports Daily.*

Punishments

China announced that nine coaches would face one-year bans and fines. Five of the coaches were swimming coaches (Zhou Ming, Wang Lin, Chen Qin, Yao Ying, and Yao Zhengjie), one was a track and field coach (Liu Shuqian), one a cycling coach (Li Hongqing), and one was a canoeing coach (Wang Boqing). In addition, the coach of the weightlifters was suspended. China announced that in the future, coaches promoting drug use and individuals supplying banned substances to athletes would face criminal charges.[79]

In contrast to the internationally dictated two-year bans for the athletes, the one-year bans for the coaches meant that they would be allowed to attend the 1996 Olympic Games. Indeed, swimming coaches Zhou Ming and Yao Zhengjie were listed as members of the 1996 delegation.[80] There is some indication that the bans were not strictly enforced. The five banned coaches were not present at the Chinese national swimming championships in Baoding in April 1995, but Zhou Ming was present at the short course championships in Rio early in 1996, while supposedly under suspension. The *Arizona Republic* reported that he had been instructed to tell reporters that he had been suspended—and to say that he had been instructed to say so.[81] It is hard to know how to interpret this cryptic remark, which sounds like it might have been the result of poor interpretation from Chinese. Furthermore, if his suspension had begun retroactively with the 1994 Asian Games, it would have expired by then.

It appears that the head coach of the national swimming team, Chen Yunpeng, who led the swimmers to four golds in Barcelona, retired quietly at the end of 1995. The position remained vacant in early 1997, and Guo Qinglong said that it would remain so for a long time.[82] For those who understand Chinese politics, it is possible to read between the lines. Two of the four assistant coaches, Zhou Ming and Yao Zhengjie, were tainted in the Asian Games scandal. However, even if they were not,

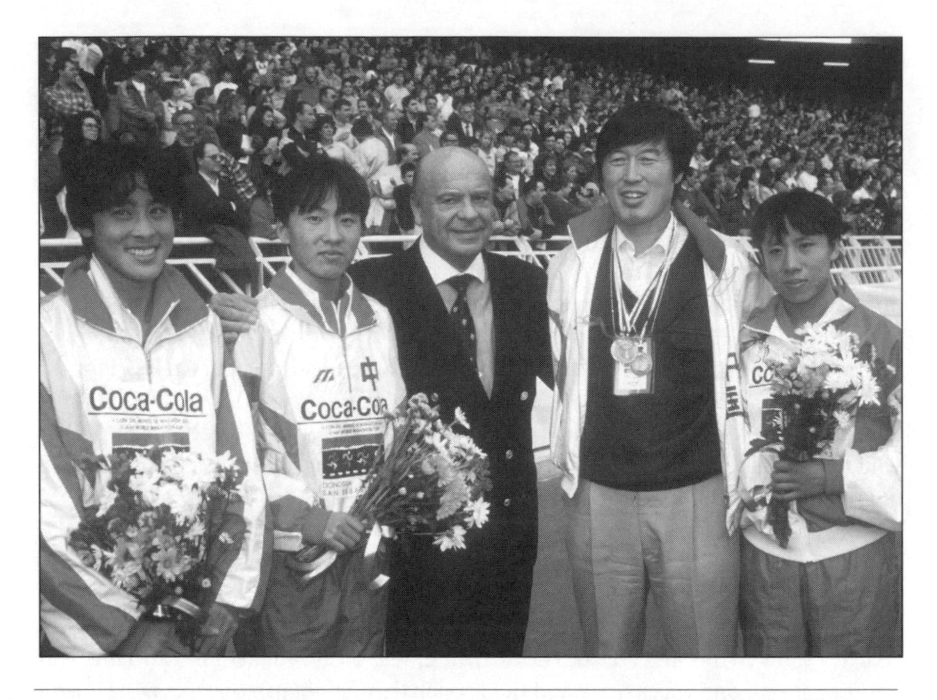

Coach Ma Junren and Chinese women marathoners who placed first, second, and third in the 1993 World Cup Marathon, with IAAF President Primo Nebiolo (center).
© Anton Want/Allsport

it would be a huge career risk for anyone to assume the vacant position, because in so doing he would assume responsibility for maintaining a clean record of drug tests. The fact that everyone agrees that the position will remain vacant may well indicate that everyone knows it will be impossible to control drugs in the sport.

New Policies

In the wake of the uproar in the international swimming community, and China's exclusion from the Pan Pacific Swimming Games, the State Sports Commission was compelled to act in order to save face. In March 1995, the *People's Daily* announced a new policy against drugs in sport. This is extremely important because the *People's Daily* is a nationwide newspaper that serves as the official mouthpiece of the Communist Party and the State Council. The fact that the new policy was announced here shows the importance placed upon it by the Party. Not every new sport policy would rate such exposure. It is also important because such a public announcement shows that the Party believed the drug scandal was widely known. It would not have drawn attention to it if it had been possible to repress knowledge about it.

The policy was announced by Wu Shaozu, director of the State Sports Commission, at an anti-doping conference. It was labeled the "Four Nos and Five Unsuitables" policy, and read as follows: (1) No drugs even if it means no gold medals. (2) No drugs even if others use them. (3) No drugs even if they are not detectable. (4) No drugs even if other people allow you to use them. Drug use does not suit (1) Marxism-Leninism, (2) socialism, (3) the people's best interests, (4) the athlete's best interests, or (5) the nation's best interests.[83] The State Sports Commission also announced that the coaches of athletes testing positive would be suspended, temporarily or for life. Doctors and officials would be punished at least as severely as the guilty athletes. China would discipline the athletes according to the individual international sporting federation's rules. A foreign news agency reported that they would be jailed, but the Commission denied it.[84]

The Standing Committee of the National People's Congress, which in theory is the highest-ranking elected body of government, passed the National Sport Law of the People's Republic of China on August 29, 1995, and it was then promulgated by Order number 55 of the president of the People's Republic of China, and became effective on October 1, 1995. This was China's first national sport law, and was a part of the continuing effort to develop a codified legal system in China. The law also contained the first statement against drug use issued by the State Sports Commission that would have the force of law behind it. Article 34 read,

> The principle of fair competition shall be followed in sport competitions. Organizers of competitions, athletes, coaches and referees shall abide by sportsmanship, and may not practice fraud or engage in malpractice for selfish ends. Use of banned drugs and methods is strictly prohibited in sport activities. Institutions in charge of testing banned drugs shall conduct strict examination of the banned drugs and methods. It is strictly forbidden for any organization or individual to engage in gambling activities through sport competitions.

In addition, Article 50 read,

> Whoever resorts to banned drugs or methods in sport activities shall be punished by the relevant public sport organization in accordance with the provisions of its articles of association; State functionaries who are held directly responsible shall be subject to administrative sanctions in accordance with law.

Beijing Evening News reported in October 1995 that Yuan Weimin, vice-director of the State Sports Commission, had announced that if two teammates tested positive, the entire team would be disqualified from competition for a year. This rule had been used in the recent National Municipal Games if four teammates in a single event tested positive. Yuan also said fines for drug use had been increased, but did not offer more details.[85]

By late 1996, China had also signed mutual testing agreements with Norway, Australia, Canada, and Sweden. In these agreements, athletes could be tested while competing in each other's countries.[86]

Ineffectiveness of Policies

Despite the new policies, it seems that drug use did continue. In September 1995, sprinter Du Xiujie tested positive after winning the 200-meter event and taking second in the 400-meter event at the World University Games in Fukuoka, Japan. Strychnine, a stimulant, was found in her system.[87] Du served a three-month suspension, the standard IAAF penalty for stimulants, and was a member of China's 1996 Olympic team less than a year later. Once again, a Chinese official claimed, "It's an isolated case and Du Xiujie is not a member of the national team."[88] Also, four Chinese swimmers tested positive at the national swimming championships in January 1996 and were suspended by FINA. Steroids were detected in three female swimmers, and elevated testosterone was detected in one male. Three unnamed coaches were supposedly banned from domestic and international competitions for one year. This particular case was suspicious because the Chinese did not report the findings to FINA until January of 1997. FINA had no record of a national championships in January 1996, although a national championships had been reported for April, and there was some doubt as to whether the Chinese had changed the dates on the competitions to predate the new, stricter drug policies that came into effect just after the claimed competition date.[89] The indications were that the State Sports Commission realized it still had not achieved control over drug use among swimmers. In April 1997, officials announced that the anti-doping campaign had been further strengthened. If two swimmers from a single province tested positive, the whole team would be banned from taking part in the Eighth National Games in fall 1997. Any swimmer who tested positive would be banned for four years.[90]

Drug Testing at the 1996 Atlanta Olympic Games

Anti-doping policy became extremely strict in preparation for the 1996 Olympic Games. Members of the Chinese delegation told me that the State Sports Commission was determined that there would be no positive tests in Atlanta because they felt their international loss of face keenly and could not risk further humiliation. Therefore, the Chinese delegation was the cleanest, most tested delegation at the Games. This was despite the fact that the delegation was under tremendous pressure to at least match the number of medals won in Barcelona, which were generally conceded to have been drug-aided. If China's performance was sub-par, top leaders in the State Sports Commission knew their jobs were in danger. But for the first time it became more important to have a clean slate of drug tests than to win gold medals. Intensive out-of-competition sampling methods were adopted. Wu Shaozu later reported that in 1996, 2,298 drug tests were carried out on Chinese athletes. Only ten were positive, or 0.5 percent, lower than the world average of 2 percent. The tests were carried out in and out of China, and in and out of competition. He hailed the figure as a result of China's commitment to wipe out drugs in sport.[91]

The State Sports Commission had engaged in intensive "thought education" with respect to drugs. It distributed anti-doping flyers and videotapes, and classes and examinations were held among team leaders, coaches, doctors, and athletes. Only those who passed the exams were allowed to go to Atlanta. The State Sports Commission and scientists examined 1,416 urine samples by June 18th. Famous athletes underwent multiple examinations—Wang Junxia 12 times, Le Jingyi eight times, and Shan Ying seven times. Le Jingyi stated at the games that she was tested four times a week, domestically and internationally.[92] Within a week before the athletes left for Atlanta, every one of the 310-member delegation was tested for drugs, according to He Huixian, publicity director for the Chinese Olympic Committee.[93]

A high-level official said, "We hope that the IOC and international sport federations will take the same attitude toward each and every delegation on the matter of drug tests. We welcome them to come test, but we think it is not fair to treat China differently. If we find any drug use on the China team, we suspended them. And still, some people are talking about China. We treat drug use more severely than any other country. Why blame us?"[94] After arriving in Atlanta, Chinese officials said that the accusations of drug use were "ideological discrimination" resulting from prejudice against a Communist country. There were no positive tests in Chinese swimming after the 1994 Asian Games and through Atlanta.

During the NBC coverage of the opening ceremonies of the Atlanta Games, Bob Costas made a brief reference to drug use among Chinese athletes, which incited an uproar in the Chinese community. When he introduced the Chinese team during the parade of athletes, he mentioned ". . . their female swimmers, possibly using performance-enhancing drugs. None caught in Barcelona, but since those Olympics in 1992, several have been caught." Much of the outrage in the Chinese community was carried out over the Internet, and from this it is possible to gauge Chinese sentiment toward and awareness of drugs in Chinese sport. For the most part, people writing into the editors of the online list service, *China News Digest,* were quick to point out that no athlete on the 1996 Chinese Olympic team had ever tested positive for illicit drugs. This was not true, since at least Du Xiujie had, and possibly some others. Writers also argued, correctly, that no Chinese had ever tested positive at an Olympic Games. At the same time, however, there were two writers who expressed some doubts. Changqing Yang wrote on July 29 that Donovan Bailey redeemed Canada after Ben Johnson's humiliation, and Ye Qiaobo redeemed herself in the 1992 Winter Olympics after missing Calgary as the result of a suspension. "Following this line, Chinese women's swimming team is still at probation period. Several of its members are on prohibition, and the team has not reached its previous level of performance. We certainly don't feel comfortable when people mentioning [*sic*] the doping incident two years ago. But we can't blame others for mentioning it and saying [*sic*] the others evil-minded."[95]

Fred Liu wrote on July 22,

> . . . The Chinese couches [*sic*] and officials are just too dumb to make any good explainations [*sic*]. Those people don't know how to develope [*sic*] good relationships with the media and the public other than simply denying the charges. . . . Chinese officials must prove to the American public that drug use was not allowed by the government when the problem was first found a few

years ago. Simply denying the charges won't work, because people still feel that the emerging of the Chinese swimmers is a result of the drug use. Even [*sic*] I don't like the NBC comments, I don't know the truth of the incidents a few years ago when many Chinese female swimmers were found using drugs. There have been no convincing explainations [*sic*] about those cases.[96]

Scandal at the 1998 World Swimming Championships

As the Chinese swim team passed through customs in the Sydney airport for the 1998 World Swimming Championships, customs officials found 13 vials of human growth hormone (human somatotrophin) in the luggage of one of the swimmers, Yuan Yuan. Yuan said her coach, Zhou Zhewen, had packed the bag, which he confirmed while stating that he did not know the contents of the vials. A team official told the customs official that the bottles were for Yuan's friends in Australia, and Zhou Zhewen later said that he was to bring the vials to a friend in Australia.[97] Zhou Zhewen was not one of the coaches previously implicated in drug scandals. Yuan Yuan and Zhou Zhewen were withdrawn from the team. Subsequently, four female swimmers were reported to have tested positive for a diuretic based on samples taken by FINA on January 8, after some resistance by the Chinese team. The human growth hormone was traced to a Danish biotechnological firm, which said it had sold it to a Chinese state import agency.[98] Again, Chinese officials denied that there was systematic doping in China, and FINA officials concurred after sending a team to China to investigate.[99]

In the wake of the scandal, eleven new articles were issued to deal with the problem. These included the following: any swimmer who tested positive for a class I drug would be suspended for life; any local association or club with two positives within a 12-month period would be banned from domestic and international competition for a year and would pay a fine; if four positive tests occurred within four years, the local association or club would be banned from the following National Sports Games and the Municipal Sports Games; sport teams were forbidden to directly award bonuses but must go through the Chinese Swimming Federation, which would hold them in trust (earning interest) until after the athlete retired; if an athlete tested positive for drugs, all bonuses, performances, and awards would be eliminated; coaches could only receive bonuses after a four-year waiting period in which none of their athletes tested positive.[100] Clearly, these drastic measures were aimed at the area that was considered the motivating force behind drug use: personal bank accounts.

In contrast to previous scandals, the Chinese Olympic Committee's reaction was swift and public. In part, this may have been because the scandal occurred in the midst of the annual national meeting of the State Sports Commission, and with all of the sport leaders already assembled, the scandal caused a serious loss of face that had to be defended against. On January 16 the annual Anti-Doping Conference was held, which was reported in *China Sports Daily*. The Director of the State Sports Commission, Wu Shaozu, complained that "some people are not conscientiously opposing the use of performance-enhancing drugs, but are searching out loopholes, damaging our sport endeavor, and after the fact refusing to speak honestly."[101] Yuan Weimin, director of the Anti-Doping Committee, also complained that "true opposition to drug use or faked opposition to drug use has not ultimately been resolved in the brains of some people." Yuan announced the promulgation of 10 more articles against drug use and the formation of a five-person investigative group that would pry into the latest scandal.[102] The seriousness of the scandal was indicated by the fact that it was addressed by Li Tieying in his closing address to the State Sports Commission meeting—a member of the Central Administrative Bureau and State Council, he had been the highest-ranking official at the meeting. This got a headline in the January 17 issue of *China Sports Daily.*

The February 7, 1998 issue of *China Sports Daily* contained a long interview with Shi Kangcheng, Office Director of the Chinese Anti-Doping Committee. He outlined the structure for doping control in the Chinese sport system.[103] Ultimately, it is funded and administered by the State Sports Commission, with the Anti-Doping Office (Fan xingfenji chu), a section of the Science and Education Department (Kejiao si), responsible for coordinating efforts among the provincial departments and the departments and bureaus of the State Sports Commission. This effort is in tandem with that of the Anti-Doping Committee of the Chinese Olympic Committee (a redundant parallel structure that results from the IOC's mandate that Olympic Committees must be autonomous from government structures). From 1985 to 1998, the State Sports Commission and the Chinese Olympic Committee issued 25 rules against drug use. Shi named the 42-article "Provisional Regulations Prohibiting the Use of Performance-Enhancing Drugs in Sport" as the most comprehensive (date of promulgation unknown). He noted that the Anti-Doping Committee of the Chinese Olympic Committee conducted 1,914 tests (708 outside competitions) in 1995; 2,080 (1,115 outside competitions) in 1996; and 3,540 in 1997. Since 1994, the State Sports Commission has convened an Anti-Doping Conference annually.

In the West, especially in the U.S. and Australia, there has been a great desire to find out exactly what is going on in China with respect to doping. Non-Chinese have wanted to go in and do the kind of investigative exposé that is not even permitted to Chinese journalists (witness the case of Zhao Yu). Even if we succeed in revealing a clearer picture than what is outlined here, it is not likely that outsiders will be able to intervene and solve China's doping problems. As this chapter shows, Chinese sport leaders have engaged in a continuous effort to control doping since 1989. This effort was perhaps mere lip service at times, and has probably been taken more seriously since the 1994 Asian Games scandal—but in this respect, were Chinese sport leaders any different from sport leaders elsewhere? If the U.S. cannot completely control drug use within its boundaries, even with many more years of experience to draw on, then it cannot expect to march in and solve China's problems. We need to recognize that sharing experience in solving problems may be more effective than punitive measures. One idea that has not yet been explored is that of pushing for greater openness in media reporting of positive drug tests. President Clinton's successful insistence that his recent meeting with President Jiang be televised live suggests that this kind of pressure may produce results. Grassroots support for cleaning up sport, such as we have seen in American and Australian swimming, can only occur when information is openly exchanged. The conditions for this are a long way off in China, but there may be ways to encourage their development.

Conclusions

The differences among these three national experiences appear with far greater clarity than do the similarities. Canadian, Russian, and Chinese officials have all expressed proper dismay when scandals have occurred in recent years. All three nations now have domestic mechanisms in place to catch transgressors before international bodies do. None of the sport leaders involved here appears willing to bear the brunt of public scorn from their peers. As international players, it is best for their careers and for the interests of the bodies they represent that they enjoy the respect of the international community.

On the other hand, official reactions to doping scandals very much reveal the broader attitudes of each nation toward the rest of the world. The Canadian willingness to put its house in order may seem similar to that of the Russians. Transparency has become a larger part of sport activity in post-Soviet Russia, but the current chaos and lack of funds make any desire to behave properly difficult to act upon. Chinese denials of wrongdoing, coupled with accusations of racism and promises to do better, have been seen in a number of areas of life other than sport. Canada's insiders contrast with the Chinese outsiders. The Russians find themselves somewhere in the middle. Eager to please but incapable of doing so, they have their noses pressed against the glass but can find no way into the house of respectability they crave in the post–Cold War world. Incidents of drug use in sport thus become a way of marking each nation's diplomatic position. They tell us more about particular cultures than about the practices of doping. In recent decades, high-performance sport may have become what some have called a global monoculture, but attitudes toward the use of performance-enhancing drugs remain highly particular.

Notes

[1]Canadian Centre for Ethics in Sport, *1996-97 Annual Report.* These numbers were higher before the recent round of federal budget cuts. In 1996, there were almost 2,500 tests.

[2]Canadian Centre for Drug-Free Sport, *Doping Control Standard Operating Procedures* (Ottawa, 1994).

[3]International agreements have been signed with Australia, Britain, New Zealand, and Norway, and the CCES has reciprocal testing agreements with the Australian Sport Drug Agency and the United States Olympic Committee.

[4]Decima Research, *A Report to the Ministry of Fitness and Amateur Sport: Ethics and Values in Canadian Sport,* March 1991. In 1994, the Canadian Health Monitor found that 76 percent of respondents to a national telephone survey said that the use of banned substances is a "somewhat serious" to a "very serious" concern among amateur athletes. Twenty-six percent of respondents said that they would be unwilling to have their child participate in sport because of the presence of drugs. In 1997, drug use by athletes was identified as the most important issue in sport by a poll of athletes and coaches at the Canada Games.

[5]Bruce Kidd, "The Philosophy of Excellence, Class Power and the State," in Pasquale Galasso, ed., *Philosophy of Sport and Physical Activity* (Toronto: Scholars' Press, 1988, 11-31), and Donald Macintosh and David Whitson, *The Game Planners: Transforming Canada's Sport System* (Montreal: McGill Queen's, 1990).

[6]Bruce Kidd, "'Seoul to the World, the World to Seoul'... and Ben Johnson: Canada at the 1988 Olympics," in Koh Byong-Ik, ed., *Toward One World Beyond All Barriers* (Seoul: Poong Nam, 1990), Vol. 1, 434-454.

[7]Sandra Martin, "The Race Card: After All These Years, We Are Still Blaming Ourselves for Disowning Ben. But We Did Nothing of the Sort," *Globe and Mail,* August 17, 1996.

[8]For example, John MacAloon, "Steroids and the State: Dubin, Melodrama and the Accomplishment of Innocence," *Public Culture,* 2 (2), 1990, 41-64.

[9]Charlie Francis, *Speed Trap: Inside the Biggest Scandal in Olympic History* (New York: St. Martin's, 1990), and Angela Issajenko, *Running Risks* (Toronto: MacMillan, 1990).

[10]See also Varda Burstyn, "This Sporting Life," *Saturday Night,* March 1990, 42-49, and Line Beaushesne, "The Dubin Inquiry's Political Purpose," paper presented to the conference: After the Dubin Inquiry: Implications for Canada's High-Performance System, Queen's University, Kingston, Ontario, Sept. 27-29, 1990.

[11]Canada, *Report of the Commission of Inquiry Into the Use of Drugs and Banned Practices Intended to Increase Athletic Performances* (the Dubin Commission) (Canada: Supply and Services, 1990), 520.

[12]For example, the 1990 session of the Olympic Academy of Canada was devoted to a discussion of the Dubin recommendations; see also Rob Beamish and Bruce Kidd, eds., *Conference Proceedings: After the Dubin Inquiry: Implications for Canada's High Performance System,* Queen's University, Kingston, Ontario, September 27-29, 1990; Canada, House of Commons, *Report of the Sub-Committee on Fitness and Amateur Sport,* Standing Committee on Health and Welfare, Social Affairs, Seniors and the Status of Women, December 1990; and Canada, *Sport: The Way Ahead, the Report of the Minister's Task Force on Federal Sport Policy* (Ottawa: Supply and Services, 1992).

[13]An independent testing authority was also one of the obligations of the International Charter Against Drugs in Sports.

[14]Joseph de Pencier, "Law and Athlete Drug Testing in Canada," *Marquette Sports Law Journal,* 4 (2), 1994, 261. The contractual nature of the Canadian system makes it vulnerable to challenges on the basis of athlete consent. For this reason, the CCES persuaded Athletes CAN to adopt its procedures and penalties at its annual forum in 1995, and it is currently undertaking to obtain similar agreements from athletes in the bylaws of participating national federations.

[15]Paul Melia, Andrew Pipe, and Leslie Greenberg, "The Use of Anabolic-Androgenic Steroids by Canadian Students," *Clinical Journal of Sport Medicine,* 6 (1), 1996, 9-14.

[16]Despite these major gains, the system can still be considerably improved. To date, athletes' representatives in Canada have generally conceded the accuracy of the tests to the scientists commissioned by the CCES. It would appear from the presentation to this conference by David Black, who indicated considerable scope for challenging the scientific protocols and results, that this approach ought to be reconsidered. More important, more effort needs to be devoted to the rehabilitation (to full good health) of those athletes who have been discovered to have used steroids and other drugs.

[17]Dubin Report, 527.

[18]Heather Clarke, Dan Smith, and Denis Thibault, "Athlete Centered System," discussion paper prepared for the National Planning Framework for Sport, Federal-Provincial-Territorial Sport Policy Steering Committee, Ottawa, 1994.

[19]Canadian Sport Council, *Constitution,* Ottawa, 1993.

[20]On the other hand, the Canadian Olympic Association has been unwilling to allow athletes an independent voice: while it, too, has created a position of "athlete representative" on teams, it has insisted upon appointing the representative itself.

[21]Paul Tomlinson and Dorothy Strachan, *Power and Ethics in Coaching* (Ottawa: Coaching Association of Canada, 1996).

[22]For instance, Peter Donnelly, ed., "Sport and the Media," *Taking Sport Seriously: Social Issues in Canadian Sport* (Toronto: Thompson Educational Publishing, 1997), 287-313.

[23]These arguments are elaborated in Bruce Kidd, *The Struggle for Canadian Sport* (Toronto: University of Toronto Press, 1996) and Donald Macintosh, Tom Bedecki, and C.E.S. Franks, *Sport and Politics in Canada: Federal Government Involvement since 1961* (Montreal: Queen's McGill, 1987).

[24]*Komsomolskaia pravda,* July 24, 1992.

[25]Yelena Vaitsekovskaia, "Doping," *Sportekspress Zhurnal,* 1(1) December 1996, 52-59.

[26]Yelena Vaitsekovskaia, "Doping," *Sportekspress Zhurnal,* 1(1) December 1996, 52-59.

[27]Yelena Vaitsekovskaia, "Doping," *Sportekspress Zhurnal,* 1(1) December 1996, 52-59.

[28]On a June, 1996 documentary broadcast on the American cable company ESPN, Portugalov estimated the use of performance-enhancing drugs by Soviet athletes at 90 percent.

[29]*Komsomolskaia pravda,* December 14, 1993.

[30]*Komsomolskaia pravda,* July, 24, 1992 and November 16, 1993.

[31]*Komsomolskaia pravda,* October 22, 1993.

[32]Among those caught in track alone (and the list is by no means complete) were Marina Shmonina (see Reuters World Service, May 20, 1993), Natalya Voronova (Reuters World Service, August 9, 1994), Yelena Lysak (Reuters World Service, September 21, 1994), Liubov Kremlyova (Reuters World Service, March 30, 1995). Other Russians caught in track included Andre Yalin, Serei Kirmasov, and Olga Bogoslovskaia in 1994; Dmitrii Shevchenko, Vasilii Sukov, and Larisa Peleshenko in 1995; Olga Nazarova and Natalya Shekhodanova in 1996. See (1) Association of Track & Field Statisticians, *Athletics 1995 The International Track & Field Annual*, Peter Matthews, ed., Surrey, England: SportsBooks Limited, p. 13; (2) Association of Track & Field Statisticians, *Athletics 1996 The International Track & Field Annual*, Peter Matthews, ed., Surrey, England: SportsBooks Limited, p. 128; (3) Association of Track & Field Statisticians. *Athletics 1997 The International Track & Field Annual 1997*, Peter Matthews, ed., Surrey, England: SportsBooks Limited, p. 66.

[33]Reuters World Service, March 12, 1993. The four-year ban was announced by the IAAF on April 28 after a second test in March proved positive.

[34]Reuters World Service, January 5, 1993.

[35]Reuters World Service, January 5, 1993.

[36]Reuters World Service, December 1, 1993; *Komsomolskaia pravda,* December 7, 1993.

[37]*Komsomolskaia pravda,* October 30, 1993.

[38]*Komsomolskaia pravda,* November 8, 1993.

[39]*Komsomolskaia pravda,* 14, 1993.

[40]Reuters World Service, March 14, 1996.

[41]Reuters World Service, July 17, 1996.

[42]Reuters World Service, May 1, 1996.

[43]Reuters World Service, July 27, 1996.

[44]Reuters World Service, July 17, 1996.

[45]Reuters World Service, July 30, 1996.

[46]Yelena Vaitsekovskaia and Maria Savchenko, "Diskvalifikatsia," *Sportekspress Zhurnal,* 1 (8): 50-55.

[47]For a full record of the proceedings see Court of Arbitration for Sport, Ad Hoc Division, Games of the XXVI Olympiad-Atlanta, 1996, Arbitration No. 003-4.

[48]Reuters World Service, February 27, 1997.

[49]*Sportekspress,* June 11, 1997.

[50]Yelena Vaitsekovskaia and Maria Savchenko, "Diskvalifikatsia," *Sportekspress Zhurnal,* 1(8) 55.

[51]State Sports Commission Research Division, *Tiyu wenjian xuanbian, 1949-1981,* [Collected Physical Culture Documents, 1949-1981], *Renmin tiyu chubanshe* [People's sports publishing house], 1982, 498.

[52]Zhao Yu, "Qiangguo meng" [Superpower dream], *Dangdai,* [Contemporary Times], February 1988, 163-198.

[53]The stimulant is identified as *benbing'an,* the translation of which I have been unable to confirm; perhaps it is benzedrine.

[54]Mark Zeigler, "China's Sports Machine: The Great Wall of Secrecy is Falling," *San Diego Union-Tribune,* December 26, 1994, C-1.

[55]*Zhongguo tiyu bao* [China Sports Daily], November 4, 1994.

[56]Yang Zeyi, "Recent Advances in Sports Physiology and Sports Biochemistry," Howard G. Knuttgen, Ma Qiwei, and Wu Zhongyuan, eds., *Sport in China,* (Champaign, IL: Human Kinetics Books, 1990), 169-181.

[57]Xinhua Press wire, "Zhongguo Aoweihui shengming" [Statement by the Chinese Olympic Committee], *Zhongguo tiyu bao* [China Sports Daily], December 5, 1994, 1.

[58]John MacAloon, "Steroids and the State: Dubin, Melodrama and the Accomplishment of Innocence," *Public Culture* 2 (2), 1990, 41-64.

[59]"Special Issue: A CND Interview with Wei Jingsheng, Part II," *China News Digest* (Internet news service), January 20, 1998.

[60]"Dihui Zhongguo yongjiang kebei" [Slandering China's top swimmers is lamentable], *Zhongguo tiyu bao* [China Sports Daily], *Xinhua* press wire, October 14, 1994, 1.

[61]Ming Zi, "Wo siyuan tianjing nüjiang yuanhe wei di Guangdao?" [Why didn't four of our outstanding female athletes go to Hiroshima?], *Zhongguo tiyu bao* [China Sports Daily], October 12, 1994, 3.

[62]Elliott Almond and Rone Tempest, "The Crooked Shadow," *Los Angeles Times,* February 12, 1995, C1, C9, C16.

[63]"Asian Games: China Takes Hard Line: Drugs Cheat Faces Life Ban," *The Irish Times,* October 15, 1994, 47.

[64]Elliott Almond and Rone Tempest, "The Crooked Shadow," *Los Angeles Times,* February 12, 1995, C1, C9, C16.

[65]Alexander Wolff and Richard O'Brien, eds., "Great Fall of China," *Sports Illustrated,* December 19, 1994, 19.

[66]Agence France Presse, May 13, 1997.

[67]Agence France Presse, May 13, 1997.

[68]Steven Mufson, "China's Leap Backward: Swimmers' Positive Drug Tests Cast Pall," *The Washington Post,* December 6, 1994, B-1.

[69]Alexander Wolff and Richard O'Brien, eds., "Great Fall of China," *Sports Illustrated,* December 19, 1994, 19.

[70]Elliott Almond and Rone Tempest, "The Crooked Shadow," *Los Angeles Times,* February 12, 1995, C1, C9, C16.

[71]Alexander Wolff and Richard O'Brien, eds., "Great Fall of China," *Sports Illustrated,* December 19, 1994, 19.

[72]Alexander Wolff, "The China Syndrome," *Sports Illustrated,* October 16, 1995.

[73]*China News Digest* (on-line listserve), February 13, 1995.

[74]Elliott Almond and Rone Tempest, "The Crooked Shadow," *Los Angeles Times,* February 12, 1995, C1, C9, C16.

[75]*China News Digest,* March 31, 1995, quoting Agence France Presse quoting *Xinhua.*

[76]"Position for Chinese Swimming Coach Remains Vacant," *Xinhua,* January 10, 1997.

[77]"Zhongguo tiyujiede yiguan lichang shi jianjue fandui shiyong xingfenji" [The consistent standpoint of the Chinese sport world has been to oppose the use of performance-enhancing drugs], *Zhongguo tiyu bao* [China Sports Daily], benbao pinglun yuan [this newspaper's commentators], December 21, 1994, 1.

[78]Elliott Almond and Rone Tempest, "The Crooked Shadow," *Los Angeles Times,* February 12, 1995, C1, C9, C16.

[79]*China News Digest,* March 31, 1995.

[80]*China Sports Delegation to the 1996 Atlanta Olympic Games*. Publication of the Chinese Olympic Committee.

[81]Norm Frauenheim with Jeff Metcalfe, "Snapshots of the Road to Olympics," *Arizona Republic*, January 14, 1996.

[82]"Position for Chinese Swimming Coach Remains Vacant," *Xinhua,* January 10, 1997.

[83]Ma Yihua, "Zhongguo fan xingfenji da xingdong" [China's anti-doping program], *Zhongguo tiyu bao* [China Sports Daily], February 7, 1998.

[84]*China News Digest,* March 5, 1995, off Agence France Presse.

[85]*China News Digest,* October 25, 1995, off Associated Press.

[86]*Financial Times,* London, November 25, 1996.

[87]*China News Digest,* September 19, 1995.

[88]Agence France Presse, September 19, 1995.

[89]"Timing is Everything," *Sports Illustrated,* May 12, 1997, 15.

[90]"Swimming—China Says Anti-Doping Rules Much Tighter," Reuters, April 30, 1997.

[91]*China News Digest,* January 8, 1997, off Agence France Presse.

[92]Jere Longman, "Chinese Women Falter, But Still Strike Gold," *New York Times,* July 21, 1996, Sec. 8, 1.

[93]*China News Digest,* July 17, 1996.

[94]*China News Digest,* July 17, 1996.

[95]*China News Digest,* July 29, 1996.

[96]*China News Digest,* July 22, 1996.

[97]*China News Digest,* January 10 and 11, 1998, based on Associated Press, Reuters, and Nanyang Siang Pau.

[98]*China News Digest,* January 15, 1998.

[99]*China News Digest,* January 18, 1998.

[100]Cao Jianjie, Li Jiazan, "Guoji yonglian daibiaotuan juxing xinwen fabuhui" [FINA delegation convenes press conference], *Zhongguo tiyu bao* [China Sports Daily], February 20, 1998.

[101]Xu Jiren and Li Jiazan, "Zhongguo Aoweihui, zhaokai fan xingfenji dahui" [Chinese Olympic Committee convenes an anti-doping conference], *Zhongguo tiyu bao* [China Sports Daily], January 17, 1998.

[102]Xu Jiren and Li Jiazan, "Zhongguo Aoweihui, zhaokai fan xingfenji dahui" [Chinese Olympic Committee convenes an anti-doping conference], *Zhongguo tiyu bao* [China Sports Daily], January 17, 1998.

[103]Ma Yihua, "Zhongguo fan xingfenji da xingdong" [China's anti-doping program], *Zhongguo tiyu bao* [China Sports Daily], February 7, 1998.

7 CHAPTER

Drugs, Sport, and National Identity in Australia

Tara Magdalinski
University of the Sunshine Coast

Throughout the 1990s, the use of performance-enhancing drugs in sport has become an increasingly contentious international issue. Within Australia, the consumption of drugs to enhance sporting prowess has been publicly condemned by various sporting organizations and media campaigns. Magazines such as *Inside Sport,* Australia's foremost sports monthly, regularly discuss drugs in sport and cast aspersions on those organizations, such as FINA, the international swimming federation, and the International Olympic Committee (IOC), that have taken what the media see as a "weak" stance against performance-enhancing substances. Young athletes are told to "Just Say No" to drugs in sport through educational programs, and the Australian sporting fraternity has declared itself a "world leader" in the fight against doping. Before major sporting events, opponents are regularly accused of illicit drug taking and are labeled "drug-cheats," while national coaches publicly affirm that Australian athletes are "clean."

Since late 1997, the Australian media have been saturated with reports and commentaries on the issue of drugs in sport. Australians were positioned as adamant supporters of "clean" sport, and alleged "drug-taking" nations were publicly condemned. The positioning of a clean "us" against a cheating "them" can be read as part of a process of developing an understanding of the Australian self through the lens of sport. The Australian media seem obsessed with performance-enhancing drugs, particularly in the lead-up to the Sydney 2000 Olympic Games, and an analysis of media reports can assist scholars of sport in interpreting the significance of sport in generating a national identity. Observers who question the legitimacy of public outrage over drugs in sport are marginalized and castigated as "un-Australian" and popularly perceived to be a threat not only to the 2000 Olympics in Sydney, but to Australia's reputation as a whole. In this way, a study of the Australian media's reporting of performance-enhancing drugs reveals how sport and sports-related issues contribute to the process of nation-

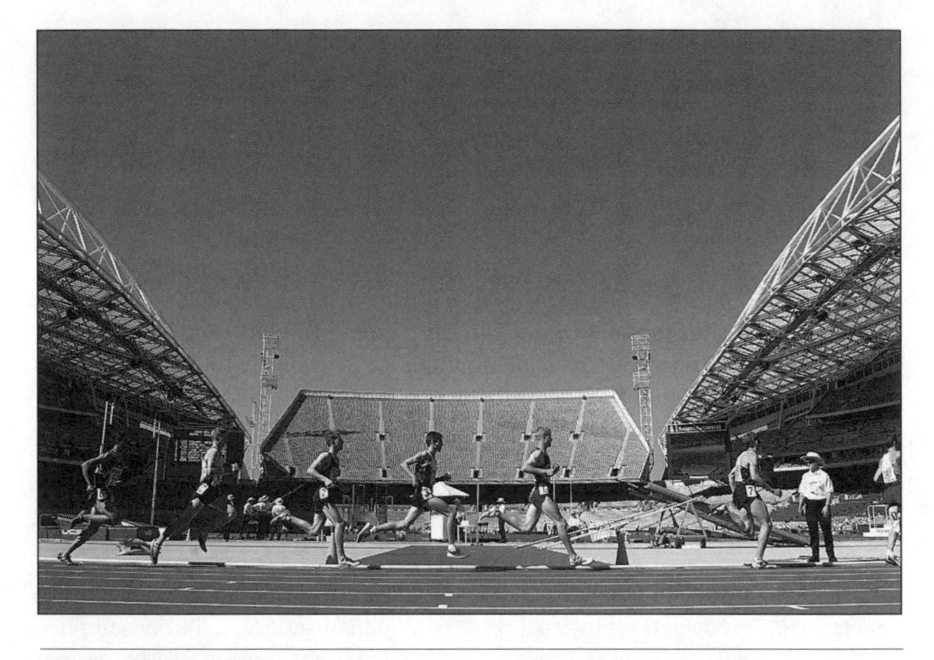

Runners at Homebush Bay, central site of the 2000 Sydney Olympic Games.

building, particularly in the lead-up to international sporting events such as the Olympics.

Since Sydney won the right to host the Games in 1993, the 2000 Sydney Olympic Games provided Australians with an opportunity to strengthen their sense of national unity through the construction of unqualified public support. Unqualified support for this event, however, was threatened in a number of ways. Scandals surrounding Australian IOC member Phil Coles, alleged improprieties of the Sydney 2000 Bid Team, and questions concerning the public funding of the Games began to adversely affect public endorsement of the event (Lehmann, 1999; Cameron, 1998). With fewer than 500 days to go until the Sydney 2000 Games, Olympic tickets on sale, and an expected shortfall of funding, the Australian government increasingly relied on positive and reaffirming images of a healthy nation at "play" to ensure positive public support and thus the success of the Games. Furthermore, the notion of "fair play" as a premise on which sport and the Olympics are founded was brought into question by the scandals surrounding elite performance sport and doping. In this chapter, I argue that a singular Australian national identity is repeatedly articulated through the careful juxtaposition of "clean" Australian athletic bodies against "drug taking" Others.

Since the advent of international competitions in modern sport in the late 19th century, athletic bodies have come to symbolize the nations that produce them (Jarvie and Walker, 1994). Athletes are viewed as representative of political ideology, economic superiority, and cultural value. Australia, for example, has used international sport as a means of demonstrating independence from an imperial center (Nauright, 1992). In the late 19th and early 20th centuries, competitions in cricket and rugby became markers of colonial strength and success, and more recently, international sporting events, particularly within swimming, have been used to validate the status of the Australian nation. This chapter argues that the development of an Australian identity, positioned within the conceptual framework of Australia as sporty nation is incomplete without the location of sporting Others on the fringes of that identity. In the case of Australia, sporting Others are embodied in the physical exploits and, more importantly, the "chemically enhanced" bodies of Chinese and East German swimmers.

Building the Nation: Australian Identity

The issue of drugs in sport in Australia increases in significance when contextualized within a broader discussion of Australian identity. The geographical, political, and cultural peculiarities of the Australian nation and its relationship to sport clarify the ways that debates surrounding performance-enhancing drugs can be employed to shore up a sense of nationhood at a time when the world's sporting attention is turning towards Australia. The recent Australian media coverage of drugs in sport can be read as part of a larger process of positioning Australia as a deserving recipient of the Olympic Games and as a legitimate leader in an international (sporting) hierarchy. This process culminates in efforts to (re)assert a sense of Australian identity in the lead-up to the Sydney 2000 Olympics (Magdalinski, 1998b).

"Australian identity" has become increasingly fragmented in recent years as a result of the rise of an extreme right-wing political party, sustained debates about the ethnic and racial composition of the Australian population, and concerns about indigenous land rights. This is, of course, not to argue that Australian identity has ever been cohesive and uncontested, but it does suggest that in periods of social upheaval there are concerted efforts to promote an image of the nation as unified.

Reading Australia through the lens of sport replaces many contentious issues with a focus on another kind of "them" and "us" binary. National identity is a fragile construct and is subject to (re)negotiation. Competing identities struggle for acceptance by presenting citizens with images designed to secure consensus about the nation and about what that nation *means* (Hall, 1992). History in general can provide a nation with a foundation that presents the nation as not only unified but as inevitable (Magdalinski, 1998a). Further, meanings about the nation are often explained in historical figures who become rallying points for the nation. According to Anthony Smith (1991: 161), a nation must be able to "unfold a glorious past, a golden age of saints and heroes" who are recognized as the foundation for the present. Australian sports history is replete with designated heroic events and people, which effectively supply a plethora of apolitical, sanitized heroes. Meanings about the nation are thus increasingly located within the realm of sport and are symbolized by the success of athletic bodies. Athletic heroes, such as Dawn Fraser, epitomize rags-to-riches scenarios and evoke images of the Aussie battler struggling to overcome obstacles. Thus, the sporting past, symbolized by the success of past athletic heroes, is reclaimed, revitalized and recast as a largely uncontested foundation for national identity.

Yet history in general and sports history in particular cannot develop a national identity. In order to establish the desired image of the nation, it is crucial to contrast Australia with other, less acceptable nations. Images of Australia as a unified, successful, and sporting nation, as denoted by its athletic representatives, are juxtaposed against images of "despicable," "drug-cheating" nations. A collective national stand against drugs is symbolic of the desired unity of the nation, despite the realities of a nation divided by debates about multiculturalism and immigration, indigenous land rights, and the rise of ultraconservative political movements. Over the past two centuries, nation-building in Australia has rested on attempts to construct an homogenous national identity based on oppositional cultural positions. On the one hand, the Australian nation is contrasted with other nations in order to stress its uniqueness, particularly when it comes to the environment (Walter, 1992); on the other, internal differences are minimized through the presentation of the nation as a unified, coherent structure. As a relatively isolated geographic entity, it has been much easier to maintain the unity of the discreet Australian nation compared with nations with more fluid national boundaries, such as European states. The integrity of Australian national borders, however, is popularly perceived to be under the threat of penetration by outside forces, such as Asianization, American popular culture, and disease. Consequently, Australia national borders are monitored and regulated with vigilance. Penetration of these borders is, firstly, a national concern and, secondly, a personal one, as can be seen with the regular unannounced arrival of boatloads of illegal Chinese immigrants. In one instance, the arrival of these illegal aliens on Australian shores was announced with great alarm by a newsagent (Meade, 1999). Even national citizens police the geo-political borders, establishing a correlation between the macro and micro social: the nation stands for the individual and vice versa. The threat, in the form of the illegal immigrant, is contained, and borders both personal and geographical are re-established. This type of containment is not reserved for illegal immigrants alone. Refugees, even those personally welcomed by the prime minister, such as the Kosovar refugees, are isolated and quarantined in a manner similar to foreign plants, foodstuffs, or anything that may cause the introduction of dis/ease and thus threaten the health of the Australian nation and the security of its borders.

The health of the Australian nation has been a concern for many since the foundation of a white settler colony in the late 18th century. The colonial settlers, upon arrival in Australia, encountered a hostile environment, and many observers feared that the colonial British would physically deteriorate as a result of the harsh Australian bush (Nauright, 1992). Yet, it was the bush and the vigorous outdoors lifestyle that began to clearly delineate an emerging Australian nation from its imperial core, if only in the minds of the urban dwellers (White, 1992). Given the successes of colonial troops in the Crimean and Boer Wars and in international sporting events, British leaders recognized that colonial bodies were thriving, and fears of racial degeneration began to focus on British bodies at home. By the early 1900s, physical activities in the form of institutional sport were considered primary in efforts to prevent the "enfeebling" of the British nation through the strengthening of individual bodies (Wohl, 1983). International sporting contests became moments in which physical national strength could be demonstrated to the world (Nauright, 1992). Success based on physical or sporting performance gradually supplemented and replaced success based on other forms of international competition. Athletic bodies became potent symbols of national strength/unity/health. In Australia, the distinctive national body, produced by a hostile and foreign environment, modified and improved in battle, tested against the imperial center in sporting contests, and cemented in a love affair with the great outdoors became central to an understanding of the nation. In this way, nature, and the composition of the natural Australian body, has been intrinsic in the construction of the Australian national identity.

When Sydney won the bid for the Olympics in 1993, its success was, in part, based on its commitment to an "environmentally friendly," "athletes' games," that is, a Games that was unpolluted and unpolluting (McGeoch and Korporaal, 1994). Selling the 2000 Olympic Games as the "Green Games" clearly links athletic bodies through sport to a bush mythology that regards the "Australian spirit" as "somehow intimately connected with the bush" and thus with the natural/national environment (Ward, 1992: 179). The Olympic vision promulgated by the Sydney bid team (later SOCOG) was of Australia as a natural and unpolluted environmental paradise, where the youth of the world could gather to celebrate in play without the threat of contamination. This "freedom to play" in a healthy, natural environment forms the basis of efforts to "clean up" not only the dioxin-contaminated Homebush Bay Olympic site, but also the wider Olympic movement through the removal of the corrupting influence of Phil Coles in particular and other IOC members in general as well as other "scourges" such as drugs (Lehmann, 1999; Magnay, 1999a). By removing these "snakes" from the Olympic "Garden of Eden," the unpolluted home/bush is in turn reproduced in assurances about the purity and naturalness of those Australian athletic bodies that intend to occupy this site. By constructing the nation as "clean/sed" and "natural," Australian athletes are signified as rightful heirs to the utopian psychosocial space of the home/bush.

The significance of the bush, the environment, and nature is magnified in efforts to present Australian athletes as "natural," that is, representative of the purified nation/nature. Foreign athletes, just like the illegal boat people who seek to penetrate Australia's shores, threaten the purity of the natural home/bush that has been constructed for the purpose of establishing Australia's global, sporting position. Thus foreign athletes who threaten the success of Australian athletes have been accused of variously breaking the Olympic Charter through state-sponsored training regimes or through the illicit ingestion of performance-enhancing substances.

Thus foreign athletic bodies represent an Other against which Australian athletic bodies can be tested.

Pitting bodies against each other in sporting competition to demonstrate relative national superiority is significant in this case study. Although they appear to be discreet biological entities, bodies are not natural phenomena. Sporting bodies in particular are inscribed with the symbols and rituals of nation through costuming, endorsements, tattoos, and demonstrations of patriotism such as carrying flags and singing anthems (Jarvie and Walker, 1994). Individually and collectively, sporting bodies stand in for the nation by representing "us," the people. In Australia, sports commentators regularly link the nation through its people to the sporting bodies on display:

> Kieren Perkins epitomises the Australian who lives in so many of our hearts. He is the face of Australia. Kieren is the Australian we want to hang on to. The Australian so many of us admire. Kieren Perkins made me feel not only extremely proud to be an Australian. Kieren Perkins made me feel both privileged and proud to have an Australian of his calibre out there representing me. If the world is going to see what an Australian is like, if there is a picture of an Australian we'd like shown around the globe, Kieren Perkins represents that image (cited in *Ironbark Legends*, 1997: 46).

In this way, individual bodies symbolize the collective aims and goals, characteristics and ideals of the nation.

Graeme Turner suggests a relationship between forms of national identity in Australia and sporting competition in which patriotism is embodied in the spectator, the sportsperson, and the spectacle (Turner, 1994: 68). Although this proposition may have some merit, these sporting events can also be read as attempts to produce a false vision/version of national unity. Through sport and sports-related entertainment, citizens are encouraged to take pride in the nation through the achievements of the nation's representatives (Brooks, 1996: 50). In addition, as David Sibley (1995: 15) points out, "the self is associated with fear and anxiety over the loss of control" and these fears and anxieties are "projected onto bad objects," anything that threatens the national borders, including foreign bodies. This correlation between the body/individual and the nation/social self is extremely significant in the discussions of how the issue of drugs in sport is used in nation-building.

Drugs in Sport

Analyzing the public focus in Australia on anti-doping campaigns can assist in interpreting ways in which an accepted (singular) national identity can be generated through sport, and specifically through elite, Olympic sport. In Australia, the drugs-in-sport issue has increased to immense proportions in the popular imagination. Regular debates appear in sporting magazines, and news and current affairs shows focus on cleaning up sport's "tarnished image" in time for Sydney 2000. The drug scandals at the Seoul Olympics and the Australian Senate Inquiry into Drugs in Sport were landmarks in anti-doping debates during the late 1980s, yet more recently focus has turned to swimming, a sport in which Australia prides itself on being historically internationally competitive—over half of Australia's Olympic medals have been won in or on the water. Since the late 1980s, the discourse has shifted slightly, however, from one of identifying drug cheats within Australia (the Senate Inquiry) to identifying cheats outside Australia's national borders, with attention focused on the Chinese swim team. The identification of foreign drug cheats contrasted against clean Australian athletes reduces the relationship to a binary arrangement that revolves around the concept of "natural" versus "unnatural" bodies.

Casting Australian athletes as "natural" and contrasting them with "unnatural" foreign athletes becomes important in the process of constructing the right of Australia as a legitimate leader in an international (sporting) hierarchy, particularly as these types of configurations form a nostalgic link between Australia 2000, the 1956 Olympics, and a romanticized ideal of a pure and noble ancient competition. This oppositional framework also works to legitimate the competition. Regardless of the outcome, Australia as a pure, natural nation will always be the winner; thus boundaries are maintained that clearly place the "loser"/"unclean" bodies/nation outside the geographical, political, and imagined nation. Boundary consciousness is a characteristic of modern Western society that is particularly prevalent in times of crisis. There is particular effort to sustain a cultural homogeneity that contains the self and expels the other (Sibley 1995: 38-39). Sporting events are indicative of this. Sporting competitions are regulated by rules, and competitors are placed in direct competition with an/other. The winning individual/team is constructed within the discourse of competition as a self; the losing individual/team as an other that is expelled. This boundary consciousness, however, also applies at the level of the body where spatial boundaries equate with moral and ethical boundaries and where what constitutes an acceptable human embodiment is strictly policed (Cranny-Francis 1995: 96). The rules that structure competition also govern what a body can and cannot ingest, and the ways that a body can be modified and manipulated in order to improve performance. Methods and substances, however, differ over time and between sports. The penetration or violation of the individual body by drugs threatens the integrity of the athletic body, the sporting body and its laws, and ultimately, the nation. Drug-taking destabilizes these firmly monitored borders, turning them into a "heterogenous" and "dangerously unstable zone" (Donald, 1988: 36). The expulsion of drugs and the body/ies that ingest them reaffirms the oppositions that maintain cultural and social homogeneity.

Scientific Training, Drugs, and Identity

Throughout the 1990s, Australia has been (re)positioned as a nation that is "drunk" on sport and as a community that is particularly concerned with the "naturalness" of physical achievement. Yet, the concept of "natural" sport or "natural" sporting bodies has adjusted over time to accommodate changing training methods. In Australia, before the 1980s, the Soviet model of elite sport was denigrated for its overt professionalism, popularly known as "shamateurism" and anathema to the "true" nature of sport that promoted ideals of "fair play" or of playing for the "love of the game." The Soviet system was accused of violating, if not the law, then the spirit of the Olympic Charter, and, by implication, of sport itself. The rejection of scientific training methods in favor of a more natural "amateurist" approach classified training methods according to the binary categories "physical/technological" or "natural/artificial." In this way, the distinctions made between the two training regimes meant that despite a lack of international athletic success, particularly in the 1970s, the Australian system of elite sport was justified as more wholesome, more "natural," and thus, more legitimate. Despite widespread criticism, Soviet scientific training methods proved to be highly successful in the development of elite sport, which led to rapid international success for the Eastern Bloc. Australia's more "natural" approach, however, was not as successful, and following the 1976 Montreal Olympics at which Australian athletes won no gold medals, Eastern European training methods were quickly adopted by the Australian sporting fraternity. Despite public reservations about the appropriateness of "communist" style sport, the Australian Institute of Sport, opened in 1981, was founded on the principles of "scientific" training (Daly, 1991; Semotiuk, 1987). Training according to efficient scientific methods was now a "natural" approach to extending physical capabilities, whereas physical enhancement through drugs increasingly became regarded as unnatural or artificial. Despite this slight shift in focus, "Othering" remained centered on the manipulation of the body not at a gross anatomical level, but rather, at a cellular level.

The drug-taking foreigner has therefore been constructed as antithetical to the essential character of Australians while the application of sophisticated sports science and training methods in Australia are accepted as a necessary part of contemporary sport. Australia's role as anti-drug crusader is more important than simply shoring up a sense of contemporary identity. Australia's "glorious" sporting past is reclaimed through the evocation of Australia as a nation of legitimate/natural athletes who resist the temptations of "cheating" or gaining "unfair" advantage. Past sporting failures, particularly those in the 1970s, are viewed in light of allegations of Eastern Bloc drug-taking. By branding certain athletes as drug cheats, images of the beleaguered "Aussie battler" are evoked, and Australia's (non-)successes in sport are represented as more legitimate and thus worthy of recognition. Heightening Australia's image as a crusader for clean sport reinforces the battler amateurist ethos surrounding Australian sport and sporting heroes, and this battler image is extended into the past as some athletes have sought to have medals awarded or upgraded because they lost to Eastern Bloc athletes who were accused of being "drug cheats."

In 1997 and 1998 references were repeatedly made to athletes who had their medals "stolen" by "drug cheats" (Kitney, 1997; Black, 1998). Lisa Curry-Kenny and Raelene Boyle both were "robbed" of their medals by "steroid-fueled" athletes from East Germany, and thus Australia was denied part of its place in golden Olympic history (Kitney, 1997). In order to prove this point, the Australian current affairs show, *Sixty Minutes*, took Curry-Kenny and Boyle to Germany to search for evidence against, and then hunt down and confront, the women who had "stolen" *their* medals (*Sixty Minutes*, 1997). Raelene Boyle, who believes she "lost to drugs," was defeated by East German sprinter Renate Stecher in the 100 meters and 200 meters in Munich, and Lisa Curry-Kenny finished fifth behind three East Germans in the 100-meter butterfly in Moscow in 1980 (Evans, 1997; Gatt, 1997; Black, 1998). These athletes demanded that the women who defeated them admit that their victories were drug-induced. With this information, they hoped to be able to reclaim from the IOC the medals that were "rightfully" theirs.

The Natural/Unnatural Body

Signifying athletes or even nations as "natural" is not an exclusively Australian practice. Within sport in general, bodies are presented as "natural," uncontested entities. Tim Armstrong (1996: 10) argues, however, that "the body . . . is an open text that is constantly rewritten and reinterpreted." As a result, athletic bodies need to be regularly re/presented to the public through advertisements, current affairs programs, and campaigns against drugs in sport to confirm their status as clearly natural entities. Laurel Davis and Linda Delano (1992: 4) have argued in their study of campaigns against drugs in sport that "media texts assume, reinforce, and help to naturalize the notion that the human body is or can be purely natural." Further, readers of these texts are "encouraged to assume that the body is [always] purely natural unless disrupted by artificial substances" (Davis and Delano, 1992: 4). Other texts, such as advertisements for "natural" foodstuffs, reinforce the link between the "natural," "healthy" body and sport, through the use of former "Olympic legends" such as Shane Gould, who promotes a nongenetically engineered soy drink product.

Despite the fact that external intervention may threaten a body's "natural" status, as indicated before, some procedures are recast as legitimate and in fact desirable for elite sports performance. In this instance an interesting paradox emerges. Sport is supposed to compare "natural" bodies with one another, yet bodies cannot remain in an unaltered state if they are to succeed at an international level. Of course, training and the ingestion of performance-enhancing substances, such as carbohydrates, may be regarded as a necessary part of any training regime. Nowhere is this paradox more clear than in the *Report of the Working Group on the Legal and Political Aspects of Doping* presented at the 1999 World Conference on Doping. This report suggests that doping be defined, in part, as "the use of an expedient (substance or method) which is potentially harmful to athletes' health and capable of enhancing their performance" (Mbaye, 1999: 3). With such a broad definition, training itself becomes "unnatural."

Chris Shilling (1993: 5) suggests that the body can be read as an ongoing project in which bodies "become malleable entities which can be shaped and honed with the vigilance and hard work of their owners." Within sport, bodies require constant monitoring, regulation, and programming to achieve optimum physical performance. In other words, they must be "shaped and honed" into a fit and proper athletic specimen to compete against equally fit exemplars. The Queensland Department of Tourism, Sport, and Racing highlights the notion that the "fundamental ethos of sporting competition is the rivalry between highly skilled athletes who have attained their expertise through *hard work* and *natural ability*" (Information Paper No. 1, 1998; emphasis added). Performance-enhancing drugs, by contrast, represent some kind of simplistic avenue to physical success. They appear to be an "easy option" or "quick fix," one that negates the vigilant "shaping and honing" that is required to succeed in elite sport (Slattery, 1998). However, if substances can be proven to be "natural" or even essential for health, they can be seen as appropriate for ingestion. Bordreau and Konzak (1991: 93), for example, suggest that steroids are essentially in a class of their own, since unlike (banned) drugs such as antibiotics or antiasthmatics, steroids do not "bring back health." The restoration of health is a critical element in the defense of Australian athletes who take drugs, for the condition of Australian athletic bodies symbolizes the condition of the nation, even though international sporting success usually does not correlate with national physical fitness. In the case of swimmers Sam Riley (headache), Richard Upton (ear infection), and Natasha Bowron (chronic bowel inflammation) and the Australian cycling team (immune system), the restoration of health is considered a legitimate reason for the ingestion of banned substances (Smith, 1998; Schlink, 1998). In each of these cases, the drugs were required by selected athletic bodies for legitimate health/medical reasons in order to cure the body and return it its "natural," "healthy" state.

Colostrum provides a useful example of the process for reconfiguring banned products as legitimate health-restoring supplements. At the 1998 Commonwealth Games in Kuala Lumpur, the head of the British Sport Council's drug unit revealed that Australian cyclists were taking colostrum, a product that contains the banned substance Insulin Growth Factor-1 (IGF-1) (Schlink, 1998). These allegations came soon after Australian cyclist and Festina team member Neil Stephens was accused of taking the banned substance erythropoietin during the 1998 Tour de France and the Australian cyclists were subsequently branded "drug cheats." Such allegations threatened to invalidate Australia's claim to take the toughest stance on illegal performance-enhancing drugs and expose the Sydney 2000 Olympics to potential disruption by the drug-fueled bodies of not only Other athletes but "ours" as well. Without the presence of a definite Other, the security of Australian identity is in jeopardy; thus colostrum was firmly recast as a "natural" product that represented an advance in scientific training that boosted the immune systems of representative Australian bodies. Thus, colostrum could not be equated with artificial or synthetic products, and the performance-enhancing properties of IGF-

1 were negated by the natural ingestion of colostrum *tablets*. According to Australian Commonwealth Games medical director, Brian Sando, if colostrum is taken in tablet form, the IGF-1 is "*denatured* in the stomach and cannot be absorbed into the body. The only way it can be absorbed is by injection"(Schlink, 1998, emphasis added). Colostrum tablets are thus assuredly natural, for all sustenance must come through the mouth. The *injection* of this same substance, however, represents an illegitimate penetration of the body's boundaries and thus cannot be regarded as a "natural" method of training. While negating the performance-enhancing aspects of IGF-1, the Australian cycling team doctor Peter Barnes further explained that colostrum was a "dairy product" rather than a drug and confirmed that colostrum is "produced *naturally* at the moment of birth" (Schlink, 1998, emphasis added). The "naturalness" and thus legitimacy of the product is validated through associations with "Mother" nature. Barnes is thereby linking colostrum with the purity of life and the innocence of children, and equating athletic performance enhancement with the life-giving properties of mother's milk. Thus the (national) body is strengthened by "natural" substances that prevent the penetration of infection and the nation takes on the role of motherhood in the management of the health and well being of her athletes.

The preoccupation with the drug-taking of the Chinese and East German swimmers clearly indicates how social anxieties are projected onto a concern with the body (Shilling, 1993). By focusing attention on the *abuse* of foreign athletic bodies, the correct use of Australian athletic bodies is highlighted. This displacement and "othering" of those who take performance-enhancing drugs displaces them outside not only a national discourse, but also outside the boundaries of a shared international moral discourse. By injecting her/his body with a forbidden substance the athlete incorporates, or makes part of her/his body, the other, and thus contaminates her/his self/national identity. When this occurs, a destabilization of the boundaries between self and other and nation and other occurs, introducing the notion of dis/ease and creating national and global uncertainty. The process of identifying drug abusers requires strict monitoring and surveillance that moves across individual, physical, and national borders (Whiting, 1998; Magnay, 1999b).

When the Chinese swimmers first came to international attention in the early 1990s, the media constructed their performance as spectacle. These "grotesque bodies" were labeled clearly "unnatural" and as these bodies began to dominate the international swimming scene, allegations of drug taking quickly surfaced (Carlile, 1995). They were demonized immediately by Australian competitors and commentators alike, and an emotive discourse was used to both construct and convey the unnatural state of these bodies to the viewing public. Part of the reason that these bodies appeared "grotesque" was because of the obvious gender confusion their external appearance caused. Although they were signified as female, they appeared to have male attributes that confused the boundaries between essentialist gender categories. As Chinese swimmers appeared neither wholly male, nor wholly female, they were regarded as objects of fear for Australia's female swimmers, as these "anabolic Amazons" represented what their bodies could become—masculine women (Treacy, 1998). These forms also represented further threats to the clear boundaries between east and west bodies, for the Chinese swimmers obliterated the traditional stereotype of the small, petite, fragile oriental body. Only occidental bodies were considered to be large and strong. These swimmers were the Yellow Peril manifest, a particularly potent threat in light of Australia's cultural history and anti-Asian hysteria. As a prophylactic to the dis/ease the Chinese athletes augured, Australian swimmers publicly announced their victories in the pool before races were held. This type of announcement functions as a recovery for the lost or threatened self as the other invades and penetrates by winning and taking the glory that rightfully belongs to the nation/self. By making these announcements, Australian athletes were ensuring that after a drought of Olympic swimming medals over the past 20 years, the Chinese will not rob them of "their" "rightful" medals as the Communists had done.

The search for Australian identity thus becomes a search for wholeness, yet the sporting culture, in which national identity is popularly located, cannot provide a pure, whole self. The sporting body itself is "contaminated." Australia's struggle to purify sport can be read as mirroring attempts to purify the nation. The futility of this process is clear. By closely linking Australian identity with sport, and particularly through the issue of drugs in sport, the search for a pure Australia will never end. The Australian nation has been constructed as a hard-line, vigilant campaigner, a lone ranger in the war against drugs in sport. This positioning gives the island nation standing in the international community and sets it apart from other "weaker" or more "impure" nations. However, confirmation of Australia's identity through the relentless crusade against drugs could unravel if all drug use were removed from sport. An "Aussie battler" only exists if there is something to battle. Yet despite this, increasingly sophisticated efforts are made to rid the sporting body of the "scourge" of drug use.

As the climax of the Sydney 2000 Olympic Games draws closer, the manufacturing of a specific "natural" Australian identity and associated nation-building becomes apparent. The relationship between the nation as an imagined community and the sporting body as a manifestation of this construct signifies the relevance of sport and athletic competition to national identity. In Australia, the construction of a "natural" and healthy Olympic site has focused on drugs in sport and the elimination of the drug threat as a way of excising the "unnatural" and grotesque from the nation/self. The media, the public, and a number of Australian athletes have sought to demonize athletes from other countries who have been suspected and/or found to be taking performance-enhancing drugs. These campaigns seek to specifically brand as "Other" a variety of sporting bodies, such as the East Germans and Chinese. This displacement and "Othering" creates an "us" and "them" binary in which the "us" is configured as clean and proper and the "them" as grotesque and improper. The use of these binary oppositions to support and enhance national identity functions to displace the bodies that "abuse" to a position outside mainstream configurations of national and sporting identity, and thereby reaffirm the purity of the Australian nation/body.

References

Armstrong, T., ed. 1996. *American Bodies. Cultural Histories of the Physique*. New York: New York Press.

Black, R. 1998. Cheated duo calls for action. *Sunday Mail*, 25 October.

Bordreau, F., and Konzak, B. 1991. Ben Johnson and the use of steroids in sport: Sociological and ethical considerations. *Canadian Journal of Sport Science*, 16(2): 88-98.

Brooks, K. 1996. Odysseus unbound and Penelope unstable: Contemporary Australian expatriate women writers." Unpublished PhD thesis, University of Wollongong, N.S.W.

Cameron, P. 1998. Aussies' Olympic Apathy. *Sunday Mail*, 24 April.

Carlile, F. 1995. Why the Chinese must not swim at Atlanta '96. *Inside Sport* 47: 18-29.

Cowley, M. 1998. China long day journey into drugs nightmare. *Sydney Morning Herald*, 9 January.

Cranny-Francis, A. 1995. *The Body in the Text*. Melbourne: Melbourne University Press.

Daly, J. 1991. *The Australian Institute of Sport in Canberra*. Canberra: AGPS.

Davis, L., and Delano, L. 1992. Fixing the boundaries of physical gender: Side effects of anti-drug campaigns in athletics. *Sociology of Sport Journal* 9(1): 1-19.

Donald, J. 1988. How English is it? Popular literature and national culture. *New Foundations* 6: 31-47.

Evans, L. 1997. Anger as East German gets top sport job. *Sydney Morning Herald*, 3 October.

Evans, L. 1998. Perkins: FINA must act to save our sport. *Sydney Morning Herald*, 10 January.

Gatt, R. 1997. Aussies line up for retrospective honours. *The Australian*, 12 September.

Hall, S. 1992. The question of cultural identity. In S. Hall, D. Held, and T. McGrew, eds., *Modernity and Its Futures*. Cambridge: Polity Press.

Ironbark Legends. 1997. *Kieren Perkins*. Melbourne: Macmillan.

Jarvie, G., and Walker, G., eds. 1994. *Scottish Sport in the Making of the Nation: Ninety Minute Patriots?* London: Leicester University Press.

Kitney, G. 1997. Raelene's hopes for gold dashed once more. *Sydney Morning Herald*, 22 November.

Lehmann, J. 1999. Coles case hurting good name of Games. *The Weekend Australian*, 6/7 March.

Magdalinski, T. 1998a. Organized memories: The construction of sporting traditions in the GDR. *European Sports History Review* 1: 144-163.

Magdalinski, T. 1998b. Recapturing Australia's glorious sporting past: Drugs and Australian identity. *Bulletin of Sport and Culture* 14: 1, 6-8.

Magnay, J. 1999a. Coles accused of disgracing IOC. *Sydney Morning Herald*, 5 March.

Magnay, J. 1999b. IOC backs airport drugtest. *Sydney Morning Herald*, 18 June.

Mbaye, K. 1999. *Report of the Working Group on the Legal and Political Aspects of Doping*. World Conference on Doping, Lausanne, February 1999, p. 3.

McGeoch, R., and Korporaal, G. 1994. *The Bid. How Australia Won the 2000 Games*. Melbourne: William Heinemann.

Meade, K. 1999. Life's a beach for boatload of intruders. *The Weekend Australian*, 13/14 March.

Nauright, J. 1992. Sport and the image of colonial manhood in the British mind: British physical education deterioration debates and colonial sporting tours, 1878-1906. *Canadian Journal of the History of Sport* 23(3): 54-71.

Queensland Department of Tourism, Sport and Racing (1998). *What Is Drugs in Sport?* Information Paper No. 1.

Schlink, L. 1998. "Drug cheats." Games claim rocks Aussies. *Sunday Mail*, 20 September.

Semotiuk, D. 1987. Commonwealth Government initiatives in amateur sport in Australia 1972-1985. *Sporting Traditions*, 3(2): 152-162.

Shilling, C. 1993. *The Body and Social Theory*. London: Sage.

Sibley, D. 1995. *Geographies of Exclusion. Society and Difference in the West*. London, New York: Routledge.

Sixty Minutes. 1997. Channel 9 Australia, 23 November.

Slattery, L. 1998. Steroids: Society's quick fix. *The Weekend Australian*, 27/28 June.

Smith, A.D. 1991. *National Identity*. London: Penguin.

Smith, W. 1998. Nightmare over drugs use. *Sunday Mail*, 24 April.

Treacy, L. 1998. Letters to the sports editor. *Sunday Mail*, 18 January.

Turner, G. 1994. *Making It National: Nationalism and Australian Popular Culture*. St. Leonards, N.S.W.: Allen and Unwin.

Walter, J. 1992. Defining Australia. In G. Whitlock and D. Carter, eds., *Images of Australia*. St. Lucia: University of Queensland Press, pp. 7-22.

Ward, R. 1992. The Australian legend. In G. Whitlock and D. Carter, eds., *Images of Australia*. St. Lucia: University of Queensland Press, pp. 179-190.

Whiting, F. 1998. Lie tests nab drug cheats. *Sunday Mail*, 11 October.

Wohl, A.S. 1983. *Endangered Lives. Public Health in Victorian Britain*. Cambridge, MA: Harvard University Press.

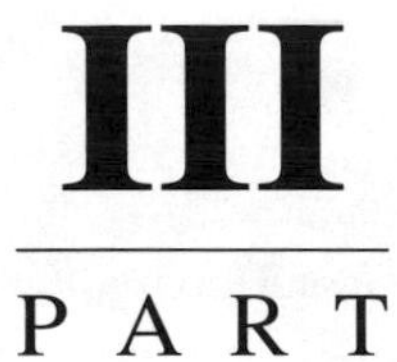

PART

The Politics of Doping

8

CHAPTER

Doping and Moral Authority: Sport Organizations Today

John J. MacAloon
The University of Chicago

At the World Conference on Doping in Sport in February 1999, International Olympic Committee (IOC) leaders were stunned by the vigorous attacks on their moral authority in the doping field made from the podium by government officials and technical delegates to the conference. The IOC should have anticipated what was coming and that it would come directly from the doping front line and not (as some IOC members and senior staff wanted to believe) as a mere spillover from the bribery and corruption scandals simultaneously afflicting the organization.

Since Max Weber, authority has been defined in modern organizational science as the socially legitimated use of power: the force of violence where state authority is concerned, the power of salvation or enlightenment where religious authority is at issue, and the force of judicial sanctions where legal authority is in question.[1] The root paradigm is the same regardless of the type of organization: if society withdraws its gift of moral legitimation, the organization necessarily falls into a crisis marked by the progressive decline of its moral authority into factionalized assertions of mere power and interest. This is precisely the process that overtook the IOC in 1998-1999.

On July 26, 1998, concurrent with the doping "busts" of the Tour de France achieved by French ministerial, judicial, and police officials, IOC President Juan Antonio Samaranch's explosive remarks on doping were published in *El Mundo* and within a day, around the world. These statements accelerated the waning of confidence in the IOC's moral commitment to the anti-doping fight, not only among a wider public (because of the press these remarks received) but within the "Olympic family" itself. In the aftermath of their president's unfortunate remarks, the IOC Executive quickly announced the Lausanne doping summit as a transparent attempt at damage control, an intended antidote to the suddenly public challenge to IOC authority.

This was still four months before the Salt Lake City scandal began to break. Hence, the summer 1998 developments in doping surely contributed more to reception of the bribery scandal in specialist, press, and public opinions than the other way around. However, there can be no doubt that by early 1999, the two imbroglios were powerfully reinforcing each other, as the IOC plunged into a full-blown legitimacy crisis from which it has a very long way to go, at this writing, to recover.[2]

However, it was already possible to foresee these developments well before the Festina team trainer was caught with his carload of erythropoietin and human growth hormone, and well before Samaranch stated that with respect to use of "nonharmful" pharmaceutical training aids: "For me that is not doping."

In the original version of this paper, presented at an April 1998 conference on doping in elite sport hosted by the Amateur Athletic Foundation of Los Angeles, I argued that any public perception that the IOC had secretly given up on the anti-doping fight would be far more damaging to the organization than its obvious and repeated failures to stop the tidal wave of drug use in Olympic sport. Appearing to throw in the towel, I suggested, would be even more harmful than if all of the critics' charges, rumors, and innuendoes about abuses of testing procedures and cover-up of results by Olympic and International Federation (IF) officials were suddenly proved true. Battles can be lost and traitors can be outed, but surrender and abandonment of the field, especially under some self-serving rationalization, would remove any claim an organization had to moral standing as a true social movement in sport.

In this published version, my original text is preserved (with superficial editing) in the following section. This original article did not of course predict the specific events of summer 1998, but it foresaw what the impact of events with such meanings in such contexts would surely be on the IOC. After presenting this material, I will further discuss what Samaranch and French minister of youth and sport Marie-George Buffet between them wrought, the World Conference on Doping in Sport, and aspects of the present situation, all of which confirm my original hypothesis that any perception that the IOC had given up the anti-doping fight would seriously damage the credibility of the organization.

Under Authoritative Eyes (Spring 1998)

Whether judged to be immoral, unethical, illegal, psychopathological, or all of these, doping in high-performance sport is everywhere determinedly invisible. That, after all, is in the essence of cheating. Under normal conditions, the moral authority of institutions also operates in a largely imperceptible manner. Indeed, structures of authority become most apparent to both their subjects and objects when their legitimacy is publicly threatened. To begin an inquiry whose purpose is to worry about the general effects on the authority of international sports organizations if they should come to be perceived as having given up on the anti-doping struggle, I therefore offer a cautionary tale about visibility and invisibility. Although it speaks directly from the experience of only one sport ethnologist, it offers a paradigm of the several modes by which many Olympic partisans can and have lost faith.

If, like me, you had a background in the sport and had attended nearly every session of track and field over the last four Olympic Games, you too might have noticed a rather strange development. By Atlanta, Olympic track and field finalists seemed to have become less thirsty.

In "Hotlanta," I observed no finalists drinking on the field immediately after their races. Had the athletes at last learned how to properly hydrate for the finals? Were they for some reason more emotionally overwhelmed by their performances in Atlanta than they had been in Los Angeles, Seoul, and Barcelona? One had to wonder, because in those Olympics, there had been a lot of odd postrace thirst-quenching.

From the Games of 1984 through the Games of 1992, an increasingly noticeable number of competitors just past the finish line—in those moments of thrilled incomprehension, horrific frustration, shocked destiny, or deepest release scarcely imaginable to the rest of us—ran to the railings and barriers separating the field from the stands, managed to find a particular coach or lover or clubmate to embrace, and somehow collected themselves long enough take a long drink from bottles of liquid pushed into their hands by these equally delirious friends and associates.

Now it's pretty hard for anyone to drink and to exult at the same time. If I'd ever finished an Olympic final, getting a drink of water would not be the first thing on my mind. Strange, too, that with the thirst so great, the plastic bottle always went back up into the stands with the colleague who'd brought it and was never taken along on the victory lap or into the mixed zone, or just dropped on the infield as the negligible object one would suppose it to be.

Was water being denied in the warm-up areas? It hardly appeared so the times I visited them during each of these Games. Had athletes become so paranoid that they now refused bottled water and sports drinks supplied by the Olympic organizing committee (OCOG)? Well, if so, they surely had their own prerace supplies of fluid. No training regimen in any athletics event, to my knowledge, actually prescribes dehydration before competition. Of course, hyped-up athletes might forget to drink, and serious dehydration could weaken an athlete for days to come. But how would their collaborators up in the stands have known this to have happened? And why would they have stopped knowing in Atlanta (where no new International Amateur Athletic Federation [IAAF] rule had come into force against such comradely succor)? Moreover, I observed this curiously urgent, postevent drinking among athletes who had just finished their final competition of the Games, not just among those with other events ahead of them. And sprinters, long-hurdlers, and multi-eventers rushed to get this apparently much-needed refreshment, more frequently than distance runners.

With respect to Los Angeles, it was pretty much after the fact that this odd behavior began to stand out in my mind. In Seoul, I didn't think to count the episodes I saw and pointed out to colleagues. (Perhaps there were a half-dozen, all surely recorded in the international-feed broadcast tapes stored at the Olympic Museum in Lausanne.) In Barcelona, I didn't want to count episodes; they'd become more numerous and more disheartening. There, the finalists and their libation-bearers had to actually get across the camera pit, a veritable moat, and break through the staff policing to meet on a narrow bridge for the exchange of a wild embrace and a carefully organized potion. Two or three times, this literally happened under a national flag being thrust into the imbibing champion's other hand for the ensuing victory lap.

I cannot prove that these so-visible drinks were filled with invisible masking agents. However, the issue here is not individual guilt but confidence in the moral authority of institutions. How could such a suspicious practice have been permitted to go on at all? What might a reasonable person conclude about the moral legitimacy of the leading international sport organizations—the IOC, the International Federations (IFs), the National Olympic Committees (NOCs)—when such public behavior went apparently unnoticed and unaddressed? The episodes I have described took place directly under the gaze of and frequently no more than 30 yards away from the entire anti-doping hierarchy of the IOC and the IAAF, not to mention officers of the various NOCs and National Federations in attendance. Moreover, I can assure from personal experience that the top athletic brass in the IOC/IF sections and the IOC and IAAF presidents' boxes are no less intensely observant of those golden postrace moments than anyone else in the stadium. Indeed, because these top officials have the best seats in the house, often have strong personal knowledge of the competitors involved and may be eager to participate in subsequent press conferences, victory ceremonies, and marketing meetings, they generally pay the very closest attention to the postevent behaviors of finalists.

Thus it is simply impossible for me to believe that the practices I've described have never fallen into the visual fields of those holding authority in the struggle against doping. On the explicit doping-control front, moreover, a tight chain of command stretches up from the OCOG athlete escorts on the field, to the doping control medical officers and technical staff waiting just offstage, through the IOC and IAAF Medical Commission members who happen to be sitting in the "Olympic family" stand, straight upstairs to Samaranch and Alexandre de Merode, chairman of the Medical Commission, sitting in the tribune on any given day, and to Mr. Primo Nebiolo, president of the IAAF, and his officers, who rarely miss a minute in their own tribunes.

It is impossible to believe that. But perhaps while ever observant, these professional authorities just never have seen, that is, have never perceived anything suspicious in these unusual drinking practices? Such a thought must strain credulity. These are *the authorities*, after all, and *by definition the authorities cannot be blind*, certainly not when mere amateurs without power or authority (and in cheaper seats) are perfectly able to see things for what they might be. Therefore, what might reasonably be concluded in the face of this contradiction between vision and authority? What are the options for interpretation and judgment?

The first would be that these are false authorities who know nothing about actual doping practices, persons so incompetent that athletes can freely dope right under these officials' very eyes. Perhaps these officials were selected for political, patronage, or commercial reasons, rather than by professional criteria.

The second interpretation would be that these are false authorities of a different, actively complicitous or passive kind, persons who are willfully and deliberately ignoring blatantly suspicious practices because they have no real wish to catch drug-users. Either there is direct reward for officials in the high performance of doped athletes, or, because officials' own careers are dependent on the goodwill of a sports organization's leadership, they turn a blind eye to this kind of doping. After all, the IOC and IF leaderships answer to no one, save occasionally a judicial court and the even weaker "court" of public opinion. Where would underlings turn for support if the leaderships are suspect of complicity?

In a third possible explanation, the authorities are neither incompetent nor venal: they are simply afraid to act. One can so easily hear them saying: "What would you have us do? Run up into the stands after the guy and confiscate the bottle? Then test that? Can you imagine the legal problems we'd open ourselves up to? We've got lawsuits enough over doping controls already, without publicly seizing ordinary citizens' property! And there could be a public incident, a brawl, and with the world media watching. Imagine the furor."

Furor is precisely what real morality would welcome. If any of these scenarios is true, it is deeply disheartening. True moral authority (never to be confused with mere moralism, much less mere management) anticipates, even cultivates furor; that, after all, is why there are social movements in the first place. True moral authority must always and automatically issue the order to itself: "The second you see such a thing, go up into the stands after them." If you observe, you must act, and you must act spontaneously whenever collective values and sentiments held sacred, are outraged, much less in such a brazen fashion. Such is the very nature of moral authority, and if you do not act in this way you are demonstrating in the clearest possible way that these values are not sacreds to you. If all you do is calculate the practical costs and benefits, the utilitarian wisdom of a counteraction, or the effect on public peace, then you demonstrate precisely that moral authority has been forsaken in favor of legal, administrative, and commercial interests and considerations.

It is an iron law of sociology, as Durkheim and Weber taught earlier in this century, that power and moral authority cannot be confused with one another without ensuring that one of them will eventually be lost. So if the authorities have reduced themselves to being lawyers and public relations managers, mere utilitarians, they have effectively surrendered any legitimate claim to wider social and moral legitimacy. This is even more so when they have surrendered out of fear for their own positions and perquisites. No pious chatter about Olympism, the glories of sport, and the dangers of drugs could ever compensate for such an abnegation.

The fourth alternative interpretation is interrelated in complex ways with the other three. It surmises that the authorities are not so much incompetent, venal, or cowed, as that they are now resigned at some very deep level to the continued presence of what they recognize, refuse, and morally despise, but cannot any longer imagine how to stop. In a nutshell, the authorities know they have lost against doping and have lost permanently. They may theoretically say, "Why even bother with a few athletes taking masking agents on the very field of play before a stadium and a worldwide television audience? The doping monster is so hydra-headed now; stop one practice, and the dope-cheats will just find four or five others. And there are far worse things going on in sport doping than having a few of the usual suspects confirming their guilt in such a visible way. At least they are obviously doing it to themselves, rather than having others surreptitiously doing it to them."

With respect to preserving the moral authority of sports officials and organizations, and not just in medical but in all sporting and social matters, this last conclusion would have the worst possible outcome. Incompetence can always be rooted out, official coconspirators can be found, embarrassed, and exiled (if rarely convicted), and ways can at least be sought to raise the voices of true authority above the legalists, public relations specialists, and marketing managers. But if there no longer are any such voices and convictions in these organizations, if the public and the rest of the international sport community come to believe that their leaderships and their organizational cultures have thrown in the towel in defeat over drugging in sport, then the effect on the overall legitimacy, prestige, and deference afforded these bodies will surely be devastating.

Sports leaders should make no mistake: as the performing body is the center of everything in sport, so the problem of the body being performance-enhanced by drugs can never be forced away from the moral center of sport authority. If the leaderships have resigned themselves to doping as an ineradicable element of contemporary elite sport practice, they have simultaneously and necessarily admitted that their authority over international sport now derives solely from the profits of the spectacle and from political control over the athletes and OCOGs who produce them. Besides these resources, only a precarious status under international and various national laws (in the relatively weak areas of transnational labor and trademark law) stands between an organization like the IOC and dissolution of institutional structures into naked power struggles it is very unlikely to win.

Given such stakes, what might lead sports leaders to resign, however unconsciously, from the fight against doping? It is not so much the impact of big public scandals, as many people believe, nor the professional frustration of specialists in sport medicine and anti-doping inside sports organizations. Rather, in my observation, the chief threat turning doping into an unconsciously normalized practice for sports officers is the moral weathering and withering that result from the grinding everyday flow of discourse on drugs in sport. Information fatigue can render officials no longer able to perceive, with moral accuracy, what is right before their eyes. Possible doping in the Olympic stadium and right in front of the television cameras? What an outrage! But why get outraged all over again, knowing that at best you'll end up stymied in some lawsuit somewhere? Why go through all that once again to no good end? Thus may outrage die of frustrated, legalized, melodramatized outrage.[3]

The IOC *Press Review* goes out several times a week to IOC members and key staffers, IF presidents who are not IOC members, OCOGs, many NOCs, candidate cities, strategic partners, and a few independent scholars and Olympic studies centers. A typical issue of the *Press Review* contains four sections: (1) selected articles from the world press on any and all Olympic topics thought to be of interest to the sports leadership; (2) digests of world political and economic news taken from Agence France Presse (AFP), Reuters, the *Financial Times,* and *The Wall Street Journal*; (3) newswire dispatches (AFP, Deutche Presse-Agentur, Agencia EFE, Reuters, Kyodo) from which the actual newspaper articles are often derived; and (4) official press releases and communiques of the IOC and other sports bodies.

I can offer no systematic information on how thoroughly sports leaders attend to these documents. I know IOC members who pore over them daily; I also know IOC members and OCOG chiefs who claim never to have looked at a single issue. In some cases, leaders with large staffs leave it to underlings to spot articles of specific interest to the person or organization. There are also linguistic considerations with these documents, as well as the very predictable biases toward the Northern hemisphere in the newspapers and wire services sampled, conventions which make these press summaries of less interest and value to sports leaders in certain parts of the world than in others. On the other hand, among IOC members and IF and NOC officials distant from the centers of world media production (which are typically congruent with the centers of sport power), among press and public relations specialists inside of organizations, and among the campaign managers of aspirants for higher office in the IOC and IFs, these documents are often closely scrutinized.

Still, with all the limitations and uncertainties attendant upon their production, distribution, and consumption, the IOC *Press Review*s, offer valuable resources for international researchers interested in characterizing public and popular discourses. As a thought experiment, let us imagine that key sport leaders are skimming all of the press reviews for a stated period of time. What would be the volume and shape of the information on doping they are receiving from these documents?

My colleague Jeanne Haffner and I surveyed the 88 editions of the *Press Review* that arrived in my office during a period of 11 months, from March 1997 through January 1998. (It must be kept in mind that these months included coverage of several weighty nondoping topics, including the bid campaigns for and selection of the host city for 2004, extensive political developments with respect to the Sydney Games, and the run-up to Nagano.) The results of this convenience sample show that of the 6,468 items contained in the published article and wire service dispatch sections of these 88 issues, 773, or over 11 percent of the total, concerned themselves with doping cases, problems, issues, and events. Of the 725 wire service dispatches in the sample, fully 232, an astonishing 32 percent, contained at least some coverage of doping issues. Of the 5,743 actually published newspaper articles in the sample, 501, or around 9 percent, treated doping matters at least to some extent.

It is not entirely obvious why wire service editors are so remarkably preoccupied with doping developments, such that they form nearly one-third of the major wire service output on Olympic and international sport in all its aspects (assuming that *Press Review* is representative of all these aspects, for purposes of argument). Editors and writers at the major international and national newspapers sampled by the IOC press office and its contractors clearly do not devote as much attention to doping, but given the volume of 2004 host city, Nagano, and Sydney news articles during the study period, we might still judge that nearly 10 percent of their output being devoted to doping is not inconsiderable either.

Content analysis of these wire service dispatches and press articles shows that they fit a pattern well known to mass communications researchers.[4] The stories are carried not by institutional, historical, scientific, or policy analyses of doping issues but by accusations, denials, test findings, court cases, and commentaries surrounding particular named individuals and coaches in the various sports and in over two dozen national contexts. In our sample, there was an average of nearly 13 alleged cases surrounding named individuals each and every month (not including the horses)! In other words, the mass circulation press finds no lack of new doping events of the sort it most prefers, with the result that the issue is front and center month after month.

This thought experiment shows, in my opinion, why a sports organization leader—who may or may not be directly involved in the specialized medical committees, in making policies regarding doping, or in concerned legal and commercial agencies, but who does assiduously follow the mass media—might be led to conclude that the battle against doping is not being won and probably cannot be won. We find actual sport officials characterized in a highly patterned way in these hundreds of articles. Their statements portray sports leaders as reactive (the story leads are case-driven), cautious and guarded (for legal reasons), and defensive (for sport in general as opposed to the "exceptional" cheaters). Thus, their proclamations of commitment to the struggle are undercut time and again by their actual portrayal in these stories as ineffective, reticent gradualists, hopelessly waiting for science to "catch up" and the courts to turn helpful. Writers of critical books and editorials who have no other source of data than newspapers simply pick up, amplify, and generalize these characterizations of international sports leaders for their own purposes. As keenly alert as sports leaders are to their own images, it is understandable how demoralized they have become by this journalistic discourse. Meanwhile, abrading them from below is a professional discourse within sports organizations that is progressively denaturing the doping issue into managerial talk about powers and interests, legal briefs and testing budgets.

The effect of such a slow but irresistible process of grinding down the resolve of sports leaders to continue the fight, wholeheartedly and on the basis of moral conviction rather than on the practicalities of power struggles, legal exposures, and organizational income, is what I am trying to insist they and we must fear most today. If no one goes up into the stands after the guy with the suspicious bottle, Olympic sport has indeed reduced itself to just another branch of the sports industry.

Events of Summer 1998

In the summer of 1998, both positive and negative events clearly demonstrated the plausibility of such fears.

The actions of the French (and later Dutch and Italian) state authorities during the Tour de France delivered the most important blow against doping since the 1988 Ben Johnson case and the subsequent Dubin Commission hearings. These actions reflexively demonstrated the impotence of the sports authorities and their testing programs from the purely practical point of view of successfully catching drug cheats. Overnight, from this one perspective, the magistrates and police took over anti-doping leadership from the sport agencies, at least in Europe.[5] Indeed, the Tour bust was considerably more important than the Johnson case, because it provided incontrovertible evidence that a complex doping practice was "normalized" throughout an entire sport and was not just the exceptional practice of a handful of bad apples. Thus the police, with the assistance of the press, did much to expose insider knowledge to the public and thereby to set off the discourse of "abnormality" and "exceptionality" of the sports organizations. Yet the sports organizations remained trapped in this discourse, because it is absolutely necessary under an individual athlete testing-and-sanctions strategy of deterrence.

Had Samaranch not said a word, these practical developments alone would have represented a momentous challenge to the IOC and its partners, the IFs and NOCs. But the challenge would probably have remained on the strategic level of debate: testing of athletes versus police action against entire entourages for "trafficking, possession, and paraphernalia." However, by clearly, if inadvertently suggesting that the IOC was about to throw in the towel—or perhaps already had—Samaranch took matters onto the moral plane. He thus helped induce a full-blown legitimacy crisis on the level of public opinion, to match what the organization suddenly was facing from the newly-triumphant political authorities, the European sports ministers and civil servants.

The IOC had long since lost the confidence of many sports anti-doping specialists and field-working academic observers. This can be attributed chiefly to the fact that no one—not the IOC, not its critics—had any real answer to rooting out performance-enhancing drug use under a testing regime which gave erythropoietin, human growth hormone, and designer drugs a free pass. But there was an additional factor. The IOC had made no more headway than anyone else, yet it kept promoting a rosy picture of its own efforts and accomplishments. In an environment of general frustration, the regular claims by Samaranch and de Merode that "we are winning the war on drugs" and "while we haven't won the war, we are winning many battles" had been taken by informed experts and activists as baseless public relations statements likely to confuse the public and comfort the dopers, no matter how effective such verbal gestures might be in reinforcing IOC image and resolve. But activists were living with their own insoluble dilemma: supporting athletes' rights meant simultaneously supporting all the legal threats, tricks, and costly procedures that dirty athletes and entourages were using so effectively to hold at bay the anti-doping agencies within the sports organizations. The situation in the 1990s was therefore almost entirely a negative one, a balance of frustrations on every side. Then Marie-George Buffet and Juan Antonio Samaranch together overthrew the status quo, the former by a great practical victory, the latter by musing whether it might not be time to give up the struggle. Things were becoming newly discernible.

Furor and Faction

The decline of moral authority into power politics reveals itself as factionalism within an organization and furor against it from without. These two processes eventually join together, as internal contenders for leadership mobilize external allies, and vice versa. In the case of the IOC, Samaranch's statement[6] on doping had the effect of releasing as sources to the press the contenders to succeed him as IOC president, their surrogates, and all those who sought to leverage the doping issue toward their own interests (which included reform of the system). These discourses, as further selected and framed by mass-media editors and writers, offer clear evidence that the suggestion that the IOC had given up on anti-doping had triggered a legitimation crisis. Let us look at *Press Review* news articles and press agency filings for July 27 and 28, the two days after publication of Samaranch's remarks.

Citing erythropoietin as an example, Dr. Jacques Rogge, IOC member in Belgium, was widely quoted regarding how impossible it is to easily distinguish between dangerous and nondangerous drugs because of variability of dosage practices. The lawyer Thomas Bach, IOC member in Germany, was quoted in *Frankfurter Allgemeine* as saying that Samaranch's statements were a "personal opinion" and not IOC policy and did not affect the integrity of the IOC Medical Code or the IOC's fight against performance-enhancing drugs. Australian IOC member, corporate executive Kevan Gosper, told a press conference, "[Doping] is where we need to regain the moral high ground. Maybe the public and the corporate world feel that the IOC leadership is not coming up with new initiatives and ideas." In collectively distancing themselves from the president, each one asserted himself precisely in terms of his own professional expertise and credentials for subsequent leadership campaigns. With outcries coming from every corner of the Olympic movement, no reformist candidate had any real choice but to get on public record as quickly as possible.

Clean Olympic athletes have for some time been the strongest and most morally influential voices against doping, and they were not long in expressing their outrage. British athletics gold medalist Steve Ovett told the *International Herald Tribune* that "the remarks showed Samaranch wanted to 'throw in the towel.' . . . I think he is saying that they can't control it which is a shame. How do you define dangerous? Is it when someone keels over and dies?" Former world marathon champion Rob de Castella expressed shock in remarks to Reuters. "It scares me to think Samaranch may be throwing up his hands and saying 'it's all too hard,' and backing away from the issue."

Many influential members of the "Olympic family"—IOC members, NOC officers, and OCOG officials—jumped quickly into the breach. Sir Arthur Gold, past president of the British Olympic Association, told reporters: "These are very unwise remarks by the IOC president. . . . To use drugs is to cheat, whether they damage your health or not." Said current British Olympic Association chair and IOC member Craig Reedie, "If these reports are accurate then it is a major change in IOC policy, and I am not aware of it being discussed anywhere. . . . Imagine what the chemical industry are thinking this morning!" In a Reuters dispatch, Australian Swimming president Terry Gathercole said he was devastated and dismayed by Samaranch's comments. SOCOG sources were quoted as accusing Samaranch of a "complete backflip" from his earlier stance that "doping equals death," and Sydney Games chief and Australian Olympics minister Michael Knight issued a statement that the banned substance list, although adjustable, must never be weakened.

On the 27th and 28th of July, the IOC issued press statements asserting that the "IOC was more determined than ever" and announcing a world anti-doping conference for the following January. But with sensational headlines such as "IOC Sets Talks on Doping as Chief's Remarks Spark Outrage" (*International Herald Tribune*, July 28) and "Samaranch's Shock Stance on Drugs" (*The Age*, Melbourne, July 28), newspapers made plain that these public relations moves would not stop the media bloodletting. The *Daily Telegraph* (July 27) in Britain did not shrink from the extraordinary headline "Olympics Chief Backs Drug Use." In an opinion piece in the July 28th *Frankfurter Allgemeine* ("Bis dass der Tod entscheidet"), Hans-Joachim Waldbroel asserted that Samaranch has "capitulated in the fight against doping." An accompanying editorial noted pointedly that only the chiefs of the cycling teams embroiled in the Tour de France busts had come forward to approve of Samaranch's remarks, while the sports doping experts had been thrown into "anger, disbelief, and despair."

There was no lack of such experts available to be quoted, particularly in a Germany mobilized by the recent investigations and trials of former East German sports officials. Professor Wildor Hollman, honorary president of the World Association for Sports Medicine and the German Sport Doctors Union, told Reuters: "I fell under the table when I heard [Samaranch's statement]. This way of thinking is nonsense. That would be an unbelievable step backwards." Deutsche Press Agentur quoted Wilhelm Schänzer, head of doping analysis at the Deutsche Sporthochshule: "Samaranch has opened a dangerous discussion which can have very negative effects." Medical expert Klaus Müller said of Samaranch's remark: "The suggestion is a slap in the face." Taking matters to the moral heart of an Olympic movement ostensibly in service to sport and youth, Professor Werner Franke asserted: "Softening the anti-doping rules would mean the end of promoting sport among young people. If Samaranch gets his way, nobody can send his son or daughter to a sport that is full of drugs." Thomas Kistner's opinion piece in the *Süddeutsche Zeitung* is worth quoting at length.

> At last the truth has come out. In gratifyingly clear words, Juan Antonio Samaranch has revealed what he really thinks on the subject of performance manipulation. . . . Put crudely, take what you like sports lovers, and don't let the best man win, but the one who is best at stuffing himself full of performance-enhancing drugs. Obviously a shameful thesis, but at least it reveals the real Olympic spirit. Samaranch's declaration is so scandalous because it does not correspond to the standard pathos, but comes from his most deeply held personal beliefs. It is an attempt at a forward defense after world sport has come under increasing pressure thanks to the unspeakable doping Tour-ture de France. While noble physical culture goes rushing on, reason can sometimes grind to a halt. Then justice decided to have a tantrum: investigations and arrests made it clear to the public that a sport stuffed full of drugs was not living in a lawless world. Medical confessions show that cheating lends itself well to methodology, and top names in the peloton admit that victories in the past are similarly worthless. . . . All that was missing was the officials. By pleading for the decontrol of medically harmless chemical substances, the IOC boss is putting in place the missing piece of the mosaic, "Big Mess in Top Sport." Now everything fits together perfectly. . . . Samaranch's attempt is part of the tradition of the cynical, misanthropic GDR [East German] sport which is currently on trial before the ordinary courts in Germany: doping under medical supervision.

Government and legal authorities were quick to assert their advantage over the sports organizations in this new journalistic discourse, half derived from Samaranch's scandalous remarks and half from the successful attack on Tour dopers by the coordinated French forces of the sport minister, magistrates, police, and customs officers. Describing himself as "gobsmacked" by the first partner to this morganitic marriage, Australian Federal Sports minister Andrew Thomson was quoted in many news services as saying: "Samaranch has put the IOC in direct conflict with the Australian Government and the Sydney Olympic organizers. We are totally opposed to the use of performance-enhancing drugs fullstop—that position is not negotiable. It's appalling that here we are doing our best to fight against drugs and our politicians should be undermined by people beyond our borders." United Kingdom Sports Council anti-doping chief Michele Verroken told *The Guardian*: "There is now a case for Government to step in. So far they haven't legislated but it is one way of dealing with the problem. If we are going to have inaction, vagueness, or wooliness, if some sport bodies can't be bothered to tackle drug-taking, then the government can."

Over the next months, as all of these speaking parts became established, many additional actors got to perform these rhetorical roles in the press. My colleague Kathryn Wycliffe and I conducted another content analysis of the IOC *Press Review* for doping stories and wire service dispatches across this period. A sample of seven reviews between June 17 and July 10, 1998, showed 11 percent given over to doping coverage, exactly the background rate found in the earlier March 1997 to January 1998 study. Between July 27, 1999—the first Tour busts and Samaranch's remarks—and September 30, 1999, in the 24 *Press Review* issues studied, a per issue average of 61 percent of the 1,144 total articles and agency dispatches surveyed concerned themselves with doping. The daily range was between 30 percent for the September 2 issue and 93 percent for the August 11 issue. Over the course of October and November (23 issues analyzed), the rate dropped off somewhat but still remained at an average of 42 percent of all articles and dispatches, nearly four times the prior year's background rate of 11 percent.

Over the course of December 1998 (15 issues surveyed), the proportion of articles and dispatches mentioning doping fell to 28 percent, despite the fact that the number of new cases kept close to the monthly background rate and the World Conference on Doping in Sport was coming up. The Salt Lake City/IOC bribery and corruption scandal had now broken and was claiming more and more of this press space. Indeed, the smooth and direct transition of press interest in the one story to the other demonstrates a deep-seated relationship between them for news agency editors and writers. If this were merely a case of generic "love of scandal" among the press, then such an ordered substitution would not likely be observed. Instead, a rhetorical equivalence became quickly established between the story lines "doping/IOC" and "corruption/IOC" in the press.

As With Doping, So With Corruption

Return to the newspapers and wire service dispatches of July 29, and we find that this rhetorical structure is already present in all its elements. Moreover, here we will discover precisely the same range of interpretive options delineated earlier with respect to officials' behavior in the matter of possible doping in the stadium. Moral authority, these stories among themselves say, has been lost through the incompetence, complicity, venality, timidity, or cynical resignation of top sports officials. But there is an added element, a familiar way of getting the system off the hook by turning tragedy to melodrama. Nearly everything in these texts becomes personalized to Samaranch.[7] This rhetorical pattern and interpretive paradigm would be repeated exactly with the bribery scandal, beginning in December 1998, and it generally governed news coverage of the IOC crisis throughout 1999.

On July 29, Associated Press and Agencia EFE dispatches citing new reactions by Olympic leaders were taken up in news articles in many countries. The overall effect was described in a headline in the Adelaide *Advertiser*: "And the Winner Is: Confusion!" For example, under the headline "Games Boss Backs Down Amidst Outrage," the Melbourne *Herald Sun*, like many other papers, cited Australian Olympics Minister Michael Knight, after a phone conversation with the IOC president, as saying "Mr. Samaranch assured me that the IOC's campaign against drugs in sport would continue with full determination and vigor. He made it clear he believed there were no performance enhancing drugs that did not cause harm to the health of the athletes." United States Olympic Committee (USOC) executive director Dick Schultz, after a similar phone call, told the Associated Press that

Samaranch supported the IOC and USOC banned drug lists "completely." Samaranch "emphasized very clearly that any drug that impacts the health of an athlete or enhances performance should be banned."

However, while likewise insisting there had been no change in IOC policy, other Samaranch defenders suggested that the president still meant what he'd said and was right to want the banned list reduced. Kevan Gosper told the Australian press (and was cited next to Knight in the very same articles) that the issue really was the definition of doping. "If you give an athlete a Panadol to fix a headache does that mean you have enhanced his performance? There is a grey area there." IOC member Phil Coles (who would soon be a center of controversy in the corruption scandal) suggested that "drugs like Sudafed, ephedrine, and whiskey could easily be removed from the list without weakening the rules." But the press was just as quick to find other voices to assert that such substances in excessive doses could have anabolic or pain-masking performance effects. That is why these drugs, together with analgesic narcotics, were on the banned list in the first place, as Professor Arne Ljundgvist, IOC and IOC Medical Commission member, told EFE.

So, was Samaranch backing down or rightly sticking to his guns? Was he cowed by bad press or simply resigned to go with the political flow? Some IOC leaders offered the rather stunning defense of their leader as morally committed but incompetent. Dr. Ljundgvist also told EFE, "Samaranch doesn't understand the principles by which [the Medical Commission] puts together the list of banned doping products." Concerning Samaranch's original interview in *El Mundo*, Dick Schultz told reporters, "I just don't think he understood at the time what he was saying." Most remarkable of all were IOC director general François Carrard's statements to the Associated Press. "[Samaranch] never meant to give up the fight against doping or to launch himself a change of policy. . . . He is not very precise in his scientific approach. Sometimes on technical issues he expresses himself in maybe an abrupt way."

But there were voices suggesting nationalist venality and conspiracy as well. Roy Masters, in the *Sydney Morning Herald,* quoted an anonymous "IOC source" as claiming that "Mr. Samaranch's softening of his stance on drugs was motivated by Spanish concerns over the future of the Tour de France. The source claimed Mr. Samaranch, a native of Barcelona, was prompted to speak by fears the gloss would go from the five tour victories of Spaniard Miguel Indurain. Several of the teams in this year's Tour de France have Spanish cyclists. 'Samaranch is coming to protect the cyclists because the French police have ripped the heart out of the Tour.'" Statements in support of Samaranch's "very good words" by the Spanish cycling team ONCE and Banesto cycling team directors were widely cited in support of this theory.

There were also writers who persisted in believing, despite the new statements, that Samaranch was indeed resigned and retreating. As Olympics editor of the *Sydney Morning Herald*, Matthew Moore will shortly become the most influential Olympic newspaperman in the world, and he was prepared to credit the pragmatism in Samaranch's original statements.

> This was no accidental slip of the tongue, despite the hopes of senior sports officials around the world, especially in Sydney. Samaranch gave his interview at a time of overwhelming evidence of widespread drug use among elite sportsmen and women. To ensure he would be accurately reported, he elected to be interviewed in Spanish, his mother tongue. With the Tour de France crippled by daily drug revelations, Samaranch knew questions would focus on doping.
>
> Drug use in sport has simply become too widespread, too commonplace, for the world to be surprised any more. That seems to be the conclusion Samaranch reached in the summer of 1998. What he is advocating is a tactical retreat to a position that can be more readily and credibly defended. . . . He will find plenty of support. Australia's response to Samaranch has been largely one of incredulity and anger. He's been condemned for chucking in the towel. But the evidence is he is responding to a more pragmatic view of drug use that appears to exist in Europe.

However, resignation of another kind and not *realpolitik* was a louder theme in the newspapers of the day. Voices from several sectors of the Olympic movement thought to simplify things in another way. Olympic athlete Lee Naylor: "If that's the attitude of the leading Olympic official in the world, then you have to question whether he's suitable for the job." Olympic contender Nicole Stevenson said, "He said he was going to retire four years ago—now, if he's making statements pro-drugs, then perhaps it's time for someone else to be head of the IOC." Commonwealth Games and Australian cycling chief Ray Godkin: "[Samaranch] is out of his tree. . . . They've got to have a good hard look at him. Use-by dates come and go." The platform was opened for more sensationalist and abusive voices. Jacquelin Magnay, reporter for Melbourne's *The Age*: "His fiefdom is the entire world of sport, his minions the hundreds of IOC lackeys who bow and scrape at his every word. He is powerful, he knows it, and expects others to respect it. . . . But in Australia, such obsequious behavior is treated with contempt." Said Australian anti-doping activist Forbes Carlisle to whomever would listen: "Now is the time for revolt . . . for Juan Antonio Samaranch and all he stands for to be thrown out. The wolf has shed his sheep's clothing. The aging dictator has in effect informed his minions they must relax their pursuit of drug cheats."

Thus, the ground was laid and the media patterns grooved for interpretations of subsequent IOC bribery and corruption scandals. The doping scandal—"the IOC has given up," said Samaranch; "The IOC will fix it" (at the World Conference on Doping in Sport), said Samaranch—set the whole rhetorical stage for reception of the bribery scandal. "The IOC is not corrupt," said Samaranch; "The IOC will fix it" (with expulsions and the IOC 2000 Commission), said Samaranch. Many more and many worse things would be charged, from November 1998 through today, as to the putative incompetence, venality, cupidity, timidity, hypocrisy, and cynicism of the entire IOC organization (regularly simplified and personalized in the figure of Samaranch and with the question of his resignation). Factionalism would likewise break out into the open and with a vicious intensity that even most IOC insiders failed to anticipate. Institutions external to the Olympic system, such as the United States Congress or the European Sport Ministers Conference, would seize the opportunity to insert themselves into the legitimation crisis of the IOC.

This too was chartered in the doping summer of 1998. On July 29, as the press was documenting and accelerating the erosion of IOC authority represented in and occasioned by Samaranch's remarks, the French police temporarily released Festina team director Bernard Roussel and hauled in instead TVM team riders and medical personnel. Meanwhile French border officials stopped and seized substances from an official car carrying Chinese athletes and officials to the world junior championships in Annency. No confusion here. No absence of authority here. The contrast between the sport organizations and the government authorities could not have become more marked.

The president of the Association of Summer Olympic International Federations and of the IAAF, and an IOC member, Primo Nebiolo felt forced to react with a press release. "We cannot leave these matters to be resolved by the police and the courts. Police action and eventual imprisonment for offenders may be necessary, but only as a last resort. . . . It is sport which must fight this battle, with the help of the institutions." It was difficult to judge which was more pathetic here: that the internationally mistrusted and reviled Primo Nebiolo, boss of a dirty sport (track and field), was the one reasserting the sports organizations' prerogatives; or, with anti-doping activists everywhere cheering on the French authorities, that the sport organizations actually imagined they would have any popular support for bringing the police to their own heel. In any case, the policy position was a loser from the beginning. The Tour busts in combination with the Samaranch flap ensured for the foreseeable future that public opinion—certainly in Europe, Canada, Scandinavia, Australia, and wherever else it might be informed—would side with the governments over the sports organizations.

Naiveté and self-delusion are further signs of an organization that has lost its authority so out of touch has it become with societies and public cultures, which alone confer the gift of moral legitimation. That IOC and IF leaders were taken aback by the degree of independence, criticism, and sovereignty expressed by government representatives at the World Conference on Doping in Sport is testimony to how out of touch with reality the sports leaders had become. Or perhaps, it is testimony to their laziness and that of their staffs. As with the exemplary case of possible doping in the Olympic stadium itself, official eyes have been blind to what was right before them on their desks, much less on their competition fields. The materials that make the situation obvious—already in July 1998, before the corruption scandal arose to reinforce the corrosive effects of the doping scandal—were right there in the IOC's own *Press Review*. Then again, if the IOC leadership, directorships, and staff no longer really care about Olympism and the Olympic Games as a social movement, then it is possible to understand how they might read public and press reaction as just so many marketing, public relations, and political problems in a rapidly growing industry.

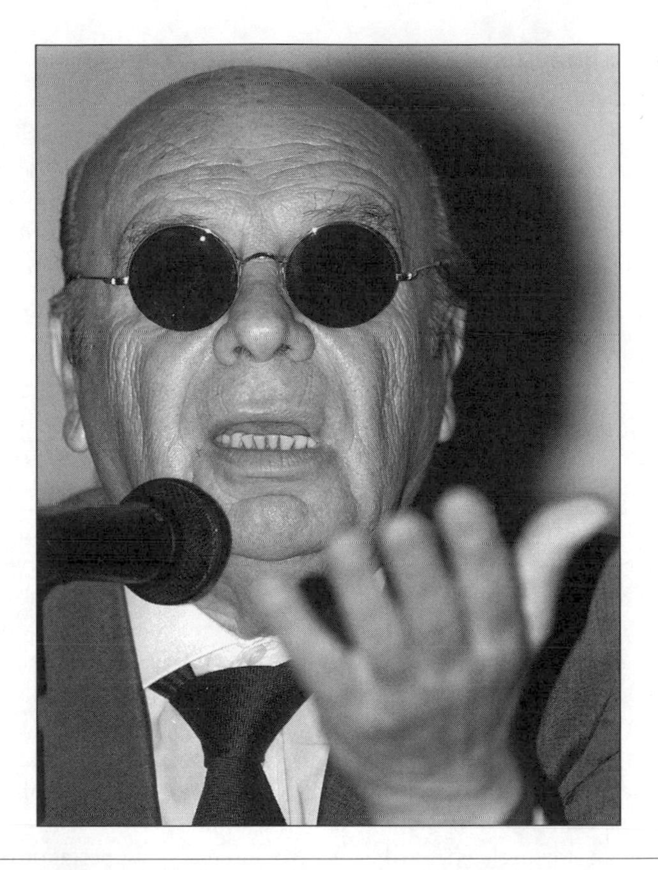

Primo Nebiolo at 1998 news conference. At the time of his death in November 1999, Nebiolo was a member of the IOC and head of the IAAF, the Association of Summer Olympic International Federations, and the International University Sports Federation.
© Craig Prentis/Allsport

Conclusions

To regain true and general moral authority in any foreseeable future, these organizations will have to clearly recognize that doping will continue to present the master ambiguity at the core of the institutional sacreds of any national and international sports organizations claiming moral status beyond mere industrial, commercial, or political power. No such organization can be anything but morally determined in the battle against doping, even if no such organization has any clear idea of how to win that battle. As clearly shown by the events and discourses of 1998-2000, this is a dilemma in the domain of practical action, but it is also a generative ambiguity in the realm of meaning for Olympic sport in the postcolonial, post–Cold War era.

Acknowledgments

Grants from the Wenner-Gren, Paek Sang, and Hewlett Foundations, and by the University of Chicago Center for International Studies helped make possible the stadium observations discussed in this paper. I'm also grateful for the research assistance of Jeanne Haffner and Kathryn Wycliffe, who carefully sifted three years' worth of IOC *Press Review*, demonstrating the research value of these documents. Of course, no one but the author necessarily shares any of the opinions in this paper.

Notes

[1]Max Weber, *Economy and Society*. 2 vols. Berkeley: University of California Press, 1969.

[2]I wish to make very clear that I am speaking of the public understanding and evaluation of the IOC here and not of the Olympic Games or of Olympic athletes. The IOC 2000 Reform Commission (on whose Executive Committee I served as an appointed "external" member) has reviewed substantive data from IOC-commissioned but professionally conducted public opinion polls, focus groups, and interviews in 10 countries, including Japan and the English-speaking countries, whose press and politicians have been most clamorous during the scandal.

The pattern of results is quite consistent. In reaction to the scandals, these sample populations have maintained or increased their commitments to the Olympic Games and to Olympic athletes, while severely disassociating these entities and themselves from the IOC. My summary interpretation of these data, as expressed to the IOC 2000 Commission in June 1999, is that "public opinion in these countries is asking the IOC to prove that *it* remains a part of the Olympic *movement*."

Unfortunately, it is not possible to separate the effects of the doping issue from those of the corruption scandal in interpreting these data. Moreover, though I suspect that negative associations between athletes and doping are suspended here in favor of the marked contrast between athletes and sports bureaucrats, especially in the English-speaking samples, this cannot be demonstrated given the limits of the data.

[3]For an analysis of this process in the Ben Johnson case, see John MacAloon, "Steroids and the State: Dubin, Melodrama, and the Accomplishment of Innocence," *Public Culture* 2 (2):41-64.

[4]For a classic study of general media practices in such areas, see Herbert Gans, *Deciding What's News* (New York: Pantheon, 1979). On the framing of doping issues as legal narrative, see John MacAloon, "Steroids and the State: Dubin, Melodrama, and the Accomplishment of Innocence," *Public Culture* 2 (2): 41-64.

[5]Such actions could only have been taken in countries with a Napoleonic legal code, notably those of Western Europe. European skepticism of the American

commitment to anti-doping is certainly well deserved. However, it is not widely realized in Europe that certain kinds of police search and seizure practices so effective in the Tour de France bust are quite impossible under the very different legal codes and practical judicial and police regimes derived from English common law, especially in the United States.

The challenge for American anti-doping activists has been to find an effective means of mobilizing state authorities in the anti-doping fight within the constraints of domestic law. (Criminalization of illegal steroid trafficking was one such step, alas of marginal effectiveness given police and prosecutorial priorities.) Until better strategies can be found, the domestic struggle will remain largely a testing regime in the hands of the American sport authorities, notably the USOC and its national governing bodies.

For these cultural and historical reasons, the gap between Europe and the United States will surely widen, and the European perception that U.S. athletes are the dirtiest in the world will likely become even more widespread than it presently is. The European perception of the American state as fiercely hypocritical has been made clear in the general reaction to the U.S. White House "drug czar's recent attacks on the IOC. General McCaffrey seems, at this writing, unaware that Europe and much of the rest of the sports world regards the United States (professional sport and the USOC) as leaders in the announced-test-to-support-tainted-performance regime.

[6]Samaranch as quoted in *El Mundo* on Sunday, July 26, 1998: "Doping now is everything that, firstly, is harmful to an athlete's health and, secondly, artificially augments his performance. If it's just the second case, for me that's not doping. If it's the first case it is." In the same interview he also suggested that the IOC list of banned substances needed to be reduced.

Samaranch's concern with a consensual definition of doping was hardly new. In a private meeting between the IOC Executive and leading human scientists of sport, a meeting arranged by the late Professor Fernand Landry in Quebec City in May 1990, Samaranch pointedly asked the scholars present to dispute a definition of doping very like that contained in his June 1998 public interview. Those of us in attendance vigorously did so and left the meeting quite uncertain whether this was a "trial balloon" or indeed represented President Samaranch's own thinking.

In 1998, it was a public statement just after the Tour de France scandal broke and but two days before two distinguished American Olympic champions were revealed to have tested positive. The IOC press office failed completely in its (somewhat half-hearted) efforts to suggest that Samaranch might have merely been thinking out loud before the *El Mundo* reporters and that it was the specific removal of codeine from the list that he had in mind, not any major reduction in banned substances.

[7]It is in one sense ironic, in another perfectly understandable, that Samaranch should be made subject 10 years later to the same process of melodramatization as Ben Johnson. In both cases this served well as a mechanism to preserve the system.

See John MacAloon, "Steroids and the State: Dubin, Melodrama, and the Accomplishment of Innocence," *Public Culture* 2 (2): 41-64. Back issues of the *IOC Press Review* containing stories on Samaranch and other aspects of the doping issues are available in two repositories: the Olympic Studies Centre in Lausanne, Switzerland and the Amateur Athletic Foundation sports library in Los Angeles.

9

CHAPTER

Doping in Elite Swimming: A Case Study of the Modern Era From 1970 Forward

John Leonard
Executive Director American Swimming Coaches Association;
Executive Director World Swimming Coaches Association

This chapter is a case study on the sport of swimming and examines the impact of doping on the sport since 1970. I am a swimming coach and since 1985 have been the director of the American Swimming Coaches Association (ASCA), the world's largest organization of swimming coaches. I have gradually learned to practice sport politics on both the national and international levels. In 1989, I was one of three founders of the World Swimming Coaches Association (WSCA), an international attempt to bring the same independence to the ranks of international coaches that American coaches have had since the formation of the ASCA in 1958. The analysis that follows is based on my first-hand observations of international swimming over many years as a coach and administrator.

One of the key goals of the WSCA has been clean sport. Another has been the involvement of professional swimming coaches at the highest levels of our sport, in order that decisions made by FINA, the international swimming federation, might be influenced by experience directly from the pool deck, the swimmers and the coaches. These two goals relate directly to the issue of drugs in the sport of swimming.

With that brief background, the following section presents an examination of the issue of doping in elite swimming.

The Current Doping Situation in Swimming: A Brief Assessment

How much doping is there in elite swimming at present? We know that, as of 1998, there had been 58 positive tests for drugs in swimming. We know that one nation, China, accounted for 29 of those positive tests. Coaches are of the opinion that doping has been much reduced since the collapse of the Eastern Bloc. The stagnation of swimming performance times since 1990 supports this opinion.

At the same time, one of the statements that swimming coaches and athletes support strongly is "Absence of proof is not proof of absence." Swimming is a comparatively small and "close" sport around the globe. Relatively few unknown competitors suddenly emerge to prominence. The pattern of typical improvement, which coaches observe and influence every day in practice, is slow, steady, and predictable by any experienced coach. When this predictable pattern of improvement is violated, the suspicions of swimming coaches worldwide are raised, and history has subsequently supported the "gut feelings" of the coaches.

The ability of this "gut feeling" to identify drug users, and its wide ridicule by officials in the sport of swimming, is a constant source of anger among coaches. We spend our lives on the decks of pools helping young people swim faster. We know what is normal and what is assisted chemically.

So how much doping is there in swimming today? I believe there is much more than is caught. However, a study of elite performances shows that the level of doping in 1998 was far less than at any time in the previous 25 years. Support for this statement can be found by examining the top 15 times in swimming history. Nearly 80 percent (79.8 percent to be exact) of the total times on that list are pre-1990 times. Between 1994 and 1998, only 6 percent of the times were added to the list (total list—men and women together).

In the women's events, the picture is significantly different. With the Chinese athletes included in the count, only 48 percent of the top 15 times are pre-1990. With the Chinese deleted from the list, a startling 91 percent of the times are pre-1990.

Absence of Proof Means What?

Neither athletes nor coaches put much faith in the ability of drug testers to catch cheats. It is widely quoted that to be caught, even in out-of-competition tests, one must be "stupid or sloppy." Clearly, like athletes in many other sports around the world, the athletes in swimming who are doping have moved on to the hard-to-detect drugs such as erythropoietin, human growth hormone, and the insulin growth factors (IGFs). Rumors persist of exotic new "designer drugs" that have replaced the "old-fashioned" easily detected steroids. And, it is widely assumed that there is significant inaccuracy in the testing process itself, as well as significant corruption of the process by those who wish to have the drug culture continue or to escape punishment. A well-placed source has told this writer that there are only two labs in the world that the source has confidence in, and that when the source sees tests from other labs, the person regularly sees positives that have been "missed" in the process. This destroys the confidence of the "clean" athlete in the detection process.

The world swimming organization, FINA, now does a fair number of out-of-competition tests, and although this is preferable to in-competition tests, there is still substantial doubt as to the ability of these tests to clean up our sport. Repeated tests, unannounced, do seem to disrupt the cycling and use of drugs in a way that we do not yet fully understand. A correlation is evident between the number of FINA out-of-competition tests, and the apparent decline of drug use in swimming. For this reason, even though the exact cause is unknown, coaches and athletes want to see out-of-competition testing accelerated and enlarged.

"Absence of proof does not constitute proof of absence." This statement sums up the opinion of swimming coaches and athletes at the present time.

If the Absence of Proof Argument Does Not Hold, Then on What Do Swimming Coaches Base Their Concerns?

There are several key indicators that coaches look for, none of which could stand up in a court of law, but which may in fact be the best long-term indicators of something amiss.

- Too-rapid improvement. History shows that improvement in a given event at a rate far exceeding that of an athlete's peers will eventually be revealed as drug-fueled. Though the rate of improvement varies from one event to another, at the elite world level of the sport, there are predictable improvement curves that make sense for that event.
- Hidden training. In swimming, athletes improve best when consistent, progressive training is employed. When individuals or teams "hide away" for extended periods of time in exotic locations, where finding them or traveling to visit them is prohibitive because of time, money, or distance, there is a reason. When individuals or teams do this repeatedly in cycles of predictable years, it is because an increase in volume or intensity levels of training that is inconsistent with drug-free swimming is taking place. Levels of training that cannot be supported (or "leaped to") without drugs, are a clear indication that the recovery period has been accelerated by drug use.
- Coaches who cannot or will not produce credible training programs for their athletes. Historically, there have been few worldwide training secrets in swimming. Our sport culture has been characterized by a completely open sharing of methods and training regimens. This culture is how our sport made such remarkable improvements worldwide in the 1950s, 1960s, and early 1970s. It continues in many swimming nations today. The notable exceptions have been the East Germans, the Chinese, and the Hungarians. When any of these nations have been invited to present training programs at coaches' conferences, they show remarkably ordinary training plans for athletes who have performed far beyond the norm for that level of training. If two athletes

both do the same work, and get radically different results, the question must be asked, "Is the talent level that different?" Coaches worldwide laugh at this presumption.

- Coaching history. Who was taught to coach by whom? What is the derivation of coaching thinking? Where was the coach taught? What philosophies were followed by the teacher? This is indeed guilt by association, and the cliche has often proven to be correct. These questions also are related to the issues raised in the first three points in this list.
- Physical status of the athlete. When a coach looks at an athlete, what does the coach see? Does the athlete one day look cut and lean, prepared to race? Three months later, does the athlete look soft and bloated? Or, do we not see the athlete except at the most major competitions? Are the results from minor competitions "off the scale" below the level of championship performance? Is performance from one championship level meet to another radically different? Swimming is not that type of sport. Clean athletes retain a major part of their ability to swim fast at all times of the year, and differences in championship form may differ by minor percentages when an athlete is deemed to be "way off." In doped athletes, the differences in performance level can be remarkable.

Also, of course, with some drugs of choice, there are the typical physical signs of drug use, but in today's drug environment, absence of muscular bulk, deep voices in women, or the other traditionally telltale signs is not proof of absence. This has a historical basis that we shall explore shortly.

History of the Doping Problem Since 1970

At the 1972 Munich Olympic Games, rumors circulated around the pool deck of strange new things happening in East Germany. To my knowledge, this whispering did not extend beyond conversations on the pool deck among coaches.

By 1976 in Montreal, as the East German women nearly swept the pool, the rumors had become a rising tide of voices from athletes and coaches in protest against what they saw as clear evidence of cheating. Shirley Babashoff, whom history later proved should be the woman crowned the queen of Olympic swimming, was vilified as a "crybaby" and "surly Shirley" when she stated openly that she felt like she was swimming against men, and that what she was seeing in the locker room confirmed those feelings. Comments about deep voices, and retorts claiming "we came to swim, not to sing" began a deep divide between the athletes and coaches, and the administrators who simply turned a blind eye to all this, and decided that the defeated were simply "bad losers" and "bad sports."

The lifetime effect on both coaches and athletes was profound. The head coach of the U.S. women's team was deemed an outright failure. He was never again offered an Olympic coaching position, largely because of his perceived failure in Montreal. In fact, delete the now-proven German cheats, and the U.S. team, under his leadership, had one of its top Olympic performances of all time in the women's events, one that nearly would have matched the men's near sweep of events. Canadian Swimming, which enjoyed its heyday in Montreal, would have gained significant additional medals, and elevated even higher a program that was progressing nicely.

The battleground, though, was set—the athletes and coaches on one side, the "Blazerati" on the other. Officials of the International Olympic Committee (IOC) and FINA said nothing, literally nothing except that we could not possibly be anything other than poor sports. That division between the Blazerati and the participants continues to this day and increasingly becomes more antagonistic and adversarial.

The effect on the U.S. swimming program was dramatic. As the East Germans continued and even accelerated their dominance in the later 1970s and 1980s, endless meetings in the United States centered on the questions, "What are we doing wrong?" "How can we compete?" "What has gone wrong in our society?" "Why are we losers? Has America lost its edge?"

Careers in both swimming and coaching were ruined. Talented athletes retired early; talented coaches who could see clearly the impossibility of competing in the drug scene left the sport for other opportunities in business. The national angst over our performance was enormous. All the while, we were putting up the finest national swimming performance in history, if the known cheaters are removed from the results, rankings, and record books.

The same effect was seen in other nations, but the United States, because of the quality of its performances, was most affected; Australians were the second most affected.

Is there any question about why the response later in the century has been so vehement and angry when the same problem re-emerged in China?

What About FINA During This Period?

One of the most aggravating of circumstances was the fact that FINA included as the second ranking member of its Medical Committee, one of the architects of the East German Doping Program, State Plan 14.25. Although coaches did not know exactly what position he held in the East German hierarchy, we did know that he was part and parcel of the conspiracy. In individual, personal contact with this man, he would laugh and deny any doping involvement at all by his nation, and simply refer to the genetics of the German nation in producing big, strong, "masculine looking" women. His laughing at the world while he was a part of the inner circle of the FINA Committee supposedly charged with keeping doping out of our sport, was absolutely infuriating to coaches worldwide. And no one would listen. At least five members of the FINA Bureau were approached on this issue by coaches between 1984 and 1988, and not one response or action was ever taken. This failure of FINA to make even the most tentative gesture to keep drugs from our sport, was a clear and unambiguous indictment that they were not interested in solving the doping problem.

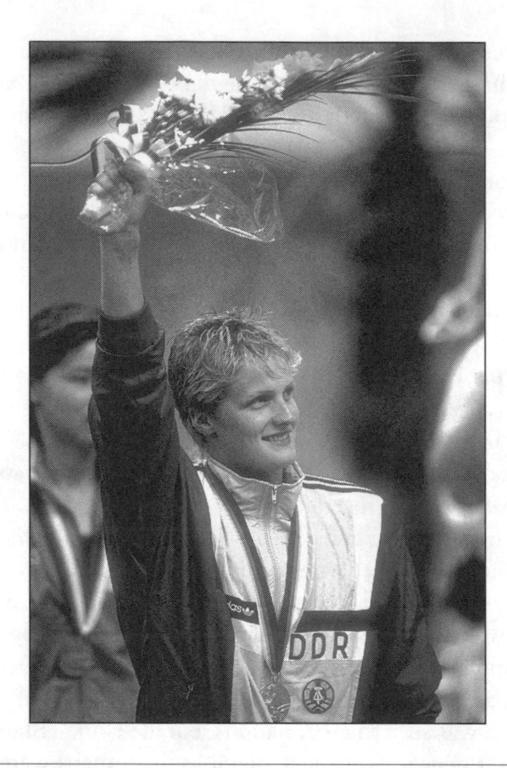

Swimmer Kristin Otto celebrating one of her six gold medals at the 1988 Seoul Olympic Games. Documents released after German reunification named Otto as one of many East German athletes who had been given banned substances as part of their training regimens.
© Mike Powell/Allsport

From around the time of the boycotted 1984 Olympic Games and culminating at the world championships in 1986 in Madrid, an ominous new problem became evident. The old stereotype of the German "superwoman" with her five o'clock shadow, her huge build, and her deep voice to match her magnificent musculature, went away. A new generation of German swimmers emerged, highlighted by the very attractive and "feminine" Kristen Otto, the star of the 1986 world championships and 1988 Olympic Games. Certainly at the same time some other German swimmers exhibited some strange facial features and strange features of their hands and feet, which we later learned resulted from use of human growth hormone, but the old stereotype was gone.

And with it, much of the growing suspicions of the world press. If you couldn't see it, it must not be there, seemed to be the attitude. The drug use must be over.

But the world's coaches knew better. If anything, the incredibly (and I use the word with full intent) rapid improvement of the new generation, and their enormous ability to dramatically "shift gears" in mid-pool, looked like powerful male swimming, not female. If anything, their physical prowess in the water was even more fearsome than that of the previous versions of East German swimmers. The classic specific example was Kristen Otto's 100-meter freestyle in Madrid, when, in mid-pool at the 75-meter mark, she unleashed a finishing kick never before seen in an world-class race by a male or female. No experienced observer had ever seen anything like the aggression and power of her final 25 meters to set a world record. She went from being even with her competitors to a body length victory in the final 25 meters, a huge margin of victory in world swimming.

Later, we learned from the Stasi (East German secret police) records, that her testosterone to epitestosterone ratio on that day was a remarkable 18:1, shattering the "accepted limit" of 6:1. The aggression had a physical basis.

Last Gasps of a Dying Monster

In the final years of the 1980s, rumors were heard and later confirmed that as the Eastern Bloc was heaving its death coughs and rattles, they had also exported their doping techniques to Asia. We know now that one key former East German doctor and two key East German coaches went to work in China, officially sponsored by the East German government, from 1986 to 1989. They made lengthy stays and return visits, helping the Chinese set up their own drug use system. It also was reported but not confirmed that the East Germans established their own "experimental station" in remote northern China.

Again, coaches heard of the visits, warned members of the FINA Medical Committee and Bureau, and were ignored. No investigation took place. It was all dismissed with a wave of the hand and a "You guys are paranoid" attitude. And still, FINA officially denied that there was a doping problem in East Germany. (The "There is no proof" excuse.)

A person can be convicted of murder on circumstantial evidence, but FINA could not launch a real investigation when the most damning of circumstantial evidence existed. The ostrich still had his head stuck firmly in the sand. Not one East German athlete ever tested positive in FINA tests.

The Involvement of Other Nations

Although the focus of the swimming world in the 1970s and 1980s was clearly on the East Germans, other nations were also suspected of doping. Circumstantial evidence was convincing in other cases as well.

The Soviet swimmers in particular attracted attention because with techniques that could most charitably be described as "from an older era," Soviet athletes in backstroke, breaststroke, and at least a couple of freestyle events, set world records. The coaching community noted that only by extraordinary training, training beyond the level that anyone else had been able to do unassisted by drugs, could those times have been achieved. And rumors and tales of unusual drug use occasionally left the Soviet Union with its defecting citizens. With no smoking gun, and no results as completely obvious as those of East Germany, the focus did not fall as strongly on the Soviets.

From 1956 on, Hungarian swimmers were suspected. Long absences from public view during training, sudden departures from competitions where drug testing was unexpectedly announced, and radical physical changes in appearance and musculature in periods of rest and relaxation versus those of the athletes when in training all pointed to drug use. In addition, the flawless ability of the Hungarians to be "perfectly on" at the world's major competitions also fueled the fire of speculation. No Hungarian swimmer has ever tested positive for drug use. Tales persist of the use of human growth hormone and insulin growth factor use, in primitive forms early, now in more sophisticated form. Mothers and fathers of swimmers, years after the retirement of their child-athletes, have spoken "off the record" of the "assisted means" used in Hungary. Other circumstantial evidence has also at times cast suspicion on Italian swimmers and most of the old Eastern Bloc swimmers, including Rumanian and Czech swimmers.

The United States is an unusual case. At times, individual swims have caused suspicion. Most frequently mentioned among these were Mary T. Meagher's historic swims in the 100- and 200-meter butterfly, records that have now stood for close to 20 years, an eternity in our sport. Those who know Mary T., and her family, this writer among them, angrily reject any possibility that this most moral of swimmers would ever have used any performance-enhancing drug. Later, she was a repeated victim of East German cheating at championship after championship. Had she cheated to set her records, surely she would have ended her frustration at losing major title after major title by using once again. The opinion of most of the swimming world is that Mary T. was clean. As Bob Beamon shattered the long jump world record in the 1968 Olympics, so too are her records considered the "Beamonesque" event in swimming history.

However, the United States is often painted with a broad brushstroke, as a "dirty" nation. This is not difficult to understand. Without a doubt, certain sports in the United States are among the most drug-dirty in the world.

For a European or an Asian, where track and field national offices often sit "down the hall" or in the same building as swimming offices, there is constant interaction between coaches and administrators. There is good reason to expect that "if a nation is dirty in one, it's dirty in all." The organization of most national Olympic Committees around the world follows this centralized model, at least to some extent.

In the United States, however, even the most elite swimming coaches live in a world isolated from the rest of the sports environment. An American swimming coach might well not have a conversation, much less form a relationship, with any coach outside swimming, in their lives. American swimming coaches talk to other U.S. swimming coaches, even in the relatively sheltered university community. National offices for various sports may be a half a continent apart, and the administrators may have no more than a "handshake at meetings" relationship.

American swimming has developed independently, and has treasured that independence and nurtured it, after decades of perceiving that the sport of swimming was being used by the old AAU. For the casual observer, because the United States is dirty in some sports, it is suspected of being dirty in swimming. Swimming coaches and other knowledgeable observers view the two documented doping cases in American swimming, during the last 20 years, as probably the *only* doping cases at the elite level in our sport. A final factor working against doping in American swimming is the highly competitive and jealous nature of swimming at the local level. Any sudden or unsubstantiated improvement in the better athletes will be widely known, noted, and suspected by other local coaches and observers. The free-enterprise nature of the sport in the United States is an effective deterrent to drug use.

Free Enterprise Runs Amok in China

In the early 1990s, following the work of East German coaches and doctors in China (all of whose identities we now know), we found an unprecedented rise in Chinese performance in women's world swimming. The astronomical increase in Chinese women in the world top 25, 50, and 150 swimmers had never been seen before.

At the same time, several highly ambitious Chinese coaches spread out around the world to learn more, and were invited to lecture. Again, what was revealed in public was not extraordinary training. What was discussed later, over beverages, was truly extraordinary training that could only be supported by drug use. And, of a much more sinister nature, the sudden appearance of completely unknown athletes at the world level, to an extent never seen even in East Germany. From 1990 to 1994, suspicions were rampant, and information was gained slowly.

In 1994, in Rome, after the most noticeable demonstration of sudden superiority in the history of swimming, coaches around the world had had enough.

Petitions circulated asking for FINA investigations. FINA reacted angrily, again using the tired "no proof" argument. And the Chinese themselves, through the same coach who had been hosted all over the world at swim clinics, accused his former hosts of being "racist" and of "not understanding Chinese swimming culture." This last charge was a signal for the world's coaches to work hard to gain that understanding.

At Rome, the WSCA formally adopted an action plan to put high priority on ridding our sport of drugs. For the previous five years, since its formation, the WSCA had informally taken over this role, but now, in Rome, that action became the major priority of the Association.

In October 1994, FINA tests at the Asian Games in Hiroshima caught seven Chinese swimmers, bringing the total number of Chinese swimmers who had tested positive between 1990 and 1994 to 19. That was the highest single-nation total in history, and, at that time, exceeding all other nations combined, in positive drug tests.

WSCA investigations in 1994 and 1995 began to get to the heart of the Chinese problem. We discovered the following:

- The financial engine that drove the drug use was outside of the Chinese swimming federation. It was driven by local political and municipal money.

- Coaches and athletes were being rewarded in phenomenal financial ways for top performances first at the Chinese National Games, and secondarily at the world championships and Olympic Games. When Chinese coaches told us that the National Games were their top priorities, and the world championships and Olympic Games were secondary, we thought they were kidding us. They were not.
- Chinese coaches were "buying athletes" from sports schools in northern China, identifying good body types for swimming, and purchasing the services of these children as early as age 10 and 11, then taking them from their families to the south of China for training. Parents were signing consent forms to give their children drugs to help them perform, and the agreements were set up so that the financial rewards would not flow to the families if they ever revealed the agreements.
- Single or multiple government-sponsored research institutes existed from approximately 1987 to 1990 in northern China, in close proximity to the sports schools, to do research on usage, doping levels, and related items for sports performance. Persistent rumors tell of many deaths, physical deformations, and later reproductive disruptions that resulted from these researches. Finally, a government unit shut down the research stations in 1991, out of fear of discovery. The doctors and technical persons employed there scattered throughout China.
- This scattering of the medical personnel resulted in several key events. First, centralized control of doping in China, which had been so successful in East Germany (and was never caught in a drug test) had ended in China. (It is important to note that the first Chinese athlete testing positive occurred during a test done by the Chinese in April of 1990, though this was not revealed by the Chinese until 1994. Three other positives quickly followed.)

This end to central control resulted in unemployed medical personnel scattering to the provinces and cities in southern China where the sports clubs and swimming teams were centered. They took their knowledge of doping and sold it to the highest-bidding coach. This was a temptingly lucrative practice for doctors, who do not receive the high pay and status that doctors are given in other countries. Fast swims at the national games brought money to the coach and athlete. A portion of that money could purchase, on the open market, more medical support to help swim even faster. The coach got richer, the athlete got richer, and the doctor, if the athlete was not caught, also go richer.

Not only that, but doctors could sell their knowledge and information to other doctors, who could also then sell this expertise. Naturally, there was some "slippage" between teacher and pupil. Not all the doctors and medical personnel to whom the information was passed on, were perfect receptacles. The doping sophistication of the East German system was lost, and China has, from 1992 through 1999, registered an astronomical 29 positive drug tests in swimming, leading to a loss in credibility of international swimming.

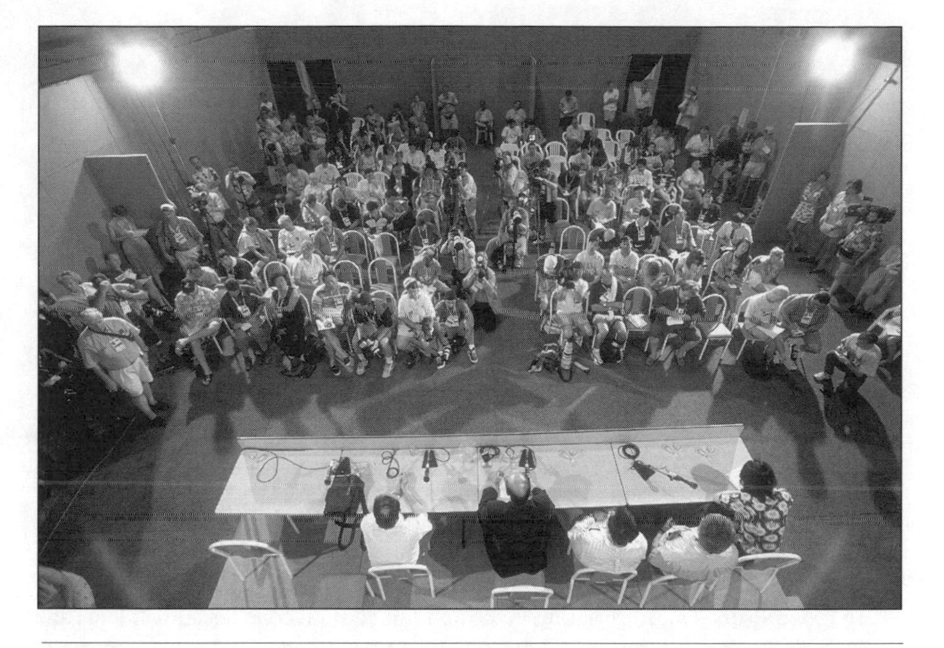

Press conference at the 1998 World Swimming Championships in Australia following the announcement that four Chinese swimmers had tested positive for banned substances.
© Ben Radford/Allsport

I reported another 17 points regarding the Chinese situation in early 1995. These 17 cases were confirmed many times by sources around the world in the following three years. FINA finally accepted these points in February of 1998, after its own investigation into the Chinese problem. WSCA had given its full report to FINA in May of 1995. FINA did not take any action except to continue to castigate the world's coaches for their "unproven suspicions" and "troublemaking" in the world of swimming. Relations between FINA and the WSCA became frosty after initial good relations. (A FINA vice president had actually helped draft the original WSCA constitution and bylaws.)

The WSCA took action, following a year's effort to understand "the Chinese swimming culture." That action did have some positive results: it exposed FINA's double-talk, no-action policies in the press; and the pressure forced FINA to change to an action mode.

Doping as a Sport Political Problem

In the 1970s and 1980s the naive view of most swimming coaches was that once FINA and the IOC saw and understood the problem of doping in swimming, they would swing into serious action and work to end the problem. During the 1970s, not a single official word was noted about doping in FINA minutes. Not a single out-of-competition test was conducted by FINA, and the Medical Committee of FINA, which in the later 1970s and throughout the 1980s was to include one or more of the architects of the East German doping program, typically ignored the doping situation.

Finally, during the late 1980s, FINA took note of problems of doping within the sport in its official newsletters. Before 1980, FINA suspended exactly four athletes in the aquatic sports for doping, all from tests at competition. When FINA did begin to "see" the doping situation, they constantly rebuked anyone asking for action with the comment, "There is no proof; there can be no action." That approach continued up until the mid-1990s.

One of the most frustrating and aggravating points in discussion with FINA became the ritualistic insistence that the complaints of coaches and athletes were simply "poor sportsmanship" on the part of losing participants. Meanwhile, coaches walked the deck, swimmers saw doped athletes in locker rooms, and every participant in the sport who paid attention knew that there were two types of swimming going on: "clean" swimming and "dirty" swimming. Being told that they were "poor losers" was infuriating in the extreme to both coaches and athletes and created severe animosity and a clear delineation between administrators and participants. Gradually, the obtuseness of FINA in recognizing the problem created an adversarial relationship between athletes and their coaches, and FINA.

Accelerating the antagonism is FINA's penchant for posing as a leading anti-doping organization while at the same time dragging their feet on every occasion and having to be forced into every minor action that should be taken. The perception is that when FINA takes action, it is too little, too late, and too ineffective. Although FINA puts out "good talk," its actions do not come close to matching that talk. An example is the 1999 grand gesture of "revealing to the swimming world" the extent of FINA's out-of-competition testing program, a step that WSCA has been asking for since 1994. When FINA did reveal its numbers of tests for each nation in Perth, under extreme duress from the media, they "looked good" with 178 tests in China. What FINA failed to tell anyone was that only eight of these tests were done before the October 1997 National Games of China, when Chinese athletes dominated the world rankings again, with absurdly good performances. FINA, then under pressure from the world swimming community to investigate, did 170 out-of-competition tests *after* the major training period that resulted in the improvements. As a result, two more dirty records appear in the world record books, and the Chinese disastrous performance at the Perth Championships reinforced the idea, "No Dope, No Hope," just as at the Atlanta Olympic Games. Despite this, FINA presented the numbers of tests as if they had performed a great service to the swimming world. Only alert journalists forced the issue of when the Chinese tests were conducted. The WSCA knew in September that only eight tests had been conducted before October and demanded that FINA account for its spending. Only the media responded, with intense questioning of FINA representatives.

The Role of Sponsors

During the early 1990s, coaches have finally caught on. Repeated IOC statements regarding the five rings as the "Olympic brand"; countless statements regarding the fact that the IOC was "bigger than the Catholic Church"; and continued rumors of Nobel Prize efforts on behalf of Juan Antonio Samaranch; and exposure of the plans of major corporations to expand behind the use of the Olympic Rings into China, the largest market on earth, finally woke up the coaches and athletes.

Drug use discredits the Olympic brand. Discrediting the Olympic brand hurts sponsorship potential. So the interests of the marketing corporation that is now the IOC, and, by extension, FINA, are to protect the brand. If protection means discarding positive test results, so be it. If protection means not testing, so be it. If protection means manipulating test results and names, so be it. If protection means saying "Yes, we have a problem, and we care to solve it," but then not spending the money to fix it, so be it.

The IOC Medical Commission rests in the hands of a nonmedically qualified sport politician, Prince Alexandre de Merode. In FINA, the hamstringing of the Medical Committee is more subtle. Although in this decade the Medical Committee has been in the hands of properly prepared medical professionals who truly want to clean up our sport, the money to do so has come only reluctantly, and bureaucratic delays have proliferated.

In 1995, one of the most absurd chapters of FINA's history in the drug wars took place when FINA sent four lawyers to investigate the Chinese doping problem. They stayed for four days, had six "formal dinners," interviewed a handful of people, and came home to tell FINA that they found nothing substantially wrong in China, and that the Chinese Swimming Federation was solidly behind the anti-doping effort. In the most bizarre report from this "Potemkin visit," the group interviewed Coach Zhou Ming, whose athletes tested positive in 1994 in Hiroshima. Ming claimed, and the FINA investigators accepted, that he could not answer their questions because he could not speak English.

This same Zhou Ming solicits speaking engagements all over the world and in May 1994, lectured for two hours in flawless English, to the World Swimming Coaches Association Gold Medal Clinic in Hawaii. The FINA investigation team was so completely out of touch with what happens on the pool deck that they accepted this explanation without question.

The overall effect of this "investigation" was summed up by this writer as "sending bakers to investigate a nuclear accident." Coaches and athletes smiled at the accuracy of the comparison.

The Real Information Is Passed

In April and May of 1995, I visited Hong Kong and the southern provinces of China on my own investigation. The result was a 19-page report detailing the Chinese doping problem, including sources of money, sources of doping information, procedures, and processes used by Chinese Coaches in doping their athletes. Seventeen key points were noted, including the fact that the Chinese Swimming

Federation, despite its reported interests in stopping the doping, had absolutely no control over what was happening with its coaches and athletes in the provinces. This report was hand-delivered to FINA President Mustaapha Larfaoui by the author, in November of 1995 in Rio de Janeiro, Brazil, site of the short course world championships. FINA now had the complete story on the reasons, methods, and details of operation of the Chinese system at that time. Absolutely nothing happened.

The disgust of the participants (clean athletes and coaches) deepened when FINA appointed a doping panel to hear all doping cases, and selected an individual, Mr. Harm Beyer of Germany, as the chairman of the Committee. Since the late 1970s, Mr. Beyer has waffled with his views on doping, suggesting several times that the quest to rid the sport of doping was impossible and that dope should simply be allowed in the sport. His public statements since that time have wavered back and forth between support for the official FINA anti-doping position, and acceptance of drugs in the sport. This is the person chosen to lead the Doping Panel of FINA. This is not surprising for an organization that included one of the architects of the East German doping program on its Medical Committee.

Coaches and athletes have described FINA's consistently absurd pursuit of anti-doping action as "the fox guarding the henhouse." The tag is most apt. FINA's actions, and the inaction of the IOC, would be funny if not for the horrendous effects that this incompetence has had on our sport, and on individuals within it. Lives have been dramatically altered, economic opportunities have gone to cheaters and been denied to honest athletes, and the basic fabric of sport has been torn.

Sport's guardians, the administrators, are in fact guarding nothing but their own perks, power, and prestige. It has been left to the coaches, essentially powerless because of the deliberate exclusion of their profession from the FINA bureau and committees, to holler, shout, disrupt, question, and attempt, by using the power of the press and the public, to get FINA's administrators to simply do what is right.

None of the world's cheated athletes and coaches from the past three decades of ineffective FINA leadership are laughing. And our sport, once a magnificent centerpiece of sport, is now the subject of scornful editorial cartoons. In one, a child sits on his father's lap watching the news stories break of the Chinese drug busts in Perth, and Dad says, "Be a rock star, son, at least they're not ALL on drugs."

The IOC, FINA, and their sponsors, in attempting to cover up and ignore a problem, have begun the death watch for the sports programs that are their raison d'etre.

Solutions

There are no lightning solutions to the problem of drugs in sport. Where there are financial gains to be made, human beings will attempt to cheat. This is sad, but true.

Some things can be done to restore credibility to our sport. Coaches and athletes, want to see them done. The overwhelming majority of athletes and coaches in swimming want clean sport.

- Step to solution: Transparency. Every out-of-competition drug test done should be posted on the Internet as it is taken, identified by the athlete's name, date, and site of test. When analyzed, the results should be immediately posted. If blood tests are scientifically valid, they should be taken in conjunction with urine. Athletes from five nations endorsed this concept at the Perth World Championships. Athletes realize that some personal liberties must be given up in order for their sport to be clean.
- Step to solution: Get ahead of the cheats. Its time for the IOC to spend some of its billions and turn over drug testing and drug research to an independent international body. IOC funds, put into an independent fund, can be used to clean up sport. Get quality scientists excellent labs and let them work ahead to anticipate the next moves of the dirty chemists—then get there first, and prepare tests to check athletes for illegal substances.
- Step to solution: Turn it inside out. Put the cash on the reward side. Make swimming at the world level so lucrative that athletes will choose to participate in whatever level of testing is necessary to ensure clean sport, and pay for it themselves, in order to have a clean, verifiable "drug passport," which is necessary for them to enter major cash-reward events. Spend less money on tests, more money on independent labs, let the athletes at the highest levels pay for their own tests, and require the level of testing necessary to keep the sport clean.
- Step to solution: Involve participants in decision making. The time has come for athletes and coaches to sit on the FINA Bureau, at the highest levels of decision making in the sport. This will ensure that current, active athletes and coaches will participate in all action concerning drug affairs, and the tired excuses of "We didn't have the information" will cease. Communication will be enhanced at all levels of the sport.

The old British Empire definition of and concern for "amateurism" is long dead. Let's bury it and allow participants some input and control over the sport they love.

Note

Supporting documents and information for all statements made in this paper are available at the office of the American Swimming Coaches Association, 2101 N. Andrews Ave., Fort Lauderdale, FL 33311. (1-800-356-2722).

10

CHAPTER

How Drug Testing Fails: The Politics of Doping Control

John Hoberman
University of Texas at Austin

Over the past 30 years illicit drug use in Olympic sport has reached epidemic proportions. The widespread and largely undetected use of potentially dangerous synthetic hormones such as anabolic steroids, human growth hormone, and erythropoietin has provoked a crisis of confidence in track and field, swimming, cycling, weightlifting, and even canoeing that may eventually threaten their existence as Olympic sports. In fact, signs of demoralization among drug-free athletes and sport officials have been evident for years. In 1991, for example, the spokesman for Germany's track and field athletes claimed that highly placed officials had simply given up on the anti-doping campaign in the face of apparently insurmountable obstacles. A month later, the former president of the German Swimming Federation, Harm Beyer, called for the "controlled" use of steroids on the grounds that German sport officials had shown themselves to be both unwilling and unable to eradicate doping. Beyer, a Hamburg judge who has served as secretary general of the European Swimming Association, and is now the head of doping control for the International Swimming Federation (FINA), proposed the formation of a "circus troupe" of elite athletes "subject to different rules and laws" who would be eligible to take steroids and other performance-enhancing drugs.[1] This conflict between drug-free idealism and hormonal realism is now a global phenomenon. Indeed, a "circus troupe" of hormonally boosted gladiators already exists in some sports. All three medalists in the shot put at the 1992 Barcelona Olympic Games were convicted steroid dopers, as is the 1996 Olympic champion and world-record holder, Randy Barnes. The Russian super heavyweight lifter and steroid smuggler Alexander Kurlovitch, arrested in Montreal in 1985 while carrying $20,000 worth of drugs, went on to win gold medals at the 1988 Seoul and 1992 Barcelona Olympic

Games. Banned for life by the Soviet weightlifting federation, he was reinstated in 1987.[2] Having tested positive for steroids in 1995, he was permitted to participate in the Atlanta Games a year later while the International Olympic Committee (IOC) and the International Weightlifting Federation (IWF) looked the other way.[3]

In fact, there is only so much even an honest federation official can do about the doping practices of elite athletes and the coaches and doctors who develop them. In May 1995, six months before his drug testers caught a staggering total of 64 lifters steroid doping, the president of the IWF, Gottfried Schödl (Austria), told an interviewer, "What are we supposed to do with these idiots? The ambition to stand on top of the victory stand will make the athletes do anything. I have the feeling that the coaches are behind these manipulations, because their contracts are frequently tied to the results they get. It's an impossible problem."[4] Among the international federation leaders, Schödl is exceptional for his honesty. The International Canoeing Federation (ICF) is more typical. Its 78-year-old Italian president, Sergio Orsi, is one of the federation dictators who have blocked reforms and fended off challenges from the ICF's anti-doping faction. Although the ICF has been on the doping defensive for years, its national affiliates have stonewalled the doping issue in their own way. Dozens of national federations have threatened a boycott of the next world championships if the ICF requires them to make their athletes available for doping control.[5] On every level—international, national, and individual—the will to eradicate doping from Olympic sport is lacking. "Hair-raising things are happening in elite sport," the (now retired) German anti-doping official Hans Evers said in 1996, "but nothing can be done without concerted international action."[6]

An effective international anti-doping campaign was never a major priority of the IOC before the 1998 Tour de France scandal. Between 1968 and 1996 approximately one in every thousand Olympic athletes tested positive for a banned substance at the Games.[7] The Olympic testing program was widely regarded as a sham, and more effective enforcement was expected from national and international federations. For Juan Antonio Samaranch and his closest associates, doping was primarily a public relations problem that threatened lucrative television and corporate contracts that are now worth billions of dollars. Even before the Ben Johnson scandal of September 1988 shocked Samaranch into a redoubled "campaign" against doping, he had devised an anti-doping rhetoric (in response to an American blood doping scandal) that sometimes took on a liturgical flavor. "Above all," he proclaimed at the 1988 Calgary Winter Olympic Games, "such behavior makes a mockery of the very essence of sport, the soul of what we, like our predecessors, consider sacrosanct ideals."[8] "Doping," he added, "is alien to our philosophy, to our rules of conduct. We shall never tolerate it."[9] Samaranch went on to address the corrupt minority among Olympic athletes: "As means of detection have improved, they now attempt to cheat scientifically by using artificial means to provoke natural physiological reactions, or by attempting with various tricks to hide the irrefutable evidence of their dishonest actions."[10] In September of that year, in his opening speech at the 94th IOC session, Samaranch intensified the rhetorical assault against the doping evil. "Doping equals death," he proclaimed, calling drugged athletes "the thieves of performance" and denouncing the medical personnel who assist them as unprincipled people who "attach little importance to their oath or the code of ethics they are supposed to respect." "Yes," he went on, "doping equals death. Death psychologically, with the profound, sometimes irreversible alteration of the body's normal processes through inexcusable manipulation. Physical death, as certain tragic cases in recent years have shown. And then also the death of the spirit and intellect, by the acceptance of cheating. And finally moral death, by placing oneself de facto outside the rules of conduct demanded by any human society."[11] Almost a decade later, Samaranch revived this approach on the eve of the 1996 Atlanta Games. "Doping is the negation of sport and its role as we understand it. Athletes who use banned substances to improve their performance commit a series of acts that transgress and violate certain immutable principles."[12] These deadly serious recitations of doping's mortal sins recall Samaranch's notorious (and apparently serious) televised claim that the IOC is more important than the Catholic church.[13] His rhetorical style on these occasions is the Olympic world's version of the transcendental language that emanates at regular intervals from the Vatican.

The head of the IOC Medical Commission, Prince Alexandre de Merode, addressed the doping issue in a less spiritual idiom during the IOC's *annus horribilis* of 1988. In February, in the wake of the blood-doping scandal at the Calgary Winter Games caused by the Nordic combined athlete Kerry Lynch of the United States, de Merode announced he would seek sanctions against two employees of the United States Olympic Committee (USOC) whose involvement with the case had become known. De Merode professed to find it odd that Jim Page and Doug Peterson had not been fired immediately by the USOC and raised the prospect of a lifetime ban for both. Lynch was eventually disqualified for a year after he confessed to blood doping. "It is quite abnormal," de Merode commented, "as if you are keeping as a team physician someone who prescribes drugs. People involved in doping should not be allowed to keep working for national Olympic committees or sport federations."[14] But why should such conduct by the USOC have surprised de Merode at all? Three years earlier, after the world had learned of a horrific blood doping scandal involving seven American Olympic cyclists, including four medalists at the 1984 Los Angeles Games, the USOC had done next to nothing to discipline the guilty parties. Seventeen other members of the U.S. cycling team had refused to undergo the illicit blood transfusions. Instead of presenting these honest athletes with the ethical conduct (or common-sense) medals they deserved, the USOC simply ignored them in favor of temporizing and damage control.[15] In a similarly absent-minded vein at his Calgary press conference, de Merode also denounced drug dealers as an offense against the Olympic ethos. "There are no excuses for trafficking," he declaimed. "We must act against dealing—it's worse than taking drugs."[16] But if this was the IOC's position, then why had it permitted the triumphal continuation of Alexander Kurlovitch's Olympic weightlifting career after the Canadian police found him carrying commercial quantities of steroids? Similarly, if doping personnel should not be allowed to work for national Olympic committees or sport federations, then why have neither Samaranch nor de Merode lifted a finger to stop or even comment on the worldwide export of documented former East German doping experts (see discussion later in this chapter) into top positions in many sport federations?[17] Are they aware, for example, that the personal "performance-diagnostician" and trainer of Hermann Maier, the Austrian double-gold medal winner at the 1998 Nagano Winter Games, is none other than Dr. Bernd Pansold, who as of March 1998 was on trial in Berlin for administering steroids and causing bodily harm to former East German female athletes under his supervision?[18]

The Roles of Samaranch and de Merode

The unofficial division of labor in the IOC's doping publicity campaign has cast Samaranch as the moralist and de Merode as the sometimes cynical and occasionally clumsy pragmatist. For example, when nine positive drug tests appeared to implicate finalists at the 1984 Los Angeles Games, the urine samples were sent to de Merode and subsequently disappeared. Dr. Craig Kammerer, associate director of the drug testing laboratory in Los Angeles, later commented, "We were totally puzzled initially and figured that something must be going on, politically or a cover up." Professor Arnold Beckett, a member of the IOC Doping Committee for the Los Angeles Games described how de Merode claimed at the time that the test results were destroyed without his knowledge. Beckett stated: "We took the responsibility of not revealing this publicly," and he speculated that the samples were destroyed to avert the sort of public relations disaster that would unfold four years later in Seoul. "It would have done quite a lot of damage if five or six . . . of the positives . . . had led to the medal winners, as undoubtedly it would have done. Some of the federations and IOC are happy to show that they're doing something in getting some positives, but they don't want too many because that would damage the image of the Games."[19]

In 1991, as the IOC carefully distanced itself from the flood of doping revelations emanating from the newly reunified Germany, de Merode cautioned against extrapolating the German situation into a global crisis and added pragmatically, "What we are dealing with here is a certain kind of public relations issue. The public must be persuaded that something is being done." The situation, he said, was really not so bad, and he recommended against precipitate action. What is more, he saw no financial obligation on the part of the IOC, asserting that its role was to lend its "moral credit" to the anti-doping campaign.[20] In December 1994 de Merode called the steroid positives implicating Chinese swimmers at the world championships in Hiroshima "accidents that could happen anywhere."[21] In April 1995 this view was seconded by the IOC president himself: "We are carrying out a decisive struggle against the doping evil, but there can be no sweeping condemnations of individual nations."[22]

In December 1996, de Merode appeared to show signs of the bureaucratic fatigue that has produced widespread cynicism about doping control among sport officials when he argued for two-year rather than four-year sanctions for serious doping offenses: "The level of sanctions is, in my opinion, excessive. In some respects, it is completely obsolete and, if we really want to be realistic today, it is necessary to reform sanctions. Strict sanctions were appropriate when we were dealing with top amateurs, but since sport has become a profession, we are faced with a major social problem. These sanctions have deep repercussions on people and their standard of living."[23] In other words, the professionalization of the Games inaugurated by Samaranch and Horst Dassler, son of the founder of the Adidas athletic shoe company, required a pragmatic attitude toward doping.

In 1981, a year after Samaranch's election to the presidency of the IOC, the word "amateur" was removed from the Olympic Charter, and over the past 15 years Samaranch has presided over an almost total commercializing of the Olympic Games that has converted the "Movement" into an advertising vehicle for the multinational corporate sponsors and American television networks that are the foundation of his power. Anyone who doubts that Dassler provided Samaranch with his blueprint for commercializing the Olympic movement need only read Dassler's article on "Sport and Industry" which appeared in the official *Olympic Review* in 1980.[24]

The strategy of public moralizing about doping has concealed the IOC's longtime underfunding and delay in implementing drug testing that might really work, since real controls would expose major athletes, alienate Olympic corporate sponsors, and put an end to record breaking in certain events, such as the throwing events in track and field, which suffer when athletes reduce their performance-enhancing drug consumption in anticipation of improved testing procedures. As if to acknowledge the IOC's lack of initiative in this area, the IOC president has recently attempted to demonstrate a new level of commitment on the doping front. On February 6, 1998, at a press conference that preceded the Nagano Winter Olympic Games, Samaranch launched a preemptive strike against longstanding criticism of the IOC's campaign against doping. "We are going to invest $50,000,000 in the doping struggle," he proclaimed. "We have won many battles, but not the war. Yet that, too, we will win. I just don't know when."[25] On this occasion the IOC president managed to stifle the poorly concealed irritation that had been evident at previous press conferences during which he had heard criticism of the IOC's inability to prevail against the doping menace. Yet this financial gesture revealed much about an inefficient past even as it promised a more efficient future. Let us pass over the fact that Samaranch did not care to specify the time period during which this money would be invested, or that in April 1997 he had inexplicably singled out the International Amateur Athletic Federation (IAAF) and the international swimming organization, FINA, for special praise even as he lambasted the other international federations for inaction on the anti-doping front.[26] More important is the record of performance that had produced the malaise he was attempting to address.

Responding to the Calgary blood doping scandal, de Merode stated in February 1988 "There is always evolution [of cheating techniques], and we are trying to develop an effective, practical test."[27] Five years later, no initiative having come from the IOC, the newly formed International Biathlon Union took blood samples from all of the 184 athletes competing at Badgastein—a path-breaking step.[28] Ten years later, reacting to pressure from the international skiing federation and the international biathlon and modern pentathlon union (UIPMB), the IOC finally announced that blood testing for elevated hemoglobin counts would be performed at the Nagano Winter Games by these federations.[29] (No positive tests were announced.) The International Ski Federation (FIS), in turn, had announced its blood testing program, establishing maximum allowable red blood cell counts for men (18.5 grams/liter) and women (16.5 grams/liter), after the Norwegian cross-country skier Trude Dydendahl Hartz published a warning that blood doping was destroying the sport.[30] Before the 1997 skiing world championships in Trondheim, the Norwegian Olympic star Bjørn Dæhlie had also demanded blood testing.[31] The Norwegian skiing official Inge Andersen had for years been demanding blood testing by the FIS.[32]

In 1992 Olympic officials backed off plans to introduce comprehensive blood testing at the 1994 Lillehammer Winter Games, deciding instead to support the limited anti-doping system already used at skiing competitions. "We are in a position to carry out the tests," de Merode announced, "but it remains to be clarified, for example, whether the blood is to be taken from the earlobe or the fingertip."[33] Dr. Wildor Hollmann, then president of both the German and World Sports Medical Federations observed that taking blood samples after obtaining oral consent raised unresolved questions about the legality of the procedure.[34] (By 1995 Hollmann, too, was calling for blood testing, even as the prominent German cell biologist and anti-doping crusader Werner Franke was calling it useless.[35]) On February 1, 1994, de Merode announced the introduction of blood testing at Lillehammer. The serious limitation of this procedure was that it could detect neither endogenous blood transfusions (transfusions of the athlete's own blood) nor erythropoietin, but only exogenous transfusions (transfusions of someone else's blood) that the dangers of AIDS and hepatitis made unlikely in the first place.[36] As we have seen, four more years would pass before more comprehensive blood testing was introduced at the Olympic Winter Games.

In November 1996 de Merode announced a breakthrough that would produce a urine test for erythropoietin by the beginning of 1997. It never happened.[37] By July 1997 German sport federations, but not the IOC, wanted to implement blood testing to detect the use of erythropoietin.[38] In March of that year, the IOC had dampened expectations that there would be reliable tests for erythropoietin and synthetic human growth hormone in the near future. Patrick Schamasch, medical director of the IOC, said at the meeting of the Executive Board in Lausanne: "We want to carry out blood tests to detect erythropoietin in Nagano in 1998, but whether we will have tests ready in time I cannot say at this point." As for human growth hormone: "A test will be developed by 1998 or 1999 at the earliest." Regarding human growth hormone testing at the 2000 Sydney Summer Games, Schamasch said he was "not so optimistic."[39] In April this gloomy prognosis was revised by a more upbeat de Merode. After consultations with leading anti-doping experts in Lausanne, he announced the IOC was "very optimistic" that tests for erythropoietin and human growth hormone would be ready by the Sydney Games.[40] A month later, de Merode was predicting that a new test for testosterone would be ready within three months for the world track and field championships in Athens.[41] However, he was already downplaying his earlier prediction that erythropoietin and human growth hormone tests would be ready for Sydney. "I cannot say when the tests can be implemented," he said. "But those who reproach us with doing nothing are mistaken."[42]

Expert Commentary on IOC Doping Policy

Among those reproaching the IOC in recent years for its failure to provide leadership have been some prominent figures in the field of doping control. Hans Evers, who left his position as head of a German anti-doping commission in October 1996, pointed out at the time that no fewer than 16 Olympic-affiliated German sport federations were not even following their own rules. A number of these federations were not testing at competitions, and some that were did not report positive tests or even keep records of those who did test positive. Among the responsible parties who minimized doping control problems, he said, was the IOC. Professor Helmut Digel, a sport sociologist who assumed the presidency of the German Track and Field Federation in 1993, has criticized the IOC's sometimes contradictory and erratic pronouncements on doping.[43] Wilhelm Schänzer, Manfred Donike's successor at the doping laboratory in Cologne, watched the IOC delay a blood-testing project and concluded in 1996 that the IOC had "missed an opportunity to show that it is interested in this matter." It should also be noted that the IOC does not necessarily control all the relevant actors in this drama. For example, at the Atlanta Games the IOC-sponsored Court of Arbitration for Sport ruled, contrary to the position of the IOC Medical Commission, that use of the Russian-made stimulant bromantan was not a violation, a ruling Schänzer called "a catastrophic decision."[44] Prof. Arnold Beckett, a former member of the IOC Medical Commission, has become an outspoken critic of the IOC's anti-doping campaign. There can be little doubt that fears of retaliation have inhibited other doping experts from issuing more frequent and harsher criticisms of the IOC's performance in this area.

The origin of the IOC's political passivity regarding doping control is its policy of delegating responsibility beyond Lausanne, so that the difficult implementation of policy is left to national and international federations whose commitment to effective doping control has seldom been evident. At the opening of the 105th IOC session in Atlanta, Samaranch proclaimed that the IOC had "spearheaded the anti-doping campaign on a world-wide scale."[45] This claim was correct only in that the IOC president has exercised an effective monopoly on moralizing rhetoric. Consequently, after the Chinese steroid positives at Hiroshima made headlines around the world in late 1994, Samaranch's director general, Francois Carrard, adroitly deflected the burden onto the world swimming body: "The IOC sees no reason to comment on a procedure for which FINA is responsible," he said. "The Chinese have problems, but they are not the only ones."[46]

Nowhere, however, has this policy been more evident (and consequential) than in the case of Germany. Reacting in late 1990 to revelations about the former East German doping policies, the IOC press director, Michelle Verdier, commented that the IOC saw no need to act and would await a report from the German National Olympic Committee.[47] Samaranch himself called the growing scandal "a German problem."[48] Unknown or perhaps irrelevant to the IOC was the fact that the (West) German National Olympic Committee could not be trusted to reveal the full scope of East German doping at the same time that West German sport officials were in the process of hiring for their own purposes the most highly regarded East German scientists and coaches who had been involved in State Plan 14.25.

Confronted with the burgeoning East German state doping scandal and an unending series of embarrassing revelations about the doping practices and cover-ups of the West Germans, Samaranch was content to preserve the imaginary *cordon sanitaire* that separated his own office from the realities of the doping underworld. An important complication, however, was the fact that this underworld and its sympathizers have always included people associated with sport federations around the world who do official business with the IOC. This circumstance has always implicated Samaranch in the doping problem despite his persistent efforts to elevate himself to a "moral" plane far above the ugly realities of doping. As chief Olympic diplomat, Samaranch made a point of forming relationships with the two most important East and West German sport officials: Manfred Ewald and Willi Daume. In 1985 Samaranch conferred Olympic Orders on both Ewald and the East German Communist Party boss Erich Honecker—the highest East German officials responsible for State Plan 14.25 and its criminal child-doping practices. In 1993 he conferred the same honor on Willi Daume.[49] In 1991 Ewald appeared as guest of honor at a party put on by the German National Olympic Committee, whose president Willi Daume subsequently procured Ewald an audience with IOC president Samaranch. Shortly thereafter Ewald also met with Thomas Bach, a German IOC member and Samaranch protégé, and Walther Tröger, general secretary of the German National Olympic Committee. In the Bundestag, the only criticism of the Samaranch-Ewald-Daume troika came from the sport spokesman of the Social Democrats, Wilhelm Schmidt.[50] As if to emphasize the grotesque character of this alliance, in March 1990 the general secretary of the East German National Olympic Committee, Walter Gitter, suggested that Honecker would have to be stripped of his Olympic Order in the event of his criminal indictment. Paragraph 7 of the Olympic Charter, he noted, provides for the removal of this distinction if the honoree damages the honor and dignity of the Olympic movement. But the initiative for such a step, he said, would have to come from Samaranch himself.[51]

In Willi Daume, too, Samaranch found a kindred spirit with whom he could do Olympic business in the confidential style to which he was accustomed. Daume, an

IOC member since 1956, had earned his status as the grand old man of West German sport and the reigning cosmopolite of the Olympic set. Like Samaranch, Daume confronted doping with the sternest sort of rhetoric, calling it "the evil of all evils" and "the moral sin of elite sport."[52] By 1991 he had been the president of the West German National Olympic Committee for 30 years, and now his reaction to the revelations from the former East Germany was appropriately somber: "The situation is grave," he said, "and we should act with dispatch." He called for an "international investigation" and announced that he had already contacted the IOC Medical Commission.[53]

As I have observed elsewhere: "These public statements were in all likelihood a charade. It is difficult to believe that the best connected man in West German sport, this popular confessor figure and all-purpose fixer, could have been unaware of doping in his own sport establishment. If anyone was in a position to expose and reform the West German doping scene, it was Willi Daume, and he chose not to act. Why, for example, was he a consistent and bitter opponent of doping critics like Brigitte Berendonk as far back as 1977? Why did he not act then on information from a German Track and Field Federation doping investigator? Why, as late as 1984, did he ignore an athlete's report about drug-test cheating? Why did he refuse to 'negotiate' Olympic qualifying norms with his own athletes in 1990? And why did he express confidence in two sport physicians, Joseph Keul and Armin Klumper, who are known to be steroid advocates?"[54]

With the passing of Willi Daume, Thomas Bach became Samaranch's German Connection. In December 1988, three months after the Ben Johnson scandal had broken and three years before Bach became an IOC member, the 1976 Olympic fencing champion already was defending the IOC president's record on the doping issue. "The IOC doesn't need any more political helpers," he declared. Samaranch, he said, had recognized the danger early and had promptly assumed a leadership role. "Already in Calgary he was calling a spade a spade, and in Seoul he said even before the Johnson scandal: 'Doping is like death.'"[55] Shortly after his entry into the IOC, Bach already was tempering his rhetoric. Samaranch, he said, had vested authority in this area to de Merode's Medical Commission. As for the IOC's campaign against doping, he conceded, "the room for maneuver is limited."[56] A year later Bach expressed his support for Dr. Joseph Keul, one of a handful of high-profile West German sport physicians, whose 20-year career as chief physician to the German Olympic team has long represented a triumph of good connections and media savvy over the integrity of high-performance sports medicine.[57] In 1987, following the horrific, pharmacologically induced death of the West German heptathlete Birgit Dressel, Keul told the Bundestag that the doping problem was being exaggerated. He added that doping did not occur in most sports, and that steroids were both safe and effective.[58] In 1970, long before anabolic steroids had achieved notoriety as potentially dangerous drugs, he had written: "Anyone who wants a muscular body and simply wants to have a more masculine appearance can take steroids. . . . This cannot be described as doping. What is more, I regard control as impracticable."[59] By the late 1970s he was a bitter opponent of the West German athlete and anti-doping activist Brigitte Berendonk, whose pathbreaking *Doping-Dokumente* (1991) revealed the full extent of doping practices in both Germanies. Bach's endorsement of Keul signified his political alignment with a sports medicine establishment that has never given up the dream of "controlled" steroid regimens for elite athletes.

Infiltrations of International Medical Commissions

A seldom-discussed obstacle to doping control has been the infiltration of international medical committees by sport physicians who have promoted or condoned doping practices, particularly when they consider these methods to be medically safe. Twenty-one years ago, for example, a heated debate occurred during a meeting of the Medical Commission of the IAAF. The subject of this contentious meeting was the introduction of doping controls to detect the use of anabolic steroids at the 1974 European Championships in Rome. Dr. Ludwig Prokop of Vienna, former president of the World Federation of Sports Physicians, expressed his concern about the future direction of high-performance athletics. The exploitation of sport as an instrument of national prestige had already led to the use of medically dangerous androgens, and he appealed for an unambiguous resolution to ban these drugs from sport. He was opposed by Dr. Joseph Keul of the Federal Republic of Germany, who argued that steroids were useful regenerative drugs that he did not want to do without and that could be safely administered in small doses. Eventually, Prokop's anti-doping resolution was severely edited and watered down by a committee consisting of himself, Keul, and Manfred Höppner, formerly the director of the East German Sports Medical Service. Dr. Prokop recalls his interaction with these high-performance sport physicians as follows: "In fact, these people just wanted to know how to minimize side effects. The whispering campaign among the physicians—so many milligrams of this and of that—was revolting. What I find just as immoral is their knowing complicity."[60]

Two decades later, we are in a position to assess the careers of these men and the doping epidemic to which they are connected in different ways. Today Joseph Keul is a holder of the Bundesverdienstkreuz, a decoration conferred by the government in Bonn, and has served as (West) Germany's official Olympic sport physician for two decades. At the same time, he has been described repeatedly in the German press as a compromised figure whose insincere criticisms of doping have concealed his membership in the medical pro-steroid lobby. Manfred Höppner is the disgraced former director of the East German Sports Medical Service who bears heavy responsibility for the practice of criminal medicine in the former East German sport establishment. Before the collapse of the East German state, Keul and Höppner had a personal relationship that was described to the East German secret police (Stasi) by Höppner. He reported in 1974 that Keul had confirmed successful West German use of steroids. Keul, he reported, had "nothing in principle" against the use of these drugs and was "not inclined" to renounce their use.[61] "The only thing that would bother him about what is going on in the GDR," Höppner commented, "is that he wouldn't be able to make money on it."[62] Ludvig Prokop has maintained his independence from elite sports medical circles, which he described in 1994 as "a Mafia." In the meantime, the campaign against steroids and other forms of doping in athletics that should have begun in earnest at that meeting in 1974 has largely failed. It is reasonable to assume that the penetration of sport federation committees by steroid sympathizers is one reason why.

It is unlikely, for example, that Manfred Höppner's long service on the IAAF Medical Commission did much to promote doping control. Manfred Donike, the deceased former head of the Cologne doping control laboratory who sat on that committee with Höppner for 15 years, said in 1990 that quite apart from where his loyalties lay, Höppner "did not understand the first thing about analytical chemistry."[63] Gunther Heinze, former general secretary of the East German National Olympic Committee, was a cofounder of the first IOC World Conference against Doping and was an IOC member until the fall of East Germany, after which he became an honorary member. By 1990 Heinze was under pressure to resign from the reunited National Olympic Committee to which West German sport officials had appointed him. As he watched former colleagues adapt to the shifting political winds, Heinze refused to play the recanting turncoat: "Otherwise I would be a hypocrite. Anyone who spits on the work he once did shows weakness of character." As for doping: "I was aware that 'supporting measures' *[unterstützende Mittel]* were being used, but none of them were on the doping list."[64] The East German discus thrower Evelin Herberg-Jahl won gold medals at the 1976 and 1980 Olympic Games as a doped athlete, then spent six years (1984–1990) sitting on the Arbitration Panel of the IAAF.[65]

Today the most interesting infiltrator of the IOC Medical Commission is the Italian sport physician Francesco Conconi of the University of Ferrara, who was put in charge of developing a test for illicit use of the red-blood-cell-boosting drug erythropoietin by athletes. In January 1998 Conconi announced a breakthrough in the detection of an antibody that can supposedly distinguish between natural and synthetic erythropoietin in urine samples. "In a certain way, we have found the right antibody," he said, "but we need to find it in a suitable quantity." The IOC called this development "a significant step" toward a practical test.[66] But in 1985 the Swedish coach Bengt-Herman Nilsson, who had served as a cross-country skiing trainer in Italy in 1968, connected Conconi with a then recent and unexpected Italian victory in a ski-relay race that took place in Sweden. "Medically and physiologically," he said, "the Italians are far ahead. Their medical organization is well developed. . . . The best known person is professor Conconi. It is no secret that professor Conconi has been doing experiments on blood transfers." So did this mean that the victorious Italian skiers had benefited from blood doping? "I don't think so," Nilsson replied. "And when you talk about blood transfers you must keep in mind that it is not prohibited by the rules governing competitions." Among the beneficiaries of Conconi's attentions had been the world-class 10,000-meter runner Alberto Cova and the world-class professional cyclist (and long-distance world record-holder) Francesco Moser.[67]

In February 1988 the successful German skier Jochen Behle suggested that the sudden improvements in Italian athletes at Olympic Games and world championships were both suspicious and somehow connected to their physician, the nutrition expert Francesco Conconi, who was reputed to be a blood doping expert, as well.[68] In December 1993 Osvaldo Fermi, vice president of the Italian Cycling Federation, stated that 60 percent of Italian riders were doped. He had spoken out (to the great displeasure of other cycling officials), he said, because certain doping practices were inducing riders to risk their lives. "There are doctors here on the riders' lists because they provide pharmacological assistance." The combinations of doping substances and masking agents were, he said, life-threatening. Although the names of these physicians had circulated for years, it was left to the interviewer to point out that Francesco Conconi had long enjoyed the reputation of a medical miracle worker and was associated with the practice of blood doping.[69] In February 1994 the head of doping controls at the Lillehammer Winter Olympic Games, professor Inggard Lereim, announced without further comment that Francesco Conconi was engaged in research on the detection of erythropoietin.[70] In April 1994 the manager of the German cyclist Uwe Ampler, who had accused the state-sponsored Team Telekom of doping him without his knowledge, observed that Telekom riders had requested in vain the "scientific" treatment for which Francesco Conconi had become famous.[71] In January 1997 the Italian track and field coach Sandro Donati issued a report, based on interviews with two dozen riders and coaches, that identified Conconi as the "central figure" of erythropoietin doping. Professor Dirk Clasing, a member of the anti-doping commission of the German Sport Federation and a doping consultant for the Association of German Cyclists, commented, "The doctor whose name begins with C is regarded within the sport as a very dangerous character." By October 1998 Conconi was under investigation by Italian authorities. In February 2000 he was being investigated on allegations of criminal association. Conconi's confiscated computer appeared to contain a list of 22 elite athletes he had treated with erythropoeitin.[72]

So who is Francesco Conconi? It is at least possible that reports of Conconi's involvement in blood doping are simply unsubstantiated rumors. It is also possible that he is one of the well-situated amoralists of the elite sport world who move easily back and forth across the line that separates "legitimate" from "illegitimate" sports medicine. Indeed, Conconi's career at the cutting edge of high-performance sports medicine may well have encouraged in him a keen, relativist, and cynical view of the often subtle differences between the natural and the artificial, between nutrients and stimulants. His insights into the somewhat arbitrary nature of these classifications may have led him to conclude that such distinctions make no sense at all. His position as head of the medical commission of the Union Cycliste Internationale (UCI), and his appointment by the IOC to an important role in its anti-doping campaign, deserve an investigation, not only of Conconi's record, but also of the procedures that permitted the infiltration of these medical commissions by a person with Conconi's reputation. These appointments indicate the lack of vigilance about personnel that is one important aspect of the politics of doping control.

SmithKline Beecham and the Atlanta Olympic Games (1996)

The integrity of Olympic drug testing was called into question in 1996 after unexplained events at the Atlanta drug testing facility resulted in reports of unannounced positive tests carried out on athletes who may have been medal winners. The Atlanta Committee for the Olympic Games had engaged SmithKline Beecham Laboratories to manage a testing procedure based on high-resolution gas chromatography mass spectrometry. This laboratory was headed by Dr. Barry Sample, who operated it in conjunction with Dr. Don Catlin, head of the IOC-accredited laboratory in Los Angeles, and Dr. Steven Horning, who represented the doping control laboratory in Cologne. The Web page posted after the Games by SmithKline Beecham was titled "No Secrets in Atlanta." "During the Games," it read, "more than two thousand samples were tested for stimulants, narcotics, anabolic agents (muscle builders), and other prohibited substances. Advanced technology at the lab detected banned chemicals in smaller amounts and over longer time periods than in earlier Olympic Games." This posting contained not a word about the reporting irregularities that made headlines around the world in November 1996. Not widely known was SmithKline's sponsorship of the 1994 Goodwill Games in St. Petersburg, Russia, in partnership with the Turner media empire, or SmithKline Beecham Consumer Healthcare's sponsorship of the auto racing driver Dennis Vitolo in the late 1990s in a state of the art Indy car.[73] One may speculate that SmithKline paid the IOC a reported $2,500,000 fee in order to secure a high-profile drug testing assignment that would lead to additional business with steady clients such as professional sport leagues in the United States. (SmithKline Clinical Laboratories also stood accused of fraud by the U.S. Government.[74]) The expiration of SmithKline's IOC approval after the Atlanta Games may have aborted this marketing strategy.[75] The fact that SmithKline manufactures androgens for the medical market adds an interesting twist to an already complicated story (see discussion later in this chapter).

On November 19, 1996, the London *Sunday Times* published an interview with Don Catlin that erupted into a major Olympic drug scandal that, like all such scandals apart from the Ben Johnson case, led to no apparent reforms of IOC procedures and was soon dropped by the news organizations that initially reported on it. Although only two steroid positives were announced during the Games, Catlin commented, "There were several other steroid positives from around the end of the Games which we reported. I can think of no reason why they have not been announced." In addition, he expressed deep reservations about the commercialization of the drug testing process: "SmithKline Beecham were in charge of testing in Atlanta. It's the first time that happened and hopefully the last time too."[76] In fact, it was not. Drug testing at the 1998 Nagano Winter Olympic Games was handled by Mitsubishi Kagaku Bio-Clinical Laboratories, which appears to be a recent spin-off of Mitsubishi-Kagaku Foods, founded as a sales division for the food ingredient business of Mitsubishi Chemical Corporation, the largest chemical company in Japan and a donor to Samaranch's Olympic Museum in Lausanne.[77] It would be interesting to know when the Mitsubishi Laboratories were accredited by the IOC, not to mention how the accreditation process actually worked. It would also be useful to know whether Mitsubishi executives, like a number of their South Korean counterparts, show up in any of the upper-echelon positions in international sport federations affiliated with the IOC. The point is that the SmithKline model from Atlanta is a deplorable precedent, and that the conflict of interest scenario was repeated in Japan without public objections from anyone.

One official who should have been informed about these unresolved test results was the Swedish physician Arne Ljungqvist, a member of the IOC since 1994 and a member of the IOC Medical Commission since 1987. In December 1996 Ljungqvist told an interviewer of his surprise and irritation upon learning about Catlin's doubts not from Prince de Merode but from a Swedish newspaper. He also reported that the laboratory results had eventually wound up, in accordance with IOC procedure, in the hands of de Merode, who in November 1996 admitted to discarding the urine samples because of "technical difficulties" with the much-heralded and expensive machines ordered by the IOC. This chain of custody was later confirmed by Steven Horning: "I give the results to Catlin, who then gives the material to Sample, and it finally winds up with de Merode."[78] This is an arrangement that virtually invites a suppression of information that has the potential to damage the commercial value of the Games and, in this special case, the image of a pharmaceutical company that could be linked in the public mind with the illicit use of drugs of which it is a major producer. In conformity with Horning's account, Catlin had told the *Sunday Times* that drug test results had been cleared by SmithKline officials before being passed on to the IOC. "Everyone understood that something wasn't quite correct in Atlanta," Ljungqvist commented. "So we want to know what really happened. I am a scientist and the head of a laboratory in Stockholm. And I have an ethical code that tells me if something is found, then it has to be reported."[79] These bold words seem to have had no effect on how drug testing is managed by the IOC. Indeed, the ethical atmosphere that seems to have prevailed in the Atlanta laboratory was conveyed in an interview Steven Horning gave just before the opening ceremony in Atlanta. Recounting a similar cover-up involving de Merode that had occurred after the 1984 Los Angeles Games, and that had provoked the suspicions of lab director Catlin, the German journalist Thomas Kistner asked Horning what he would do if he witnessed the suppression of positive tests. "I wouldn't say anything," Horning replied. "It's not my business to correct the IOC. I have to report what I find, and that's the end of it."[80]

One curious aspect of drug testing at Atlanta was the unmentioned contradiction between the official prognosis regarding the prospects of catching cheaters and the technohype spread by the press just before the Games on behalf of the vaunted high-resolution gas chromatography mass spectrometry machines that de Merode eventually decided not to trust.[81] "Drug testing is expected to be tight in Atlanta," Reuters news service said on July 11, 1996, "with the medallists to be tested, one other finalist, all national record breakers and randomly selected swimmers in the heats." "The machines are reportedly three times more sensitive than those used at the 1992 Barcelona Olympics and are said to be able to detect substances in the body months after they have been taken," United Press International said in another typical report (July 14, 1996). SmithKline, too, benefited from this sort of free advertising, as one United Press International sportswriter reported that "there was no lack of confidence in the firm's ability to conduct the testing at the Games" (July 15, 1996). Yet just before the opening of the Games, the chief medical officer, Dr. John Cantwell stated that he expected the 10,700 athletes in Atlanta to yield the miniscule total of 12 to 15 positive tests, or one-tenth of one percent.[82] In fact, this risible success rate was in line with IOC-sponsored testing over almost three decades, which included the "clean" 1980 Moscow Olympiad that produced no positives at all despite a host of East German champions whose steroid regimens have been documented to the milligram. From 1968 to 1992, IOC testing had produced only 51 positives.[83] (In 1995 the IOC reported 39,000 tests that resulted in 480 positives, 60 percent of these involving steroids.[84]) These modest ambitions for the $500,000 high-resolution gas chromatography mass spectrometry machines were seconded by Dr. Jordi Segura of the IOC Medical Commission: "The new technology has been known several months before the Games," he said. "It is very difficult to foresee what will happen but in principle we don't expect a high increase in the number of positives. . . . Our objective is to do something which prevents [*sic*] people from abuse."[85] By this account, the IOC was not out to catch the dopers so much as to dissuade them from inflicting upon themselves pharmacological harm.

SmithKline's role as a commercial producer of androgens added a new potential conflict of interest to an already complicated drug testing scenario. Before the Atlanta Games, SmithKline Beecham had donated a million dollars to the Center for Biomedical Ethics at Stanford University.[86] At the same time, by seeking and securing the assignment in Atlanta, SmithKline had virtually invented a new problem for biomedical ethics that pointed to the reciprocal and seldom-discussed relationship between androgen-consuming elite athletes and the now-swelling clinical population for which androgens can be prescribed.[87] This problem was already evident to Don Catlin: "It would be risky for any company to be associated in any way in the doping control process. The potential conflicts of interest are obvious. But it is even worse for a commercial drug manufacturer to be involved in drug testing. SB [SmithKline Beecham] make testosterone, a very effective anabolic agent. They also make testosterone patches, which administer the steroid through the skin." For SmithKline's Atlanta lab director, Barry Sample, this conflict of interest did not exist, even as he admitted that all test results were put in his hands on their way up to de Merode: "It is the physicians' responsibility for the prescribing of drugs, not the manufacturers."[88] In other words, the company's interest in the public relations aspects of its drug testing operation at a globally televised Olympiad were nil.

In fact, pharmaceutical companies have demonstrated a keen interest in the public relations aspects of androgens and other commercially valuable hormones that lead double lives as legitimate drugs in clinical medicine and as banned drugs in the sport world. For example, the author of this paper was present at a conference in 1986 when Dr. Ann Johanson, a pediatric endocrinologist and then director of medical affairs for the Genentech Corporation, assured us that the synthetic human growth hormone Genentech had just begun to produce for abnormally small children would never find its way onto the athletic black market.[89] In 1992 Genentech and Eli Lilly marketed $800,000,000 worth of human growth hormone, Genentech' s production having gone up 11 percent in one year. In 1993 the U.S. Government put human growth hormone on its list of restricted substances and made illegal possession of the drug punishable by a prison term of up to five years—an apparent refutation of the Genentech executive's claim that human growth hormone would not join the drug underground serving bodybuilders and athletes.[90] Eventually, the U.S. Government also had to issue an order restraining Genentech from canvassing American elementary schools in search of tiny customers able to pay $15,000 a year for the drug. In 1982 reports of serious side effects prompted Ciba-Geigy to stop production of the steroid it was marketing under the name Dianabol, thereby ensuring that it would not appear to be promoting doping.[91] In 1988 Searle took Anavar off the market on account of its "misuse in sport."[92] As of 1992 the German drug firm Schering AG was concerned about the public image of testosterone as a doping drug because it was investigating the potential for a testosterone-based male contraceptive.[93] In 1997 Schering executives were reading about their drug Primobolan 25 in a magazine article about doping in professional cycling.[94] In fact, even as SmithKline was gearing up for its highly publicized venture into the hormone-testing business in Atlanta, the company was expressing concern about the image of its Andropatch, a device for administering testosterone to hypogonadal males, that it had just put on the market. "So concerned is the company that thousands of men might seize on the patches as a general aphrodisiac, it has been careful to insist they be used only to treat a rare medical condition called hypogonadism, in which testosterone levels are low."[95] (The fact that SmithKline and other companies will want to test the market for testosterone as an aphrodisiac when attitudes change is another matter.) In conclusion, it is reasonable to assume that any drug company involved in the Atlanta operation would have had powerful motives to suppress steroid positives that might have tarnished the image of the Games. IOC approval of the SmithKline contract therefore demonstrated a lack of interest in the integrity of its own doping control operation. The subsequent Mitsubishi contract for the Nagano Games was only one more indication of the IOC's lack of commitment to establishing an independent, and therefore credible, drug testing system for Olympic sport.[96]

Purging the Record Lists: An Anti-Doping Strategy

Today incontrovertible proof of the systematic steroid doping of former East German Olympic champions and world record holders has opened up the possibility of stripping these doped athletes of their medals and records and reassigning them to the athletes who finished immediately behind them in the relevant competitions. Although proposals to reassign medals have come from the United States, England, and Australia, German sport officials (of varying credibility on the doping issue) have strenuously resisted these initiatives as discriminatory and unfair. "With this information we can rewrite records and send a loud message to our youngsters that you can break records without drugs," Mike Whittingham, a British coach and former athlete, said in September 1997.[97] This idea was endorsed by Dr. Werner Franke, the German molecular biologist and anti-doping expert. "It has been said that records could not be reset," he stated at seminar in London in September 1997, "because there wasn't any proof. Well, there is now."[98] But German Interior Minister Manfred Kanther angrily rejected this proposal as "absurd," claiming that Germany had dealt with its doping past in a "meticulous" manner and that German sport was now "manipulation free."[99] Even Helmut Digel, the reformist president of the German Track and Field Federation, who stands alone among German sport federation chiefs as a credible leader in the anti-doping campaign, described the foreign demands as hypocritical since doping had been a global problem for many years.[100]

However, the IOC was not interested in new information and never had been. Even as early as the doping-rhetoric offensive launched by Samaranch and de Merode at Calgary, the latter had pointedly rejected the idea of using information about doping to revise the results of tainted competitions when he stated that athletes who confessed to doping would not be penalized. "Some things belong to history," he said. "We are not going to apply sanctions from [*sic*] an event that happened four years ago. We'll never have retroactive sanctions."[101] When Samaranch was asked in December 1990 whether an Olympic champion who later confessed to doping would be disqualified, the IOC president deflected the question by saying: "Those are hypotheses. We proceed only on the basis of facts."[102] Seven years later, as those facts were arriving en masse, Samaranch declared they were irrelevant. When asked whether doped East German athletes would have to surrender their Olympic medals, Samaranch stated: "There are time limits, one cannot go back that far." IOC general-director Francois Carrard performed a diversionary maneuver by claiming that the IOC was already in the process of working out a procedure for handling such matters between Olympiads and that the IOC Executive Board would be discussing the British demands the next month in Nagano. Both German IOC members, Thomas Bach and Walther Tröger, declared that sport history simply could not be rewritten.[103]

These *ex cathedra* pronouncements about the immutability of history were matched by a similar level of concern at the IAAF. When asked in September 1997 about the possibility of changing doping-tainted world records, an IAAF spokesman replied: "We can only deal with athletes individually. The documents would mean nothing to us."[104] IAAF spokesman Georgio Reineri declared: "The rule is quite clear. After six years it is not possible to cancel any results. It is too late. At this stage there are no plans [to change the results]."[105] IAAF press officer Nick Davies referred to a six-year statute of limitations in the IAAF rules that would govern allegations of doping violations. IAAF Rule Book, Division III, Rule 55.8 reads as follows:

> An admission may be made either orally in a verifiable manner or in writing. For the purpose of these rules a statement is not to be regarded as an admission where it was made more than six years after the facts to which it relates. Therefore, any discussion about East German track and field athletes becomes redundant. The last GDR team competed at the World Championships in 1987—when [Thomas] Schönlebe set his [400-meter] mark 11 years ago.[106]

It is worth noting that the German Sports Federation has taken exactly the same position in the case of Kristin Otto, the swimmer whose six gold medals at the 1988 Seoul Games got her both an Olympic Order from Samaranch and notoriety as a doper. In October 1997 Otto was about to be inducted into the Society of German Olympians and receive a prize to boot. In addition, it appeared that rewriting the history of Otto's career was out of the question: "There is no question of taking away her victories, medals, or records. No one can do that since the general amnesty passed by the German Sports Federation in 1991."[107] Otto's candidacy for these honors provoked a storm of protest in Germany that eventually prompted her withdrawal from consideration for both German Sports Federation membership and the Sievert Prize.[108] The West German Swimming Federation released an open letter of protest, and the crusty old 110-meter hurdler Martin Lauer (fourth at Melbourne, fourth at Rome) said he would send his Sievert Prize medal back if it were given to Otto. Otto has hurt her own stature in Germany, where she works as a highly visible sportscaster, by talking circles around the doping issue. Some of her formulations are masterpieces of ambiguity and evasion, in which she always denies responsibility for ever having done anything wrong, even to the point where she has asserted the following: yes, there were pills and injections, but "I never got pimples, I never had menstrual disturbances, no depressions. I wonder why I never had any symptoms."[109] In January 1998 FINA's plan to honor Otto at the world championships in Perth was quietly dropped when officials realized that protests would ensue. The fact that FINA officials had even contemplated such a gesture to honor so compromised an athlete betrays the same unwillingness to take doping seriously that has been so evident in the IOC and in most of the international federations.

Such legalistic attempts to finesse the doping crisis by fiat were all that two of the most powerful international sport bureaucracies had to offer. The question, however, is whether the legalistic mentality shown here represents wisdom or irresponsibility. For as the 1972 Olympic marathon champion Frank Shorter pointed out: "Six years is an arbitrary statute of limitations. Also, since I maintain participation in international athletics is a privilege and not a right, it is always revocable and the federations should have total discretion in this regard. Laws have been changed in the past because of social need. 'The greatest good for the greatest number' is part of common law. Here we're talking about entities that essentially operate outside of the law. The whole point is that the users should know there is no statute of limitations."[110] Why should there be such fastidiousness about preserving the stature of compromised people whose behavior was now a matter of record?

Arbitrary statutes that are formulated and enforced by supranational entities that operate beyond any law other than their own are one of the pretensions to Vaticanlike status favored by Samaranch and other federation officials who develop delusions of ethical grandeur. Once they award the medals, discussion is forbidden. (In similar fashion, the canonization of a saint by a pope is irreversible. As Garry Wills recently noted "New information coming into the scholars' hands after the pope has spoken does not matter."[111]) But the IOC's unwillingness to rewrite history is more than grandiosity, since it also derives from a profound sense of insecurity about the history the IOC has made. For Samaranch and his colleagues, the prospect of revising medal and record lists means far more than the protracted investigations and contentious committee meetings such a reckoning with the past would have to entail. Such an investigation would probe that network of relationships between various IOC and federation officials that makes the whole Olympic enterprise possible, and this network has always operated on the premise that doping is a public relations issue that must be "controlled" primarily in the media.

So what can be done about doping-tainted world records such as Marita Koch's 47.60 seconds for 400 meters (1985)? Should it be permitted to stand, given that for some time her steroid dose was twice that of her male counterpart Thomas Schönlebe.[112] Helmut Digel has proposed to the IAAF a new interpretation of world records to commence with the advent of the new century: "I see a unique opportunity as of the year 2000 to speak of historical records relating to the past century, and to begin over again with the new century." As of January 1, 2000, Digel says, the IAAF should declare the best performances of the past two years to be world records. Better performances would earn cash prizes and recognition as new world records.[113] The historical record suggests that the most powerful IOC and federation bureaucrats will resist such reforms unless they are forced by public and media opinion to do otherwise. Restoring hope to young athletes who are demoralized by competing against steroid-assisted records is simply less important than preserving intact the egos and reputations of officials whose approach to the doping epidemic has been marked by passivity and/or complicity. As one experienced journalist put it: "It would be a miracle if Digel gets anywhere with his proposal."[114]

Doping, the IOC, and German Sportive Nationalism

Samaranch's Olympic diplomacy has always put political and commercial networking above the effective control of doping. In the case of Germany, this networking has created interests that Samaranch shares with politicians as well as sport bureaucrats. It is no accident, for example, that Interior Minister Kanther's outraged refusal to countenance any tampering with the medals and records of doped East German athletes happens to agree with the IOC's position on this issue. Nor is it by chance that it was the lone reformer Helmut Digel who challenged Kanther's remarkable claim that German sport is now free of drugs. "Cheating in high-performance sport," Digel said in January 1998, "is inherent in the system."[115] This sort of candor is anathema to the IOC and some important German politicians because they share an interest in managing public perceptions rather than the actual consumption of drugs by athletes. Whereas Samaranch is driven by his interest in preserving the IOC's brand-name entertainment monopoly, Manfred Kanther and other German politicians have been driven by the current German version of sportive nationalism—the familiar doctrine that elite athletes are a significant index of a nation's vitality.

Because the Interior Ministry is responsible for sport funding, cabinet members serving Chancellor Helmut Kohl in this capacity have also served as the most prominent federal spokesmen for the assertive sport policy favored by a majority of the Bundestag. In the case of the politician Wolfgang Schäuble, this mindset was evident long before he became interior minister. Back in 1977, when Schäuble was serving as a conservative representative in the Bundestag, he actually opposed the "Anti-Doping Charter" aimed at "every form of medical-pharmacological performance enhancement" then being proposed by the National Olympic Committee and the German Sports Federation. His rationale was openly nationalistic. "We advocate only the most limited use of these drugs," Schäuble stated, "and only under the complete control of the sport physicians because it is clear that there are [sports] disciplines in which the use of these drugs is necessary to remain competitive at the international level."[116] Fifteen years later, during Schäuble's term as interior minister, the federal government once again refused to ratify a European Anti-Doping Charter that called for a banning of all pharmacological, chemical, and mechanical forms of performance enhancement.[117] Given the prominent government support for highly publicized anti-doping initiatives such as the *Keine Macht den Drogen* ["No Power to Drugs"] and *Fair-Play geht vor* ["Fair Play Comes First"] campaigns, one might ask why the Interior Ministry would oppose ratifying a comprehensive anti-doping treaty. One explanation was provided by the sport journalist Thomas Kistner: "The striking degree of restraint in Bonn may well have to do with the fact that the Charter also prescribes procedures for dealing with those who provide doping substances. Signing the treaty would thus create a legal foundation for proceeding against physicians, coaches, and officials who practice doping. And with that, by the stroke of a pen, unified Germany—which is to say, the East German State Doping Plan—would acquire a host of problems."[118]

In 1989 Schäuble warned against both a "doping hysteria" that unfairly tainted elite sport and the use of doping as "manipulation." "The limits of human performance must be respected," the interior minister declared, even as he called simultaneously for a "new definition of the doping concept" that would not deny the athlete appropriate regenerative treatments.[119] In 1991 Schäuble demanded an end to the doping problem even as he was refusing to give up sportive nationalism as a federal priority: "I reject," he said, "the demands that the Federal Government should put an end to its promotion of elite sport on the grounds that the end of the East-West conflict means that sport has lost one of its basic functions—to express the competition between political systems." At the same time, he refused to endorse the idea that the federal government should put more emphasis on sport (read: fitness) for the masses (*Breitensport*), dismissing this egalitarian proposal behind the slogan that "mass sport and elite sport constitute a unity.[120] Five years later, Manfred von Richthofen, president of the German Sports Federation, was denouncing the federal government's refusal to promote sport (read: fitness) as a public health measure.[121]

Schäuble's successor in the Interior Ministry, Manfred Kanther, shared his predecessor's view that elite sport expresses national vitality. We have seen that this viewpoint also implies that there are necessary limits to the campaign against doping in sport, and here, too, Kanther has adhered to Schäuble's position. In May 1994 Kanther released a federal anti-doping report, surveying the period from 1989 to April 1994, that concluded that new laws aimed at doping were not necessary. Meanwhile, the indifference of conservative deputies in the Bundestag killed a Social Democratic proposal for a law punishing child-dopers.[122] In April 1997 Kanther was still opposing a change in the drug law that would have exposed doping coaches to legal penalties. He justified this position on the grounds that such a law would represent an unwarranted intrusion into the autonomous world of sport organizations that already had the doping problem under control.[123] To more skeptical observers, Kanther's refusal to support a sharpening of the drug law appeared consistent with Schäuble's position back in 1977, namely, that Germany had no obligation to practice unilateral disarmament in the area of performance-enhancing pharmacology. By the 1980s it was clear that the sheer political incorrectness of this position required a countervailing rhetoric of "clean" sport. In conformity with this political requirement, and like his predecessor, Kanther obscured the sportive-nationalist position with a series of anti-doping pledges combined with a robust discourse of nationalist self-assertion. "The successes of our athletes," he declared in September 1996, "demonstrate that the government's investment in elite sport is fully justified."[124] "Sports medals," he said in January 1997, "are a national priority. They are proof of a people's ability to compete."[125] In June 1997 Kanther and his political allies in the Bundestag opposed yet another Social Democrat–sponsored anti-doping law, and for the Social Democrat sport spokesman Eckhard Fischer the reason was clear: "The CDU [conservative party]," he said, "is scared to death that elite sport is going to crash."[126]

The sportive nationalism of important German politicians is a matter of record. Determining why they say what they say is the real challenge. It is possible, for example, that at least some politicians offer the public a feigned concern about German sporting prowess because they believe many voters are receptive to this sort of chauvinism. It is also possible that at least some of these statements are sincere, in that they express a real anxiety about the "fitness" of the body politic in an expansive sense that includes political functioning as well as public health. This elastic sense of national fitness makes possible the idea that success in elite sport is a kind of national security issue. Professor Klaus Heinemann, then chairman of the Scientific Council of the German Sports Association, stated in 1988 that "we must invest in sport because it facilitates the citizen's identification with the state."[127] More recently, several important political figures have maintained that the German state has an interest in the development of elite athletes. "[German] sport must remain internationally competitive," Chancellor Helmut Kohl declared in October 1995.[128] In May 1997 the German president, Roman Herzog, endorsed high-performance sport as a healthy influence against what he described as a sort of national malaise. "Pessimism," he lamented, "has become the prevailing mood among us," and he pointed to "a paralysis in our society." "Sport," he declared, "is dynamism. We are optimists."[129] The idea that German society had succumbed to a kind of mood disorder had appeared a year earlier in the remarks of Chancellor Kohl, as he received the German team that had just won the European soccer championship. German athletes who had rebounded from adversity, he said, set a good example at a time when "many of us at home call in sick on account of a little head cold."[130] Endorsements of elite athletic success at this political level can only encourage the tacit bureaucratic acceptance of doping that has long characterized the most ambitious sport establishments around the world.

See No Evil, Hear No Evil: The Passive Neutrality of the IOC

The IOC has frequently been ignorant of or indifferent to developments that any organization with a serious anti-doping plan would investigate and forcefully oppose. The booming export trade in former East German coaches with doping expertise is a case in point. West German hiring of such people began shortly after the Wall came down in November 1989 and proceeded to astonish many West German athletes and coaches.[131] In 1991, for example, 24 compromised coaches discussed in Brigitte Berendonk's path-breaking *Doping-Dokumente* (1991) were cleared and had their contracts extended by the German Track and Field Federation.[132] In the same year the West German swimming coach Georg Weinzierl initiated a campaign to oppose the hiring of former East German coaches who had admitted to doping their athletes.[133] This action did not prevent the German Swimming Federation from hiring, among others, people like Volker Frischke and Uwe Neumann, both of whom were convicted by German authorities of child-doping in East Germany.[134]

If the behavior of the (West) German National Olympic Committee and sport federations such as the German Track and Field Federation and the German Swimming Federation has been especially scandalous, this is due not to any special deficiencies of Germans but to the cultural and geographical proximity of an East

German talent pool that has been in demand around the world. The former head swimming coach Wolfgang Richter found work in Catalonia.[135] Austrian federations have hired Werner Trelenberg (track and field), Klaus Bonsack (tobogganing), Rolf Glaser (swimming), Hans Eckstein (rowing), Gunter Lux (cycling), Gerd Muller (cycling), Wolfgang Lange (kayaking), Rudiger Helm (kayaking), Hans Muller-Deck (judo), Bernd Kummer (biathlon), Wolfgang Kipf (volleyball), Helmuth Stechemesser (track and field), and Kurt Hinze (biathlon). Hinze lost a court case to an Olympic champion (Jens Steinigen) who had accused him of promoting doping.[136] Meinhard Nehmer (bobsledding) and Hartmut Buschbacher (rowing) work in the United States. Hans-Jürgen Tode and Alexander Schuck (both kayaking) are in Denmark. Hans Meyer (soccer) works in Holland. Eberhard Mund has been tending the French track and field team since 1991. Walter Jentzsch (toboggan), Erich Enders (bobsledding) and Theodor Körner (rowing) are in Italy. Gunter Mobius and Bernd Hahn (both bobsledding) are in Norway and Sweden, respectively. Wolfram Lindner, former coach of the East German national cycling team, has been the Swiss national coach since 1993. Others active in Switzerland are Dieter Hofmann (gymnastics), Hans-Joachim Grützner and Bernhard Riedel (both track and field), and Joachim Winterlich (ski jumping). Jochen Danneberg (ski jumping) is in South Korea, Karl Hagenberger (shooting) in Brunei, and Michael Regner, who spoke out in 1990 on doping in East German swimming, works in New Zealand. Australia has hired Heiko Salzwedel (cycling), Harald Jährling (rowing) and Bobo Andreas (boxing).[137]

Perhaps the most interesting case is that of Ekkart Arbeit, who served the East German sport establishment as head throwing coach (1982–1983) and head track and field coach (1989–1990). In late 1997 Athletics Australia hired Arbeit as chief administrator for Australian track and field with an eye to producing medals at the 2000 Sydney Olympic Games. Before the end of 1990 Arbeit had been hired by Colonel Gianni Gola, president of the Italian Track and Field Federation, to coach discus throwers.[138] As Dr. Werner Franke told an Australian journalist in October 1997, "He can't find a job in Germany so he has been to Italy and Greece. Wherever he goes there is a smell, and now the smell is in your country." "You can quote me that Arbeit was responsibly involved with giving steroids to minors," he added.[139] The Arbeit hiring created a national firestorm of controversy in Australia, but his appointment was not canceled until it was learned that he had served the East German secret police (Stasi) for 20 years as a spy.[140] The ideological cohesion of the international top-level coaching fraternity became evident when Frank Dick, the British president of the European Athletic Coaches Association, supported the hiring and stated: "Ekkart Arbeit enjoys the confidence and respect of all coaches and athletes with whom he has worked around the world."[141]

Nor does the IOC engage itself with the corruption that subverts doping control in major international federations. The political manipulation of IAAF doping control, for example, became particularly evident three years ago. On February 6, 1997, in Dortmund, Germany, the IAAF doping control agent Klaus Wengorborski was physically assaulted by a Greek coach, Christos Tzekos, after he had attempted to get urine samples from Greek athletes, including the eventual gold-medal winners Charalambros Papadias and Ekaterini Thanou. Wengoborski is supported by Staffan Sahlström, whose Swedish company has managed IAAF testing since 1992. The IAAF Anti-Doping Commission was supposed to deal with this case on February 28, 1997, at a meeting in Monaco. No decision ensued. The IAAF was then supposed to make a judgment on March 22 in Turin. It never happened because IAAF president Primo Nebiolo was determined not to cause the Greeks embarrassment before the Athens World Track and Field Championships commenced in August. Public relations took precedent over the integrity of the doping control apparatus over which the IAAF president is supposed to preside. It is worth noting that Papadias, the 1997 European men's champion over 60 meters, has made astonishingly quick progress, having cut 15 hundredths of a second off his time in an event (the 60 meter sprint) in which every hundredth constitutes an advance. Papadias claims to train a heroic eight hours a day, meaning that he is either an extraordinary talent or a doped athlete. [142]

The physical obstruction of Wengoborski in the line of duty is not the worst example of the evasive or violent behavior with which doping control officers must increasingly deal. Three weeks later, a doping control agent of the Russian National Olympic Committee, Yuri Vlovin, was assaulted on a Moscow street by assailants who beat him so badly that he lost an eye. Russian doping control is so underfunded that agents are no longer provided with cars and must use public transport, thereby exposing them to assault by criminals out to protect their investments in elite athletes. Such attacks on the doping control system reflect the increasing financial stakes involved in producing world-class athletes, a commercial escalation set in motion by Juan Antonio Samaranch when he assumed the IOC presidency in 1981.[143]

The IOC and the Doping Crisis of 1998

The IOC's relationship to doping control was changed dramatically by three events that occurred during the second half of 1998. The Tour de France doping scandal that erupted in July transformed the politics of doping by revealing that an entire athletic community—athletes, trainers, physicians, and officials—had been practicing and concealing comprehensive doping as a way of life. By demonstrating the unwillingness of a major Olympic sport to reform itself, the Tour scandal opened the door to state involvement in anti-doping activism to an unprecedented degree. In addition, the Tour debacle finally made it acceptable to say in public and without provocation what many journalists had known for a long time, namely, that long-distance cycling has been the most consistently drug-soaked sport of the twentieth century.

The Tour thus became a proving ground for a new and dramatic anti-doping strategy based on state prosecution of doping offenses in accordance with existing law, in this case the French anti-doping law of 1989.[144] Yet the unprecedented crackdown that decimated the 1998 Tour was a political as much as it was a legal

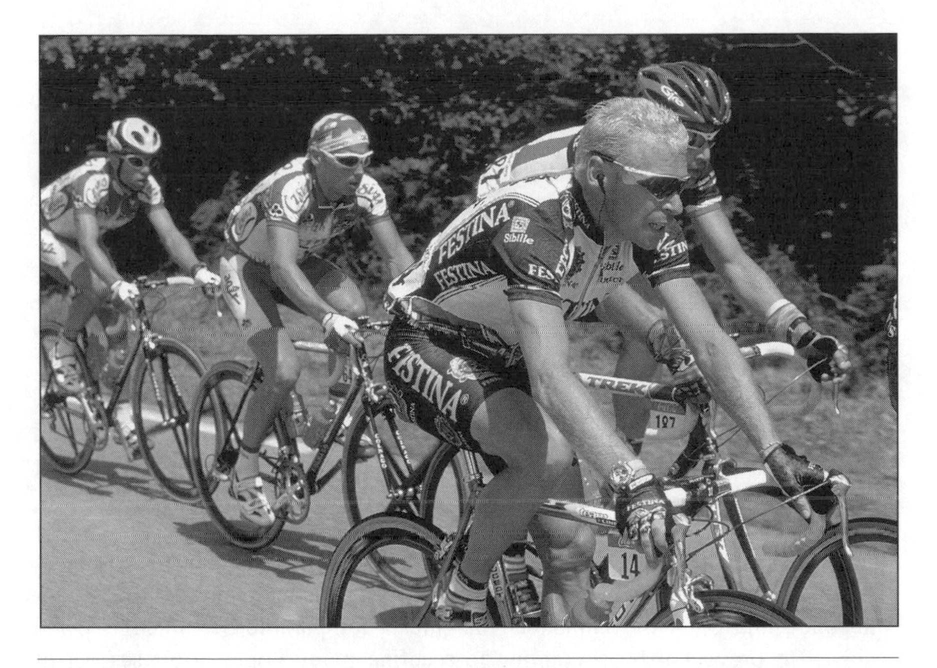

Festina team member Pascal Herve of France in the Stage 3 of the 1998 Tour de France. Tour officials later expelled Festina from the 1998 tour after riders and the team manager admitted the team regularly used performance-enhancing drugs.

event that had been waiting to happen. "For as long as the Tour has existed, since 1903, its participants have been doping themselves," one journalist noted. "No dope, no hope. The Tour, in fact, is only possible because—not despite the fact—there is doping. For 60 years this was allowed. For the past 30 years it has been officially prohibited. Yet the fact remains: great cyclists have doped themselves, then as now."[145] Indeed, the riders and their handlers were dumbfounded precisely because everyone involved, including the press, had been playing the game for so long in the interest of doing business as usual. What no one had expected was prosecutorial activism backed by politicians who meant business. It is not by chance that the Tour prosecutions had to wait for a Socialist prime minister (Lionel Jospin) who was willing to appoint a Communist minister of youth and sport (Marie-Georges Buffet). Similarly, it was a Social Democratic German interior minister, Otto Schily, who on February 2, 1999 told the IOC-sponsored World Conference on Doping in Sport that it was "not good for sport when we are dealing with a kind of constitutional monarchy."[146] For the record of the past two decades shows that left-of-center politicians have been more willing to prosecute doping offenses than their more conservative colleagues in Western European parliaments. Sportive nationalism appears to motivate right-wing politicians more than their left-wing counterparts in these societies.[147]

IOC president Samaranch opposed this threat to the IOC's authority by insisting that the sport world was still able to regulate itself. In his familiar fashion, Samaranch expressed confidence in the beleaguered federation in question by calling upon the UCI to take a "very hard and serious" approach to the anti-doping struggle.[148] The possibility that UCI inaction on doping had directly contributed to the scandal seemed lost on an IOC president who had always pursued a laissez-faire policy regarding the federations' management of doping. In contrast, Klaus Müller, chief of the anti-doping laboratory at Kreischa, pointed to International Cycling Union management of doping control, not as a solution, but as a root cause of the problems that had ruined the 1998 Tour.[149] Some sport officials were also rethinking the role of the state in doping enforcement. "Sport cannot possibly solve this problem by itself," said Walther Tröger, president of the German National Olympic Committee and a member of the IOC. "State agencies must also help."[150] The old order was dissolving, but it remained unclear what sort of new arrangement might replace it.

The second event that changed the political landscape was Samaranch's call for the responsible authorities to "drastically reduce" the number of banned substances in elite sport. Alarmed by the spectacle of Tour riders being hauled off to jail cells and police interrogations, Samaranch imagined a comparable Olympic fiasco and resolved to prevent it by attempting to redefine many doping offenses out of existence. In the July 26 edition of the Spanish newspaper *El Mundo,* Samaranch thus declared: "For me everything that does not injure the health of the athlete is not doping."[151] This apparent reversal of longstanding IOC anti-doping policy was harshly criticized by a wide range of sport officials, scientists, and physicians. Even his ally Thomas Bach distanced himself from this sort of "reform," insisting that the distinction between harmful and performance-enhancing substances was artificial and that the IOC was obligated to pursue doping in an aggressive fashion.[152] In retrospect, Samaranch's candid and heretical comments were a public relations faux pas that called into question his commitment to the campaign against doping. To repair his damaged reputation, Samaranch called for a world anti-doping conference under his leadership that would convene in early 1999, and by November the IOC had published the agenda of this hastily organized event. This strategy, however, did not restore his political stature just before the worst Olympic crisis of them all arrived to shatter his prestige and that of the entire IOC.

The Olympic bribery scandal that erupted in December 1998 weakened the authority of the IOC to the point where Samaranch eventually found it necessary to create both an IOC Reform Commission and an IOC Ethics Commission featuring celebrities such as Henry Kissinger, former United Nations secretary general Javier Perez de Cuellar, Peter Ueberroth, and the industrialist Gianni Agnelli, as well as several IOC members. A corollary effect of the bribery scandal was to push the doping issue out of the public eye before the convening of the anti-doping conference in Lausanne. And on the first day of the conference (February 2-4, 1999), it was the scandal that dominated the agenda. General Barry R. McCaffrey, the director of White House drug policy, set the tone: "Let me sadly but respectfully note," he said, "that recent examples of alleged corruption, lack of accountability, and failure of leadership have challenged the legitimacy of this institution," and several European sport ministers reiterated this challenge to the IOC's authority.[153] The eventual failure of the conference to achieve a strong, unified anti-doping strategy for world sport was a direct consequence of the IOC's diminished stature.

The inauguration of the World Anti-Doping Agency on January 13, 2000, resulted from the failure of the international sport organizations to achieve an effective antidoping system under IOC leadership. It remains to be seen whether this new organization, to be co-administered by the IOC and governmental representatives, will be able to win the confidence of honest athletes by establishing a credible global testing program. Yet even if this unprecedented initiative were to succeed, there are other looming threats to the ideal of drug-free Olympic sport. The concentrated protein powder known as creatine has already established itself around the world as a form of "soft doping" that has been accepted by the IOC. There is a burgeoning Internet market for so-called "prohormones," such as androstenedione, androstenediol, and norandrostenedione, that may well be performance enhancing. While androstenedione, the most popular of these drugs, has been banned by the IOC, American authorities have shown themselves to be either unwilling or unable to make it a controlled substance. The use of synthetic testosterone and human growth hormone is spreading beyond the small clinical populations for whom these drugs are medically indicated. In summary, the use of pharmacology to enhance human functioning will further complicate doping control in Olympic sport by making drugs accessible to athletes and by transforming what we call "doping" into socially acceptable forms of "therapy."

Notes

[1]"Zwischen Schönfarberei und Schwarzmalerei," *Süddeutsche Zeitung* [Munich] (July 26, 1991); "Beyer fordert Doping-Freigabe," *Süddeutsche Zeitung* (August 28, 1991).

[2]"Stärkster Mann der Welt unter starkem Doping verdacht," *Süddeutsche Zeitung* (March 18/19, 1995).

[3]"Peter, ein Verschwörer?" *Süddeutsche Zeitung* (May 4, 1995).

[4]"Keine Strafe reicht aus," *Süddeutsche Zeitung* (May 8, 1995).

[5]"Lücken im Netz der Fahnder," *Süddeutsche Zeitung* (August 22, 1997).

[6]"Angewidert von der Doppelbodigkeit der Anti doping-Politik," *Süddeutsche Zeitung* (October 2, 1996).

[7]On the political and ethical foundations of the IOC, see John Hoberman, "Toward a Theory of Olympic Internationalism," *Journal of Sport History* (Spring 1995):1–37; "The International Olympic Committee as a Supranational Elite." Presented at the 110th meeting of the American Historical Association, Atlanta, Georgia, January 6, 1996.

[8]"Samaranch blasts drugs and boycotts," *New York Times* (February 9, 1988).

[9]"Samaranch tough on drug abusers," *Houston Chronicle* (February 9, 1988).

[10]"IOC chief warns off drug-users," *The Times* [London] (February 10, 1988).

[11]"President of I.O.C. condemns drug use," *New York Times* (September 13, 1988); see also "Doping ist wie der Tod," *Süddeutsche Zeitung* (September 13, 1988).

[12]Associated Press, July 23, 1996. The IOC president went on in the following vein: "The principles that inspire the Olympic movement are based on justice, equality and tolerance. The International Olympic Committee spearheaded the anti-doping campaign on a worldwide scale. The battle is a difficult and complex one. Its outcome will depend not only on severe measures being taken against violations, but also on the educational and pedagogical campaigns launched at all levels to inform athletes and the general public about this despicable—and dangerous—form of cheating."

[13]Samaranch made this remark during an interview with the American sportswriter Frank Deford on "Real Sports with Bryant Gumbel," HBO Television, July 15, 1996. He soon learned that this sort of megalomania was not good public relations: "Juan Antonio Samaranch denied on Friday having said the Olympic movement was more important than the Roman Catholic Church, but said it still had more supporters than any major world religion" (Reuters, July 17, 1996).

[14]"IOC official wants blood sanctions," *Fort Worth Star-Telegram* (February 11, 1988).

[15]See Bjarne Rostaing and Robert Sullivan, "Triumphs tainted with blood," *Sports Illustrated* (January 21, 1985):12–17.

[16]"IOC medical chief criticizes blood doping," *Dallas Morning News* (February 11, 1988).

[17]See, especially, "Traum von Medaillenregen," *Der Spiegel* (November 17, 1997):206–208.

[18]"Das trube Bild der Dauerschäden," *Süddeutsche Zeitung* (March 18, 1998).

[19]United Press International, July 13, 1996. See also "IOC doping intrigue won't go away," *Chicago Tribune* (September 4, 1994).

[20]"Die Mühen mit der Manipulation," *Süddeutsche Zeitung* (September 20, 1991).

[21]"Zum Thema Doping sagt Samaranch nichts," *Süddeutsche Zeitung* (December 19, 1994).

[22]"IOC stützt Chinesen," *Süddeutsche Zeitung* (April 5, 1995).

[23]"We're too hard on drug cheats: Olympic boss," *The Weekend Australian* (December 21–22, 1996).

[24]"Horst Dassler, sport and industry," *Olympic Review* (1980):26–29. On Dassler's relationship with Samaranch, see Andrew Jennings *The New Lords of the Rings* (London: Pocket Books, 1996):43–46.

[25]"Nei til demokratisering," *Aftenposten* [Oslo] (February 6, 1998).

[26]"Samaranch rügt schärf," *Süddeutsche* (April 29, 1997).

[27]"IOC medical chief criticizes blood doping," *Dallas Morning News* (February 11, 1988).

[28]"Premiere in der Dopingbekämpfung," *Süddeutsche Zeitung* (December 10/11, 1994).

[29]COMTEX Newswire, December 5, 1997. See also "Blodtesting," *Nytt fra Norge* [Oslo] (February 10, 1998). In 1992 a Norwegian member of the international skiing federation medical commission (Lereim) stated that the available blood test had a reliability of 99.9 percent for exogenous blood and 50 percent for endogenous blood and erythropoietin. See "Keine Tests, keine Betrüger," *Süddeutsche Zeitung* (February 18, 1992).

[30]"Skal sette en stopper for bloddopingen," *Nytt fra Norge* [Oslo] (November 5, 1996); "Langrenn er en skitten bransje," *Aftenposten* (January 18, 1997). See also "Dicker Saft," *Süddeutsche Zeitung* (December 9, 1996); "Auf der Spuren in der Fingerkuppe," *Süddeutsche Zeitung* (December 18, 1996). At about this time a team of sport scientists, including prominent figures such as Manfred Donike and Arne Ljungqvist, published the results of research they had done on blood samples taken from 99 athletes participating in IAAF competitions during 1993–1994: "In conclusion, the analysis of blood samples taken during doping control indicates that blood doping or the misuse of recombinant erythropoietin or GH are not in widespread use by the athletes tested. However, the methods applied in this study may not be sensitive enough to disclose such misuse, and more sensitive and specific methods should be developed for future use." See K.I. Birkeland, et al., "Blood Sampling in Doping Control: First Experiences from Regular Testing in Athletics," *International Journal of Sports Medicine* 18 (1997):12.

[31]"IOC-Arzt skeptisch," *Süddeutsche Zeitung* (March 4, 1997).

[32]"Wer über 18,5 liegt, hat nachgeholfen," *Süddeutsche Zeitung* (December 18, 1996).

[33]"Wille und Ohnmacht," *Süddeutsche Zeitung* (December 9, 1992).

[34]"Wille und Ohnmacht," *Süddeutsche Zeitung* (December 9, 1992).

[35]"Debatte um neuen Dopingtest," *Süddeutsche Zeitung* (March 8, 1995).

[36]"EPO nicht nachweisbar," *Süddeutsche Zeitung* (February 2, 1994). See also "Zu dicke Nadeln für Vitaminspritzen," *Süddeutsche Zeitung* (February 11, 1994).

[37]"Wissenschaft der olympischen Windeier," *Süddeutsche Zeitung* (May 23, 1997).

[38]"Freiwillige im Feldversuch," *Süddeutsche Zeitung* (July 2, 1997).

[39]"IOC-Arzt skeptisch," *Süddeutsche Zeitung* (March 4, 1997).

[40]"Hoffnung dank neuer Tests," *Süddeutsche Zeitung* (April 25, 1997).

[41]"Ode an die Freude," *Süddeutsche Zeitung* (May 22, 1997).

[42]"Die Wissenschaft der olympischen Windeier," *Süddeutsche Zeitung* (May 23, 1997).

[43]"Der Doping-Betrug prospiert," *Süddeutsche Zeitung* (May 10, 1996).

[44]"Angewidert von der Doppelbodigkeit der Anti doping-Politik," *Süddeutsche Zeitung* (October 2, 1996).

[45]United Press International, July 14, 1996.

[46]"IOC stützt Chinesen," *Süddeutsche Zeitung* (April 5, 1995).

[47]"Probe 0708104 und andere 'Monster' der DDR: Doktor Höppner—Alchimist als Kronzeuge?" *Frankfurter Allgemeine Zeitung* (December 1, 1990).

[48]"Deutsches Problem," *Süddeutsche Zeitung* (December 11, 1990).

[49]"Rückgabe des IOC-Ordens," *Süddeutsche Zeitung* (March 19, 1990); "Ein Orden fur Daume," *Süddeutsche Zeitung* (May 14, 1993).

[50]"Kopf runter und durch," *Der Spiegel* (March 9, 1992):228; "Ewald trifft sich mit Samaranch," *Süddeutsche Zeitung* (November 12, 1991).

[51]"Rückgabe des IOC-Ordens," *Süddeutsche Zeitung* (March 19, 1990).

[52]"Doping als Übel aller Übel," *Süddeutsche Zeitung* (January 8, 1986).

[53]"Athleten beteuern empört ihre Unschuld: Daume will eine internationale Untersuchung," *Frankfurter Allegemeine Zeitung* (November 30, 1990).

[54]From John Hoberman, *Mortal Engines: The Science of Performance and the Dehumanization of Sport* (New York: Free Press, 1992):252.

[55]"Doping bedroht Sport," *Süddeutsche Zeitung* (December 29, 1988).

[56]"Interview der Woche: Thomas Bach (37), Mitglied im Internationalen Olympischen Komitee," *Süddeutsche Zeitung* (September 21/22, 1991).

[57]"Kein Rechtsanspruch auf einen Olympiastart," *Süddeutsche Zeitung* (March 25, 1992). On Keul's career, see John Hoberman, *Mortal Engines: The Science of Performance and the Dehumanization of Sport* (New York: Free Press, 1992): 245, 246, 252, 253, 259, 261.

[58]"Willige Sklaven," *Der Spiegel* (October 19, 1987):226.

[59]Quoted in Brigitte Berendonk, *Doping: Von der Forschung zum Betrug* (Reinbek bei Hamburg: Rowohlt, 1992):35.

[60]Thomas Kistner, "Die Stasi führt Olympia-Arzt Joseph Keul als Dopingbefürworter," *Süddeutsche Zeitung* (March 21, 1994):30.

[61]"Eine grosse Mafia," *Der Spiegel* (March 21, 1994):189, 192.

[62]Quoted in Thomas Kistner and Jens Weinreich, *Muskelspiele: Ein Abgesang auf Olympia* (Berlin: Rowohlt, 1996):194.

[63]"Es gibt kein Patentrezept," *Süddeutsche Zeitung* (December 4, 1990).

[64]"Ein Unverbesserlicher als Fehler im System," *Süddeutsche Zeitung* (December 1/2, 1990).

[65]"Dorfrichter Adams Schwester," *Süddeutsche Zeitung* (December 27/28, 1997).

[66]"Breakthrough in drug testing revealed," *Houston Chronicle* (January 22, 1998).

[67]"Professorn bakom det italienska undret," *Svenska Dagbladet* [Stockholm] (March 11, 1985).

[68]"Da müssen Sie schon Hem Conconi fragen," *Süddeutsche Zeitung* (February 22, 1988).

[69]"Der Unaussprechliche am Pranger," *Süddeusche Zeitung* (December 2, 1993).

[70]"Zu dicke Nadeln für Vitaminspritzen," *Süddeutsche Zeitung* (February 11, 1994).

[71]"Die Akte Telekom," *Der Spiegel* (April 18, 1994):224.

[72]"Von der Flüsterparole zur Gewissheit," *Süddeutsche Zeitung* (January 23, 1997); "Auch Pescante im Visier," *Süddeutsche Zeitung* (October 30, 1998); "IOC's Pescante may lose Turin seat," Associated Press (February 5, 2000); "Versteckspiel mit Cici 1 und Cici 3," *Süddeutsche Zeitung* (December 28, 1999).

[73]This information came from the following Web site postings: "SmithKline Beecham to Sponsor 1994 Goodwill Games" (August 25, 1993) (see *Team*

Marketing Report's Sports Sponsor Fact Book [Chicago: Team Marketing Report, 1994]: 206) and "SmithKline Beecham Sets the Pace With Dennis Vitolo" ("Project Indy Team returns to CART: 'Smithkline Beecham sets the pace' in Indy car racing," **http://www.speedcenter.com/news97/sc_n0102_97.html**.

[74]"Profits of SmithKline's clinical laboratories fell 5 percent. The business is under investigation over accusations of fraudulent billing of Government test programs for blood tests on kidney patients." See "Aided by newer products, 3 drug makers post higher profits," *New York Times* (July 24, 1996).

[75]"Drug-testing lab sought," *Atlanta Journal-Constitution* (July 16, 1996).

[76]Steven Downes, "Revealed: Four more Olympic drug users," *Sunday Times* [London] (November 19, 1996).

[77]This information was posted on a Web site ("Corporate Profile") by the Mitsubishi-Kagaku Foods Corporation (January 1998). Visit **http://www.mfc.co.jp/index.htm** for the English language home page.

[78]"Das Erbe von Atlanta: Vier vertuschte Dopingfälle," *Süddeutsche Zeitung* (November 19, 1996).

[79]"In Atlanta war etwas nicht ganz korrekt," *Süddeutsche Zeitung* (December 17, 1996).

[80]"Ein Anabolika-Produzent jagt die Doping-Sünder," *Süddeutsche Zeitung* (July 18, 1996).

[81]My account is confirmed by Philip Hersh, "Drug tests rate incomplete," *Chicago Tribune* (October 24, 1996).

[82]"Drug lab passes test for Atlanta drug tests," *New York Times* (July 6, 1996).

[83]Associated Press, July 23, 1996.

[84]Reuters, July 16, 1996.

[85]Reuters, July 16, 1996.

[86]"Angst vor Wildwuchs," *Der Spiegel* (June 17, 1996):175.

[87]See, for example, John M. Hoberman and Charles E. Yesalis, "The history of synthetic testosterone," *Scientific American* (February 1995):60–65; John Hoberman, "Listening to steroids," *The Wilson Quarterly* (Winter 1995):35–44.

[88]Steven Downes, "Revealed: Four more Olympic drug users," *Sunday Times* [London] (November 19, 1996).

[89]"Ethical Issues in the Treatment of Children and Athletes with Human Growth Hormone," University of Texas, Austin, Texas, April 26, 1986. This conference was organized by Dr. Terry Todd of the University of Texas at Austin, and among the participants was Dr. Don Catlin.

[90]"Turbolader für den Muskeln," *Der Spiegel* (March 15, 1993):258.

[91]"Plötzlich wahnsinnig aggressiv," Der *Spiegel* (May 25, 1992):197; "Jeden Dreck, jeden Blödsinn reingehauen," *Der Spiegel* (September 14, 1992):286.

[92]Brigitte Berendonk, *Doping: Von der Forschung zum Betrug* (Reinbek bei Hamburg: Rowohlt, 1992):49.

[93]"Jeden Dreck, jeden Blödsinn reingehauen," *Der Spiegel* (September 14, 1992):286.

[94]"Wie ein Hund an der Kette," *Der Spiegel* (June 16, 1997):122.

[95]"Gym and Tonic," *Sunday Times* [London] (November 10, 1996).

[96]A proposal for such a politically independent body was made on November 16, 1996, at the 10th assembly of the Association of National Olympic Committees in Cancun, Mexico, by Mario Pescante, an IOC member and president of the Italian Olympic Committee. In rejecting a study by de Merode's Medical Commission on anti-doping rules and procedures, Pescante stated: "We think that a world scientific organization should study these things, rather than have a commission president's report settle everything." UPI Sports, November 17, 1996.

[97]Reuters Information Service, September 17, 1997.

[98]Agence France-Presse, September 17, 1997.

[99]AP Sports, January 9, 1998. For a critical commentary on Kanther's position see Thomas Kistner, "Kanther schafft das Doping ab," *Süddeutsche Zeitung* (January 13, 1998).

[100]"Zuviel Aufwand an Moral und Ethik?" *Süddeutsche Zeitung* (January 27, 1998).

[101]"IOC medical chief criticizes blood doping," *Dallas Morning News* (February 11, 1998).

[102]"Kommerzialisierung in richtige Bahnen lenken," *Süddeutsche Zeitung* (December 21, 1990).

[103]"IOC: Rüickgabe unmöglich," *Süddeutsche Zeitung* (January 14, 1998).

[104]Agence France-Presse, September 17, 1997.

[105]Reuters, January *5,* 1998.

[106]Jim Ferstle, "East German drug revelations mount; other athletes begin to ask that sports history be rewritten" [**http://www.runnersworld.com/dailynew/archives/1998/January/980106.html**] (January 6, 1998).

[107]"Dokumente gegen das Harmonie Bedürfnis," *Süddeutsche Zeitung* (October 18/19, 1997).

[108]"Verzicht auf Posten und Preise," *Süddeutsche Zeitung* (October 21, 1997).

[109]"Der Fall Otto wird zur Nagelprobe," *Süddeutsche Zeitung* (October 17, 1997); "Kristin Ottos Beteuerungen," *Süddeutsche Zeitung* (October 20, 1997).

[110]Jim Ferstle, "East German drug revelations mount; other athletes begin to ask that sports history be rewritten": **http://www.runnersworld.com/dailynew/archives/1998/January/980106.html**] (January 6, 1998).

[111]Garry Wills, "The Vatican Monarchy," *The New York Review of Books* (February 19, 1998):25.

[112]For discussion and documentation of Koch's doping regimen, see Brigitte Berendonk, *Doping: Von der Forschung zum Betrug* (Reinbek bei Hamburg: Rowohlt, 1992):65, 151, 173.

[113]"Das Digel-Konzept," *Süddeutsche Zeitung* (January 26, 1998).

[114]Robert Hartmann, "Zuviel Aufwand an Moral und Ethik," *Süddeutsche Zeitung* (January 27, 1998).

[115]"Das Digel-Konzept," *Süddeutsche Zeitung* (January 26, 1998).

[116]Quoted in Brigitte Berendonk, *Doping: Von der Forschung Betrug* (Reinbek bei Hamburg: Rowohlt, 1992):45.

[117]"Rufschädigende Ärzte," *Süddeutsche Zeitung* (September 16, 1992).
[118]"Thomas Kistner, "Eine unliebsame Charta," *Süddeutsche Zeitung* (September 17, 1992).
[119]"Minister Schäuble warnt vor einer 'Doping-Hysterie'," *Süddeutsche Zeitung* (October 21, 1989).
[120]"Schäuble mahnt Konsequenzen an," *Süddeutsche Zeitung* (October 23, 1991).
[121]"Verärgert und enttäuscht," *Süddeutsche Zeitung* (November 27, 1996).
[122]"Gesetz nicht nötig," *Süddeutsche Zeitung* (May 14/15, 1994); "SPD-Plan gescheitert," *Süddeutsche Zeitung* (May 20, 1994).
[123]"Vertraute Vorstösse ins Vakuum," *Süddeutsche Zeitung* (April 18, 1997).
[124]"217 für den Sport," *Süddeutsche Zeitung* (September 12, 1996).
[125]"Nationales Anliegen," *Süddeutsche Zeitung* (January 7, 1997).
[126]"Blockade-Politik in Bonn," *Süddeutsche* Zeitung (June 13, 1997).
[127]"Industrie lässt sich nicht von Effekten leiten," *Süddeutsche Zeitung* (October 11, 1988).
[128]"Die Sporthilfe holt sich Hilfe beim Kanzler," *Süddeutsche Zeitung* (October 27, 1995).
[129]"Langfristige Bindung gesucht," *Süddeutsche Zeitung* (May 27, 1997).
[130]"Experten für schwierige Lebenslagen," *Süddeutsche Zeitung* (July 2, 1996).
[131]See, for example, John Hoberman, *Mortal Engines: The Science of Performance and the Dehumanization of Sport* (New York: Free Press, 1992):247–248.
[132]"Vieldeutiger Rückzug," *Süddeutsche Zeitung* (November 29, 1991).
[133]"Streit der Trainer," *Suddeutsche Zeitung* (December 9, 1991).
[134]"See "Pioniere des Vertuschens," *Der Spiegel* (April 24, 1994):236–238; "Das ist gut für die Zähne," *Der Spiegel* (August 18, 1997):126–128; "Mach' Schluss, das Thema ist durch," *Süddeutsche Zeitung* (August 23/24, 1997); "Mit Handschellen gedroht," *Süddeutsche Zeitung* (October 28, 1998).
[135]"Streit der Trainer," *Süddeutsche Zeitung* (December 9, 1991).
[136]"Wehmutige Gedanken an die Allerbesten," *Süddeutsche Zeitung* (March 23, 1992); "Kurt Hinze verliert," *Süddeutsche Zeitung* (May 30/31, 1992).
[137]"Traum von Medaillenregen," *Der Spiegel* (November 17, 1997).
[138]"Italien verpflichtet DDR-Trainer," *Süddeutsche Zeitung* (August 28, 1990).
[139]"We have hired a 'major rascal,'" *The Australian* (October 4, 1997).
[140]"Unmasked: Files reveal coach was a communist spy," *The Daily Telegraph* [Sydney] (November 19, 1997).
[141]Reuters Information Service, October 12, 1997.
[142]"Ein fatales Missverständnis," *Süddeutsche Zeitung* (February 20, 1997); "Was den Griechen schnelle Beine macht," *Süddeutsche Zeitung* (March 10, 1997).
[143]"Dopingkontrolleur verprügelt," *Süddeutsche Zeitung* (February 1/2, 1997); "Der geklonte Athlet—das Modell für die Zukunft," *Süddeutsche Zeitung* (March 5, 1997).
[144]French anti-doping legislation had been passed as early as 1964 and 1966. "A law prohibiting the use of stimulant drugs by competitors has been recently approved by the French cabinet. Fines and imprisonment for offending sportsmen,

trainers, and handlers may be imposed if use of drugs can be proved. Blood, urine, and sweat tests are permissible in order to detect the illegal drug usage." See "France bans use of drugs in sports," *Journal of the American Medical Association* 189 (September 21, 1964):977.

"The use of stimulants at athletic competitions (called in French slang, doping) was recently put under repressive legislations. Penalties are severe: the athlete must pay a fine of 500 to 5000 francs, and the directors and managers must face, beside the fine, a prison penalty of a month to a year." See "French law on doping," *Journal of the American Medical Association* 197 (July 25, 1966):306.

[145]Hans Halter, "Alles verstehen, alles verzeihen," *Der Spiegel* (August 3, 1998):97.

[146]"Europas Sportminister setzen IOC unter Druck," *Süddeutsche Zeitung* (February 3, 1998).

[147]On the relationship between political affiliation and doping policy in Germany see John Hoberman, Mortal Engines: *The Science of Performance and the Dehumanization of Sport* (New York: Free Press, 1992):237–246; "Fitness and national vitality: a comparative study of Germany and the United States," in Karin A.E. Volkwein, ed., *Fitness as Cultural Phenomenon* (Münster: Waxmann, 1998):231–247.

[148]"Die Scheinheiligkeit der Sport-Funktionäre," *Süddeutsche Zeitung (July* 25/26, 1998).

[149]"Klaus Müller: Dopingkontrolleur und Laborchef in Kreischa," *Süddeutsche Zeitung* (July 25/26, 1998).

[150]"Olympischer Radsport gefährdet," *Süddeutsche Zeitung* (July 25/26, 1998).

[151]"Kürzung der Dopingliste," *Süddeutsche Zeitung* (July 27, 1998).

[152]"Der Vorschlag ist ein Schlag ins Gesicht," *Süddeutsche Zeitung* (July 28, 1998).

[153]"I.O.C. credibility questioned as drug meeting starts," *New York Times* (February 3, 1999).

11

CHAPTER

World Conference on Doping in Sport

Jim Ferstle
Freelance writer
Lausanne, Switzerland

When International Olympic Committee (IOC) president Juan Antonio Samaranch called for the World Conference on Doping in Sport, many had hopes that it would be a historic conference, a milestone in the battle to contain the use of performance-enhancing drugs. It was certainly historic, but perhaps for reasons other than those anticipated.

Samaranch convened the conference in response to an extraordinary sequence of doping scandals during 1998, which reached a climax in July during the Tour de France. In January of that year, Australian customs agents caught a Chinese swimmer with vials of human growth hormone in her luggage before the International Swimming Federation's world championships. In Germany, prosecutors using information recovered from the secret police files of the former German Democratic Republic, continued their pursuit of East German coaches and doctors who had given anabolic steroids and other drugs to young female swimmers. The first of these trials began in March and brought into the open the secrets of the East German state-sponsored sports doping program. The following month, Irish three-time Olympic gold medal winner Michelle de Bruin was charged with deliberately tampering with her urine sample during an out-of-competition drug test. Meanwhile, the case of American middle distance runner, Mary Decker Slaney, whose drug test at the 1996 U.S. Olympic track and field trials indicated abnormal levels of testosterone, remained mired in arbitration with the International Amateur Athletic Federation (IAAF). Two more U.S. cases—those of sprinter Dennis Mitchell and shot-putter Randy Barnes—brought further scrutiny of the tests used by the IOC for detection of testosterone use by Olympic athletes.

This seemingly unending stream of doping stories was topped by revelations of doping by cyclists, uncovered by French customs agents and police, during the Tour de France. Although rumors of the use of erythropoietin and human growth hormone by cyclists had circulated for years, the Tour scandal exposed the fact that doping was widespread and systematic among elite cycling teams. The scandal threatened to destroy the Tour and erode sponsor support for other Olympic sports as well. In its midst, IOC president Samaranch added fuel to the simmering crisis by commenting that the IOC list of banned performance-enhancing substances was too large, and that perhaps only drugs detrimental to an athlete's health should be on the prohibited list. For many, this was interpreted as a retreat in the IOC's self-declared war on drugs. Publicly, Samaranch was harshly criticized for his remarks, while privately many sports administrators admitted that the statement was, at least in part, an accurate reflection of the many problems with drug testing.

Difficulties in Drug Testing

Many substances on the banned list are commonly found in popular medications and are the subject of intense debate within the drug testing community. An example is ephedrine, a stimulant found in over-the-counter cold remedies. Sports federations have struggled for years to craft rules to distinguish those attempting to cheat by using the drug from those who innocently have been treated for an illness by an uninformed physician or team trainer. Cases involving testosterone and other endogenous hormones also clearly illustrate the difficulty of establishing definitive evidence of cheating. The lack of research funding and potential legal challenges with the testosterone test have hindered the development of tests for the illegal use of erythropoietin and human growth hormone. Thus when the Tour scandal broke, the most damning charge leveled against the sporting federations was that they could not enforce their rules because they did not have tests to detect the use of substances on their banned lists. "What do sanctions do against undetectable drugs? They are 90 percent of estimated doping cases." Hein Verbruggen, head of the Union Cycliste Internationale (UCI), the international federation for cycling, said during the IOC doping conference.

World Conference on Doping in Sports Convenes

The ineffectiveness of the drug tests used by the IOC and sports federations led to the French government, not the UCI, exposing the doping practices among cyclists in the Tour. The IOC and the sports federations under its umbrella were faced with the public relations problem of having to explain why a government appeared to be more effective in rooting out drug use. Confronting these issues, IOC president Samaranch called for a World Conference on Doping in Sport to meet in Lausanne, Switzerland from February 2 through 4, 1999. Four working groups were set up to

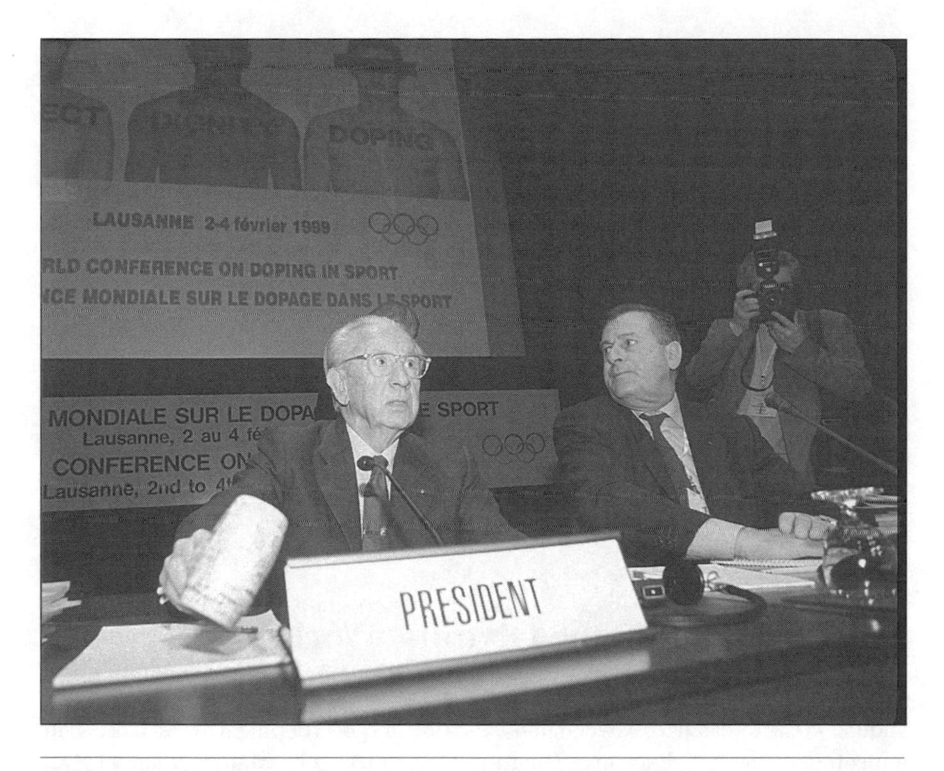

IOC President Juan Antonio Samaranch opening the 1999 World Conference on Drugs in Sport at Lausanne, Switzerland.

examine the issues and propose solutions. One obvious need was funding, and long before the conference opened, the working group on sources of funding chaired by IOC vice president Richard Pound, of Canada, proposed that a portion of the IOC's television revenues be earmarked for a new anti-doping agency. Recognizing that the IOC alone could not solve the problem, the committee invited government representatives to the conference and asked them to become "part of the solution." The sports federations of the "Olympic family" were urged to adopt uniform rules, and there was talk that those who did not conform to a strict anti-doping charter would be expelled from the Olympic movement.

As the working groups met and formulated their reports, word began circulating that the IOC would commit $25 million to create a new, "independent" anti-doping agency. With the IOC funding, the agency would be charged with developing an effective out-of-competition testing program for all sports and would sponsor research into new tests needed to combat the use of currently undetectable substances, such as human growth hormone and erythropoietin. The hope was that governments and sports federations would join in this effort, increasing the funds available and "harmonizing" the efforts of a universal anti-doping movement in sports. Pound's working group proposed that Samaranch and IOC medical commission chairman, Prince Alexandre de Merode, of Belgium, be the leaders of the new agency, which would include others from national governments, sports federations, sponsors, and the pharmaceutical industry. There was much debate within the working groups on these issues, which included questions as to whether an agency chaired by either Samaranch or de Merode could be viewed as truly independent, and over the necessity of having sponsors or drug company representatives as part of the agency.

Anita DeFrantz, of the United States, an IOC vice president who chaired the working group on the protection of athletes, said her group preferred to call the agency "international" rather than independent. She argued that the IOC should retain an important role in the agency because the IOC would provide the primary funding. "Cynics will say it's not independent, but someone has to fund it," DeFrantz noted. She suggested that the agency could be structured similarly to the Swiss-based Court of Arbitration for Sport, with a board of directors "independent of the Olympic movement."

More Scandals in the Olympic World

Before these issues could be addressed at the February conference, however, another crisis threatened to overshadow the one in sports doping. During a break in a meeting of the IOC Executive Board in December 1998, Marc Hodler, an IOC executive board member from Switzerland, ignited the scandal by revealing his concerns about corruption within the bid process selecting host cities for the Olympic Games. Hodler's comments, coming in response to documented evidence of illegal inducements given to IOC members by the Salt Lake City Olympic bid committee, touched off a media frenzy that consumed the Olympic movement. As evidence mounted in what was termed the "Olympic bribery scandal," sponsors of the Olympic movement joined others in calling for immediate reform of the IOC and its Olympic bid process. In response to this second crisis, Samaranch called another special session of the IOC for March 1999 to address reform of the IOC bidding procedures. This turmoil threatened to overshadow the doping conference.

The revelations from Salt Lake City prompted investigations by the United States Department of Justice and the United States Olympic Committee (USOC). So, while attempting to prepare for the doping conference, IOC executive committee members also were engaged with what came to be characterized in the media as a struggle for survival. Some parties felt that the doping conference should be postponed until after the IOC had resolved the issues prompted by the bribery scandal. Others called for Samaranch to resign, questioned the credibility of the IOC, and argued that the organization was in need of a drastic overhaul. On the eve of the conference, U.S. "drug czar," retired general Barry McCaffrey, said that the IOC needed to restructure and become more "democratic." He called for the IOC to open its books, be more "transparent," and hold open elections for IOC posts.

"The IOC must operate as a democratic and accountable public institution. Its procedures must be based on open books and records, open and recorded votes on issues, and an elected membership that is accountable to the athletes and the community of nations," McCaffrey said in his address at the conference. "Lack of accountability and the failure of leadership have challenged the legitimacy of this institution."

A barrage of critical press preceded the conference as journalists from around the world portrayed the IOC as an out-of-touch, corrupt empire unworthy of promoting Olympic ideals. Andrew Jennings, the British journalist who had written about Olympic bribery and improprieties in his 1992 book, *The Lords of the Rings*, became a celebrity of sorts. In a sequel titled *The New Lords of the Rings*, published in 1996, Jennings wrote: "The health of the Olympics could dramatically improve if journalists asked more questions and fans and athletes spoke up for sport not clouded by doping scandals and the sell-out to sponsors. . . . If (the Olympics) are to survive as a great international multi-sports festival based on fair play and decency, the cartel behind them needs exposing to a summer of bright sunlight, shining into every corner of the organization."

Jennings was among the more than 500 accredited journalists who came to Lausanne for the World Conference on Doping in Sport, and like most of them, he was there not to cover the doping issue, but to question the IOC about the bribery scandal and its fallout. Because of the bribery scandal, the conference drew nearly as many members of the media as delegates. To journalists and other outside observers, the atmosphere clearly was one of a kingdom under siege. It was perhaps fitting that, a short distance from the Lausanne Palace Hotel where Samaranch resides, a plaque on the wall of the downtown post office commemorates the site where historian Edward Gibbon lived while writing his historical masterpiece, *The Rise and Fall of the Roman Empire*. To many outside observers, it seemed as if the Olympic empire were crumbling under the weight of the doping crisis and the bribery scandal.

Despite the bribery scandal, however, the importance of the doping crisis was not lost on members of the IOC executive board. "The doping issue is more important in the great scheme of things than the behavior of a few of our members," said Pound, who headed the IOC corruption inquiry. DeFrantz claimed the timing of the doping conference was ideal. "I think this is exactly the right time to do this," she said. "This is the most important issue. What better time to seriously address it? We have the opportunity to do something. The athletes want a system that works. The athletes are tired of being whispered about. They are tired of the finger pointing. Enough."

Nonetheless, the main topic on the first day of the conference was the tattered credibility and stature of the IOC. European Union representatives, including British sports minister Tony Banks, as well as McCaffrey, all called for "institutional reform" of the IOC. McCaffrey said he didn't want his remarks to overshadow the terrible problem of doping in sport, but that IOC reform was the first order of business. He repeated his call for greater democracy and transparency. Without institutional reform, McCaffrey added, the IOC might lack the "moral authority" necessary to find solutions to the current sports drug crisis. Or, as Banks put it, "The system that exists does not have the confidence of our athletes. They want to know that they are competing on even terms."

Speakers Call for Changes

Most speakers called for an external, independent, and transparent body to take over doping control and education. McCaffrey repeated his pledge of $1 million as a "down payment" toward the establishment of such a body. (Dr. David Cowan, head of the IOC-accredited drug testing laboratory in London, said that any effort to do the necessary research and development for a workable doping control system would take much more than that. Cowan said that pledges of $10 million each from the United States, large European states, and others in the Olympic family would be more encouraging and a stronger signal of the seriousness of the issue.) Indeed, financial and legal issues were cited as major obstacles in setting up an independent agency.

Contained within the reports of the four IOC working groups were some other potential problems. The IOC's new proposed definition of doping, for example, raised legal issues by proclaiming doping as something "potentially harmful and performance-enhancing." This definition could force the IOC to prove that banned substances are both performance-enhancing and harmful. IOC Medical Commission Chairman Prince Alexandre de Merode attempted to address this issue by stating, categorically, that all the substances on the IOC banned list were "harmful."

Other speakers suggested that this new definition might be used to pare the current list, eliminating "benign" drugs. This might simplify potential legal problems resulting from suspensions based on the current list. De Merode argued that unenforceable sanctions were harmful to the Olympic anti-doping movement. Several speakers claimed that more scientific research was needed to combat the problem of undetectable drugs. McCaffrey said rapid technological advances made it all the more urgent to undertake such research in order to obtain results in time for the Sydney Olympics.

McCaffrey also expressed hopes that the doping agency could be in created in time for the Sydney and Salt Lake City Games, so that athletes of the new millennium would be competing in "the cleanest Games" in Olympic history. In many ways the conference debates exposed the clash of cultures at work. Government agencies, accustomed to the give-and-take of the democratic process, came to Lausanne believing they were at least equal partners in the deliberations. The IOC, buffeted by the current scandal and accustomed to operating in private, could not impose any "moral authority," as its own credibility was under scrutiny. "You can't invite government ministers to a conference and expect them to applaud politely," said Banks. The IOC had gotten its first taste of democracy, said the USOC's Dick Schultz, and it did not like it.

Among the most hotly debated of the reports was the sources-of-funding working group's recommendations for the specifics of the independent agency, dubbed World Anti-Doping Agency (WADA) by the media. The working group proposed that the agency be incorporated as a foundation under Swiss law, have its headquarters in Lausanne, and be "governed by a council headed by the IOC president." The council would consist of "three representatives each of the IOC, the international federations, the national Olympic committees, athletes designated by the IOC athletes commission, international governmental organizations, and three other persons representing sponsors, the pharmaceutical industry and the sporting goods industry."

After pointed criticism of the proposed WADA structure, Pound announced that the IOC would redraft its proposal. The announcement marked an abrupt shift in what amounted to a two-day power struggle for control over the proposed anti-doping agency. Pound said he thought the IOC plan delivered sufficient independence, and de Merode took a jab at the IOC's most vocal critics, the various government representatives, by saying, "Perhaps they do not trust us, but I ask you: Who will trust the politicians?"

Hodler said he thought the proposals for an agency independent of IOC involvement had merit "because that means the IOC will save $35 million. We won't have to pay the bill." IAAF head and IOC member Primo Nebiolo said the anti-doping agency should be free of real and perceived IOC influence. At one point, DeFrantz said she felt the IOC "had the confidence of the most important group, the athletes." Canadian representative and Olympic kayaker Renn Crichlow, however, presented a contradictory assessment. He contended that many athletes did not have the confidence in the IOC to run the new anti-doping agency, claiming, "The cynicism, the skepticism and the mistrust will go on, and it will propagate and turn into contempt, and without our support, this newly found organization is doomed from the start. In Canada and indeed throughout the world, there is a high degree of cynicism, a high degree of skepticism and a high degree of mistrust in the IOC as an organization." Even Pound acknowledged the necessity of having athletes believe in the integrity of the new anti-doping agency. "What you really have to do is win the confidence of athletes that the program you give them provides reasonable assurance that if they're in a race and not doped, no one else will be either," Pound said. "Ask athletes, 'If nobody else doped, would you?' and the answer is 'No.' There are a few who do it to get an edge. All the rest do it because it's the lowest common-denominator death spiral."

This analysis was backed by comments from a number of athletes. "To gain the trust of the athletes again I think it's important to be independent, to trust this agency to be secure," said Olympic speed skating champion Johann Olav Koss. "As an athlete you're always a bit frightened to go into a doping test. You're always afraid that those people behind the scenes there will tamper with your test. You've got to think that can always happen. There's been rumors about recent Olympics and their doping controls. You don't know if it's correctly done or not." Charmaine Crooks, a retired Canadian track athlete who serves on the athlete's commission, said that with the IOC in turmoil, it was the right time for the athletes to demand more rights. "It's an environment that's really, really receptive to our agendas. The message is there's still doping in sport and we have to put pressure on the appropriate people to make changes. . . . There's new initiatives . . . but obviously we have to move further and have athletes involved in the process. What everyone's been saying today is we need transparency and accountability [in the IOC]."

The representatives of the various governments also called for a more independent body. "We cannot at present accept the composition of the proposed new agency," said Tony Banks. He called for an independent, autonomous, transparent anti-doping group that would be charged with instituting a universal out-of-competition testing program for all Olympic sports. (As IAAF Medical Commission Chairman Arne Ljungqvist noted, only 10 of the 34 Olympic sports currently have year-round, out-of-competition testing programs, so the need for a universal agency is great.) Governments have to be involved in this process, Banks argued, because the IOC is not a legislative body, and it needs the support of governments to draft regulations that will be upheld across borders. Banks said that the large turnout of government ministers at the conference was proof of their support for societal solutions to the problem.

But independence and autonomy should not be the sole focus of the new agency, according to Canadian ethics professor, Angela Schneider. Schneider, a member of Pound's working group, contended that fighting drug abuse is essentially a problem of sports ethics, not merely a scientific war between pharmaceutically enhanced athletes and testing laboratories. This prompted Pound to respond. "We are willing to provide whatever resources are necessary to ensure doping-free sport," Pound said. "In the final analysis, drugs are not a medical or sports problem; they are an ethical problem."

Focusing on ethics is an important shift in emphasis, said Schneider, because it will allow the new agency to attack the root of the doping problem, rather than merely the symptoms. Athletes who are caught by drug tests illustrate the problem, but punishing them through sanctions does not address the key issue of stopping the athletes from using in the first place, Schneider noted, arguing that doping is an ethical dilemma that will not be corrected only by rigorous drug testing. Leeds University professor Jim Parry, a British representative at the conference, agreed with Schneider's view, adding that a punitive testing system is really an acknowledgment of the failure to properly educate Olympic athletes. He claimed that drug testing is necessary when those who govern sport realize that their efforts to create a culture of a drug-free sport through athlete education have not worked. Any new anti-doping agency, therefore, has to have an education arm that attempts to reaffirm the Olympic ideal of fair play. Punishment alone merely sets up an adversarial dynamic that pits athletes against sports administrators in a cat-and-mouse game of doping detection.

Reactions to the *Lausanne Declaration on Doping in Sport*

Debates on these viewpoints were frequent during the two-day conference and amply illustrated the complexity of the doping problem. The outcome of the doping conference was indicative of a sense of distrust and a lack of confidence among members of the Olympic community in the leadership of the IOC. Hoping to depart from the conference with a strong, unified pact to set up a new doping agency and push forward in the War on Drugs, the *Lausanne Declaration on Doping in Sport* offered by the IOC fell short of that goal.

The two-page document had six main sections: (1) Education, prevention, and athletes' rights; (2) Olympic Movement Anti-Doping Code; (3) Sanctions; (4) International Anti-Doping Agency; (5) Responsibilities of the IOC, the IFs (International Federations), the NOCs (National Olympic Committees), and the CAS (Court of Arbitration for Sport); and (6) Collaboration between the Olympic Movement and public authorities. The most controversial point of the declaration was the section concerning sanctions, which declared: "In accordance with the wishes of the athletes, the NOCs and a large majority of the IFs, the minimum required sanction for major doping substances or prohibited methods shall be a suspension of the athlete from all competition for a period of two years, for a first offense. However, based on specific, exceptional circumstances to be evaluated in the first instance by the competent IF bodies, there may be a provision for a possible modification of the two-year sanction." The European Union, represented by government sports ministers of several countries, found the sentence allowing exceptions to a two-year minimum sanction unacceptable and withheld their endorsement. Tony Banks, Britain's sports minister, served as media spokesman for the EU group. "We cannot agree with the paragraph on sanctions," Banks said. "It is both minimalist and permissive. It undermines the proposed two-year ban. . . . These issues are bigger than the IOC. It might come as a surprise to the IOC to find there is actually something bigger than the IOC, but there is." IOC President Samaranch, however, defended the proposed sanctions. "We had problems with the sanctions, we had to be very tough," he said. "Some international federations had judicial problems, but this [two-year] sanction can be changed—this was important to keep the unity of the federations inside the Olympic movement—all federations are very, very happy."

Not all federation representatives agreed, however. The International Triathlon Federation's Mark Sisson stated, "The credibility of the Olympic movement must be called into question with this language of the sanctions. The biggest winners are the lawyers of the world: we wanted to close the loopholes because the biggest issue over the years have been legal problems and we wanted to try and create level playing fields . . . but the code is now woefully inadequate."

The perceived leniency on sanctions sparked a debate pitting a few of the larger and more wealthy sports against smaller sports in the Olympic family. In defense of the Lausanne Declaration's flexibility regarding sanctions, the UCI's Verbruggen said he believed that "money could be used as an exceptional circumstance" to get a doped rider back on the road because a court might rule that a two-year ban and the accompanying loss of two years of income was disproportionate punishment for a doping offense. In response, Les McDonald, president of the International Triathlon Union, argued that sanctions need to be applied equally across the spectrum. "They've created a law for the rich and a law for the poor," he complained. "The rule seems to be that if they're rich, you can't take that away from them. Let the rich guy off and punish the petty thief. If a big-name football player is ever caught on drugs, do you think Sepp Blatter [president of the international soccer federation] would ever tell him he couldn't play in the World Cup? The rest of the bloody world backed down from soccer and cycling. When the sports federations had their last meeting in Lausanne in December, everyone agreed that if an association didn't want to play by the new rules of doping control, they should not go to the Olympic Games. We never held to that."

MacDonald's stance was reiterated by representatives from other sports. "One set of rules," said Chrichlow. "If you don't want to play by the rules, don't come to play. Why should a canoeist or a cross-country skier, who is scraping by below the poverty line be subjected to a penalty of two years and lost income, while a hockey player is not?" Helmut Digel, head of German track and field's governing body, said federations that did not accept a two-year ban should be thrown out of the Olympics. "It can't be that we have a situation three months before the Sydney 2000 Games that an athlete, a cyclist or soccer player, tests positive and can go on to the Games while others cannot," he said. "A credible fight against doping must adopt a principle that the same rights apply to everyone."

The issue of flexible sanctions involved more than just enforceability, contended Samaranch. An athlete's age might make him or her an exception. "A 15-year-old who is just starting may be manipulated by an entourage," Samaranch said. "That is different from a 30-year-old who has been to three Olympics taking drugs."

Blatter, head of FIFA, the international federation for soccer, said governing bodies should have flexibility to deal with cases. "There should be flexibility," he said. "That's all I'm asking for." Verbruggen, whose opening remarks acknowledged that many in attendance likely believed that his sport was directly responsible for the conference, said that although cycling authorities were attacking the problem, bans were not a solution. "Longer sanctions will cause a rush from athletes to the civil courts and action for compensation that we can't afford," Verbruggen said. For soccer and cycling, the support for flexible sanctions stemmed from their fears that two-year bans would not be legally enforceable. "The cases put forward by the two federations are really compelling based on their experiences before the courts," IOC vice president Richard Pound said. Blatter told the conference that "especially in the case of professional players, the courts had a record of striking down two-year suspensions using labor laws."

Debates Over Sanctions Spark More Criticism

The inability to agree on sanctions provoked further criticism of the IOC's leadership in the fight against doping. The IOC's unwillingness to at least try for a minimum sanction for doping violations, said Irish Sports Council head John Treacy (silver medalist in the 1984 Olympic marathon and two-time world cross-country champion), is another example of failure of leadership. Treacy said he was disappointed that the IOC did not realize the message this sort of action delivers. Instead of strengthening the IOC's credibility as a champion of Olympic values, he noted, it portrays the IOC as backing away from a position that has broad support within the Olympic family because of the potential legal consequences. Britain's Banks agreed. "If they are going to say, 'We're not sure we can ever get this through, therefore, we're not going to do it,' that is not the way to make legislation," said Banks. "There are those who say this has actually weakened the position on doping."

The IOC leadership presented a different view of the matter. De Merode repeated that anti-doping legislation is no good if it cannot be enforced. However, conference attendees did not unanimously support all aspects of the declaration. And it was apparent that the declaration did not represent a unified, worldwide, cooperative effort to fight doping in sport. Rather it reflected the difficulties of finding a harmonious solution to the doping crisis.

New Agency for Testing?

The Lausanne Declaration commits at least $25 million of the IOC's television revenues toward funding an agency mandated to become an independent group responsible for conducting (1) year-round, out-of-competition testing; (2) education efforts on behalf of the athletes; and (3) research necessary to develop scientifically sound testing. The agency also could be mandated to review the current list of banned substances and provide recommendations on whether the list should be pared or expanded. The structure, governance, and power of the agency remains to be decided; the declaration only commits the IOC to push forward this process.

Conclusions

In the end, although the declaration incorporated many compromises, it didn't do enough to gain full support. "This is not a declaration we accept as being an end," said Banks, "It is a first step." Don Vereen, who spoke for the U.S. delegation, echoed that feeling. Vereen said the IOC had produced a positive beginning, but the United States did not agree with all elements of the declaration and was still looking forward to working more with the IOC. Athlete representative Charmaine Crooks called the declaration "a step in the right direction" because athletes will be involved in the formation and the operation of the agency.

Aside from sanctions, the issue of control remained unresolved. "We support a totally transparent world anti-doping organization, but the IOC should not be that agency," said Banks. The IOC's Pound said the committee was ready to give governments a 50 percent role in the agency—but would expect the governments to contribute financially. "The governments must be prepared to put their money and efforts where their mouths are," he said. Eventually, Samaranch, seemed to bow to the inevitable by acknowledging, "The agency will not be run by the IOC."

For their part, a number of IOC members in attendance expressed strong anti-doping stances. "We need a repressive law to shut the door," French IOC member and gold-medal-winning skier Jean-Claude Killy said. He added that he, like Pound, considers the doping problem more serious than the Olympic corruption scandal. (The statements were something of a shift for Killy, who attempted to minimize the doping scandal at the Tour de France when the story first broke in the summer of 1998.) Princess Anne, an IOC member in Great Britain, remarked, "Athletes who choose to remain clean deserve our protection. And although I realize there are limitations here, if IFs (international federations), NFs (national federations), and NOCs (national Olympic committees) who run scared of the well-lawyered athlete or anyone else of an interested party, they are failing the majority of our athletes."

At the conference's conclusion, the IOC's revised proposal for the anti-doping agency called for an 18-member panel that would include only three IOC representatives. Other members would be athletes, government officials, sports administrators, medical doctors, pharmaceutical experts, and sporting goods executives. (The World Health Organization of the United Nations was mentioned as one possible source for the agency.)

Just as it began, however, the IOC World Conference on Doping in Sport ended with uncertainty. With an indefinite launch date, the question remained: Who will run and/or administer it? Will the governments be brought into the new agency or will some remain outside? What will the budget be? Many will be watching as the Lausanne Declaration is implemented, for after all the talk, it is action that counts. On the doping issue, as with many others, the words former U.S. attorney general John Mitchell, said during the Watergate crisis still ring true: "Watch what we do, not what we say."

Index

Note: The f and t following page numbers refer to figures and tables, respectively.

About the Editors

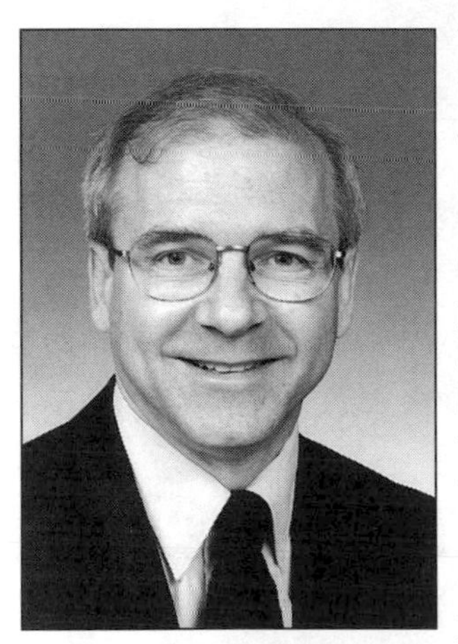

Wayne Wilson, PhD, is vice president of research for the Amateur Athletic Foundation of Los Angeles. He conceived and organized the 1998 conference *Doping in Elite Sport*, which this book is based on.

Wilson, the author of numerous articles on the Olympic movement, was the cowriter and executive producer of the CD-ROM *An Olympic Journey: The Story of Women in the Olympic Games*. Since 1990, he has edited a series of research reports published by the Amateur Athletic Foundation on race, gender, and the sports media.

He is a member of the North American Society for Sport History and the Research Council of the Olympic Studies Centre in Lausanne, Switzerland.

Currently residing in Los Angeles, Wilson enjoys cross-country skiing and traveling with his family.

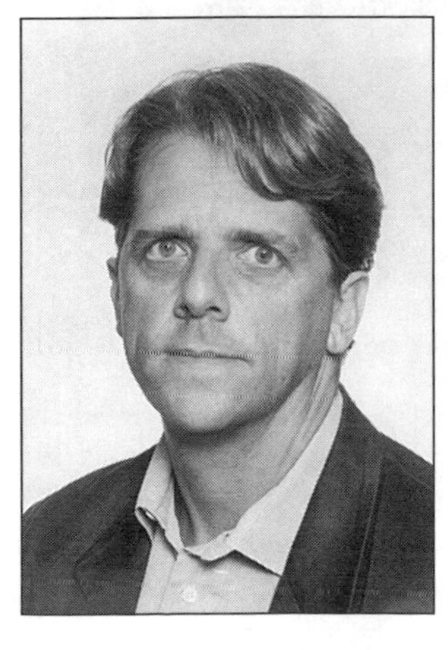

Edward Derse is senior producer for World Sports at FOXSports.com, where he is responsible for strategy, development, and production for international and Olympic sports coverage. He was previously the research director for the Amateur Athletic Foundation of Los Angeles. He also serves as vice president of the International Sepaktakraw Federation.

Derse has written or edited four books on coaching and training methods. His articles have appeared in several magazines covering a variety of sports. He also is the sports business analyst for Marketplace, a business news show airing on public radio stations across the United States.

Derse lives in Santa Monica, California and is an avid surfer.